The Rural Nurse

Deana L. Molinari, PhD, RN, CNE, Professor at Idaho State University School of Nursing, began her nursing career as a diploma graduate of Providence College of Nursing in California. She earned a baccalaureate degree from Walla Walla College in Washington, a Master's of Science degree in nursing community health care systems from Oregon Health Sciences University in Oregon, and a PhD in Instructional Psychology and Technology from Brigham Young University in Utah. She is a licensed clinical nurse specialist in Oregon and a nationally certified nurse educator. She is the current president of the Rural Nurse Organization and a researcher in the stress of learning and caregiving with several publications. She is the mother of 15 children.

Angeline Bushy, PhD, RN, FAAN, PHCNS-BC, Professor and Bert Fish Endowed Chair at the University of Central Florida, College of Nursing, holds a BSN degree from the University of Mary in Bismarck, North Dakota; an MN degree in rural community health nursing from Montana State University in Bozeman; an MEd in adult education from Northern Montana College in Havre; and a PhD in nursing from the University of Texas at Austin. She is a Fellow in the American Academy of Nursing and a clinical specialist in public health nursing. She has worked in rural facilities located in the north central and intermountain states, presented nationally and internationally on various rural nursing and rural health issues, published six textbooks and numerous articles on that topic, and is a Lieutenant Colonel (Ret.) in the U.S. Army Reserve. She and Jack, her husband, have one daughter, Andrea.

The Rural Nurse
Transition to Practice

Deana L. Molinari, PhD, RN, CNE

Angeline Bushy, PhD, RN, FAAN, PHCNS-BC

Editors

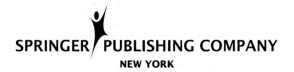

SPRINGER PUBLISHING COMPANY
NEW YORK

60 · 00

Springer Publishing Company, LLC
11 West 42nd Street
New York, NY 10036
www.springerpub.com

Acquisitions Editor: Allan Graubard
Composition: Techset

ISBN: 978-0-8261-5756-0
E-book ISBN: 978-0-8261-5757-7

11 12 13/ 5 4 3 2 1

The author and the publisher of this Work have made every effort to use sources believed to be reliable to provide information that is accurate and compatible with the standards generally accepted at the time of publication. The author and publisher shall not be liable for any special, consequential, or exemplary damages resulting, in whole or in part, from the readers' use of, or reliance on, the information contained in this book. The publisher has no responsibility for the persistence or accuracy of URLs for external or third-party Internet Web sites referred to in this publication and does not guarantee that any content on such Web sites is, or will remain, accurate or appropriate.

Library of Congress Cataloging-in-Publication Data

CIP data is available from the Library of Congress

Special discounts on bulk quantities of our books are available to corporations, professional associations, pharmaceutical companies, health care organizations, and other qualifying groups.

If you are interested in a custom book, including chapters from more than one of our titles, we can provide that service as well.

For details, please contact:
Special Sales Department, Springer Publishing Company, LLC
11 West 42nd Street, 15th Floor, New York, NY 10036-8002
Phone: 877-687-7476 or 212-431-4370; Fax: 212-941-7842
Email: sales@springerpub.com

Printed in the United States of America by Gasch Printing

*Dedicated to the many nurses making a difference in
vulnerable populations throughout the world.*

CONTENTS

CONTRIBUTORS

Nancy Asay, RN, BSN, completed her Associate Degree in Nursing at Boise State University in Boise, Idaho and her Bachelors of Science in Nursing at West Haven University in Cypress, California. Nancy is a certified Oncology Nurse and a BLS Instructor for the American Heart Association. She is also a Certified Rural Nurse Preceptor. Nancy is employed by Oneida County Hospital in Malad, Idaho as the Director of Nursing for the Acute Care Department.

Susan A. Boyer, MEd, RN, FAHCEP, completed basic education at the University of Vermont, her advanced degree at Antioch New England Graduate School, and certification at Indiana University School of Nursing. Currently, she is the Executive Director of Vermont Nurses in Partnership, Inc.

Angeline Bushy, PhD, RN, FAAN, PHCNS-BC, is Professor and Bert Fish Endowed Chair at the University of Central Florida, College of Nursing, Orlando, Florida. Dr. Bushy obtained a BSN degree from the University of Mary in Bismarck, North Dakota; an MN degree in rural community health nursing from Montana State University in Bozeman; an MEd in adult education from Northern Montana College in Havre; and a PhD in nursing from the University of Texas at Austin. She is a Fellow in the American Academy of Nursing and a clinical specialist in public health nursing.

Kathryn H. Crooks, PhD, RN, received her Associate Degree from Mount Royal College, Calgary, Alberta, Canada, her post RN BN and MEd from the University of Lethbridge, and her PhD from the University of Calgary. She is employed by Medicine Hat College, Medicine Hat, Alberta, Canada where she teaches in the University of Calgary Bachelor of Nursing Program at the Medicine Hat College Site.

Kristen Crusoe, EdD, MN, RN, completed basic education at Florida State University, receiving a BA in International Relations, returned to college to obtain her Associate Degree in Nursing at Tallahassee Community College, then went on to graduate school at Oregon Health Sciences University and Doctor of Education at Oregon State University. Her focus was on leadership in higher education and interdisciplinary collaboration. In addition, Dr. Crusoe has certifications in Legal Nurse Consultant, Forensic Nursing, and Dance/Yoga Therapy. She is employed by Southwestern Oregon Community College where she is Associate Dean of Learning, and Oregon Health Sciences University where she is an Assistant Professor of Nursing.

Linda Ferguson RN, BSN, PGD (Cont Ed.), MN, PhD, teaches at the University of Saskatchewan. Her expertise is in obstetrical nursing, inter professional education, mentorship and preceptorship in nursing practice and education, patient education, faculty development, and new nurse transition into professional practice.

Karen Louise Francis completed preservice nursing education at Armidale College of Advanced Education, Armidale, Australia. She then attained a BSN at the University of Western Sydney. Postgraduate studies include a Graduate Certificate in University Teaching and Learning from Charles Sturt University Wagga Wagga, a Master of Health Science Primary Health Care degree from the University of Western Sydney, and a Master of Education from Charles Sturt University Wagga Wagga. Karen also holds a PhD from the University of Adelaide. She is employed by Monash University as Professor Rural Nursing and Head of the School of Nursing and Midwifery on the rural campus of the University.

Quinn Grundy, PhD (c), RN, completed her baccalaureate degree in nursing at the University of Alberta. She has worked as a research assistant to Dr. Olive Yonge for over 5 years and is currently a doctoral student at the University of California, San Francisco.

Vincent P. Hall, PhD, RN, CNE, provides expertise in Adult Health Care Nursing with research in HIV/AIDS, Psychosocial and Spiritual Issues related to chronic disease. He works in North Carolina to increase education opportunities for rural nurses.

Beverly J. Hewett, PhD, RN, completed both a baccalaureate and Master's Degree from Idaho State University, and her PhD in Adult Education was received from the University of Idaho. She is employed by the Idaho State University School of Nursing as a Clinical Assistant Professor with an interest in geriatrics and nurses who care for the elderly.

Tamara Hollinger-Forrest, MHSA, RN, completed basic education at Idaho State University, with an advanced degree from Strayer University. She is employed by Idaho State University where she is the clinical coordinator of the Northwest Rural Nurse Residency.

Elisabeth R. Jacob, MEd, RN, completed basic education at Avondale College/ Sydney Adventist Hospital, certifications and advanced degrees at Deakin University, Charles Sturt University, and currently Monash University in Australia. She is employed by Monash University where she is a nursing academic.

Ashvin R. Jaiswal completed a Bachelor's of Pharmacy at Amravati University, India. Ashvin is pursuing a Master's Degree in Biomedical and Pharmaceutical Sciences from the College of Pharmacy, Idaho State University. He is employed by the Northwest Rural Nursing Residency at Idaho State University School of Nursing.

Mary P. Johnson, RN, MSN, FAAN, completed basic education at The Ohio State University, and her MSN at Duke University. She is the President and Chief Executive Officer of the Foundation for Nursing Excellence, a nonprofit organization in Raleigh, North Carolina.

Karen L. Joiner, MS, ARNP, completed basic education at Lower Columbia College and advanced degrees at the University of the State of New York and the University of Portland, Oregon. She is employed by Lower Columbia College where she is a full-time faculty member and coordinator of nursing eLearning.

Jayne Josephsen, MS, RN, CHPN, completed basic education at Boise State University, certification through the Hospice and Palliative Care Nurses Association and advanced degrees at Idaho State University. She is employed by Boise State University, where she teaches community and public health nursing in the RN to BS online degree completion program.

Helen Hing Kuebel, RN, MSN, completed basic education at the University of Michigan and advanced degrees at The Catholic University of America, Washington, DC. She is the Assistant Dean of Nursing and Allied Health at Lower Columbia College in Washington.

Dr. Beverly D. Leipert, completed a Bachelor of Science in Nursing degree at the University of Saskatchewan, a Master of Science in Nursing degree at the University of British Columbia, and a Doctor of Philosophy (Nursing) degree at the University of Alberta. She is an Associate Professor in the Arthur Labatt Family School of Nursing at the University of Western Ontario, London, Ontario, Canada. From 2003–2009, Dr. Leipert held the first and only Chair in North America in Rural Women's Health Research.

Debra A. McElroy, MPH, RN, oversees the national UHC/AACN Nurse Residency Program™, as well as managing other nursing leadership activities within UHC, including the UHC member NDNQI database. Her work with the Nurse Residency Program involves curriculum development, implementation of the program in hospitals throughout the country, and expansion of the residency model to varied nursing practice settings. At UHC she has also worked on operational and clinical performance improvement projects for UHC members.

Kathy McGuinn, MS, RN, CPHQ, received her undergraduate degree from Georgetown University and her graduate degree from the Catholic University of America. She is credentialed as a Certified Professional in Healthcare Quality (CPHQ). At American Association of Colleges of Nursing, Ms McGuinn facilitates a variety of initiatives including the QSEN Faculty Development Consortium, the Essentials of Doctoral Education for Advanced Nursing Practice, the revision of the Essentials for Baccalaureate Nursing Education, the Essentials of Master's Education in Nursing, and the UHC/AACN Nurse Residency Program. Prior to joining AACN, Ms McGuinn was on the Senior Management Team at The George Washington University Hospital as Director of Quality and Education.

Julie McNulty, MS, RN, completed her nursing degree at the University of New Hampshire School of Nursing, and her advanced degree at the University of Alaska Anchorage School of Nursing. She is a Doctoral candidate at the Oregon Health and Science University and anticipates completion in 2011. She is employed by the Alaska Native Medical Center where she is the Nursing Director of the Center for Clinical Excellence.

Christine (Tina) F. Mladenka, DNP, WHNP, RN, is a clinical associate professor at Idaho State University School of Nursing. Mladenka primarily teaches in the undergraduate program and guest lectures for nursing classes in the graduate program. She developed and co-teaches an interprofessional course, "Genetics for the Health Care Professional." She has a clinical practice in family planning services with the Southeast District Public Health of Idaho.

Deana L. Molinari, PhD, RN, CNE, is a professor at Idaho State University. She is the coordinator of the Office of Professional Development and teaches education in the graduate program. She began nursing as a nursing assistant at Elmendorf Air Force Base Hospital in Anchorage, Alaska. She attended Providence College of Nursing in Oakland, California and earned her baccalaureate degree from Walla Walla College. Her master's degree came from Oregon Health Sciences University in Nursing Community Health Care Systems, and her doctorate in instructional psychology and technology was earned at Brigham Young University in Provo. She is a certified nurse educator.

Jill Montague, BSN, CCRN, completed her nursing degree at the University of Alaska School of Nursing. She anticipates completion of her Master's of Science in Nursing Education in 2011. She is employed by the Alaska Native Medical Center where she is the Supervisor of Hospital Education.

Florence Myrick RN, PhD, has focused primarily on acute and adult critical care, specifically medical surgical intensive care nursing. She practices in Canada's north and in educational settings. Her education practice has been with all levels of nursing in health assessment, research, knowledge development in nursing, and philosophy of teaching in nursing. Her recent research was as the primary investigator of a study exploring how the provision of an ongoing structured online support program influences the teaching practices of preceptors with a view to enhancing teaching and learning in the clinical context.

Teri Peterson is a research statistician and educator at Idaho State University. She consults with faculty and graduate students about experimental designs and statistical analyses.

Cynthia J. Roleff, MS, BSN, RN-BC, completed her nursing degree at the University of Minnesota School of Nursing, and her advanced degree at the University of LaVerne, California. She is employed by the Alaska Native Tribal Health Consortium where she is a Lead Telehealth Coordinator for the Alaska Federal Health Care Access Network.

Jean Ross RN, BN, MA, PhD (c), attended the School of Nursing, North Wales, UK, obtained a Bachelors Degree from Massey University, New Zealand, a Master's Degree from University of Victoria, Wellington, New Zealand, and is currently a PhD candidate at University of Otago, New Zealand. She is employed by Otago Polytechnic, School of Nursing, Dunedin, New Zealand where she is a Principal Lecturer.

Joyce W. Roth, RN, MSN, NE-BC, completed basic education at Abington Memorial Hospital School of Nursing, a BSN at Stockton State College, and a MSN at Villanova University. She is the Manager, Organizational Development for the North Carolina Board of Nursing.

Josephine H. Silvestre, MSN, RN (JHS), completed an AAS/AND degree at Harry S. Truman College (Chicago City Colleges), and both a Bachelor of Science and a Master's of Science in Nursing from DePaul University. She is employed by the National Council of State Boards of Nursing (NCSBN) where she is an Associate in Regulatory Innovations and the Project Manager for the Transition-to-Practice project.

Nancy Spector, PhD, RN, received her BSN from the University of Wisconsin, Madison; earned an MSN at the University of California San Francisco; and earned her PhD from Rush College of Nursing. She is employed by the National Council of State Boards of Nursing where she is the Director of Regulatory Innovations. At NCSBN she is the Principal Investigator in the transition-to-practice study.

Linda A. Tieman, MN, RN, completed basic education from the University of Cincinnati, with certifications and advanced degrees from University of Florida, Fellow from the J&J Wharton Nurse Executive Program, Fellow in Hospital Administration and Managed Care, American College of Healthcare Executives. She is employed by the Washington Center for Nursing where she is the Executive Director.

Anna von Dielingen MSN, RN, Anna has been a nurse for over 30 years and has held both formal leadership and educator positions in health care. These positions include management, non-profit Board positions, New Mexico Chapter President, and Western Regional Director for the Academy of Medical Surgical Nursing, advanced practice nursing, and years of informal leadership. As the Director of the Clinical Teaching Institute at the New Mexico Center for Nursing Excellence, she facilitates leadership and preceptor workshops. She received a Master's in Nursing Education from California State University, and undergraduate degrees from Purdue and Indiana Universities.

Gary W. Wappes, MSW, completed his undergraduate studies in Health Education at San Diego State College, and received his Masters in Social Work Degree from San Diego State University. He is recently retired from a 42-year career in social service, where he worked as a Manager in public health and nonprofit agencies. For the last 16 years, he was President and Chief Executive Officer of the Oregon Health Career Center, where he developed and operated a range of programs to address Oregon's health care workforce needs.

Olive June Yonge, PhD, RN, completed basic and advanced education from the University of Alberta. She is employed by the University of Alberta where she is a Professor.

FOREWORD

Charlene A. Winters, PhD, APRN, ACNS-BC
Associate Professor
Montana State University College of Nursing

I am pleased to have been invited by Dr. Deana Molinari and Dr. Angeline Bushy to write Foreword comments for *The Rural Nurse: Transition to Practice*. Nurses have been practicing in rural and frontier settings for centuries, yet there is still much that needs to be understood about rural nursing practice. One very important area requiring attention is the transition to practice experienced by new graduates and veteran nurses alike who are new to the rural setting.

To quote one of my favorite authors, "Being rural means being a long way from anywhere and pretty close to nowhere" (Scharff, 2010, p. 251). Few people, distance, geographic and professional isolation, and scarce health care resources are common in rural settings. Rural nurses must be expert generalists when practicing in a critical access hospital, clinic, or community setting. They must demonstrate a wide range of advanced knowledge and skills and the ability to practice proficiently and autonomously across clinical areas. During a single shift, rural hospital-based nurses often care for individuals of all ages with diverse conditions who would have been admitted to a specialty unit had they been in an urban setting. When working in community health, rural nurses often experience extreme professional and geographic isolation. A case in point is the lone community health nurse in a county covering 1,700-plus square miles with one nine-bed hospital, three nurse practitioners, and lacking the services of a physician, dentist, home health care agency, hospice, or assisted living facility (Montana County Health Profiles, 2009). To be able to move seamlessly and confidently across patient populations in rural settings with scarce resources requires an independent spirit, flexibility, creativity, constant adaptability, strong networking and communication skills, and a commitment to ongoing professional development.

Transiting to rural practice can be daunting for both experienced nurses and new graduates who have an urban orientation and are accustomed to specialized practice with abundant health care resources. Since most nursing education programs and practicing nurses are located in urban settings, programs are needed to prepare nurses who choose rural practice. In their book, Dr. Molinari and Dr. Bushy provide excellent examples of practice models from North America, New Zealand, and Australia with curricula that address transition issues. This text makes a significant contribution to the discussion about how to best prepare nurses for rural practice and will be of interest to administrators, educators, and clinicians.

REFERENCES

Department of Public Health & Human Services. (2009). *Montana County Health Profiles.* Available from: http://www.dphhs.mt.gov/PHSD/health-profiles/pdf/2009%20CHPs/DPHHS_CountyHealthProfile_2009.pdf

Scharff, J. (2010). The distinctive nature and scope of rural nursing practice: Philosophical bases. In C. A. Winters & H. J. Lee (Eds.), *Rural nursing: concepts, theory, and practice* (3rd ed.) (pp. 249–268). New York: Springer.

FOREWORD

Jeri Dunkin PhD, RN
Professor
University of Alabama

The Institute of Medicine (IOM) and the Robert Wood Johnson Foundation released a landmark report titled *The Future of Nursing: Leading Change, Advancing Health* in October 2010 that provides a plan for improving health care in the United States. This plan calls for the remodeling of a health care system to achieve high-quality, patient-centered care through the leadership of nurses. This report posits several recommendations in support of nursing's role in remodeling the system and improving health care for all Americans. In order for nurses to be the vanguard in improving health care, we must prepare and enable them to lead change, and health care agencies must build and maintain an infrastructure that ensures opportunities for nurses to engage in lifelong learning.

This recognition of nurses' leadership skills must occur in all types of health care agencies across this country through the development of models, programs, and so on. This will present diverse challenges to the achievement of a system that is relatively low cost, flexible, and replicable in a variety of geographic and cultural settings. To achieve the rapid remodeling of the health care system called for by the IOM report, nurses must be prepared to lead these changes across the spectrum of agency types and settings across the country.

Rural America and rural residents present unique health care challenges that are both cultural and geographic in nature. This book (*The Rural Nurse: Transition to Practice*) presents several models that have been used successfully in rural areas that demonstrate the infrastructure and opportunities for rural nurses to meet the unique challenges of rural America. Both those just beginning their career and those changing the focus of their practice will benefit from the examples of ensuring quality in an improved health care system.

The editors of this book are to be commended for their efforts to assemble basic concepts relative to the transitions in educational and nursing practice that must occur in order to effect nurses' knowledge growth. The presentation of successful rural program examples demonstrates the creativity needed to provide safe quality practice.

PREFACE

This book focuses on national and international nurses' transition to practice and continuing education in rural settings. Medicine, economics and society are changing. The nursing profession is also changing, resulting in modifications in nursing education and practice support strategies. Consequently, nurses are encouraged to obtain knowledge through professional development programs as well as with advanced academic degrees (IOM, 2010). The purpose of the text is to provide conceptual and practical information that can be used by nurses and leaders in rural settings to develop, implement, and evaluate innovative programs designed to meet local needs and preferences.

The importance of new graduates, initial work experiences and their retention in the profession cannot be overstated. Both novice nurses and expert nurses who transfer into a new specialty area of practice adopt their leaders' attitudes about ongoing professional development. Administrators and clinical educators in a health care facility set the tone for employees with respect to development of a competent caregiver. In other words, nurses need support to develop and maintain professionalism and lifelong learning.

Recent nurse graduates usually believe the career they have chosen to be important, complex, and exciting. Those in leadership roles may inadvertently squelch an individual's motivation for self-improvement. Nourishing passion and competence requires attention to organizational and peer support and education content.

Program outcomes depend on leaders' values and the fit with an institutional culture. The rural nursing "specialty" meets the needs of rural communities. Most nursing leaders have not been exposed to rural health information or culture, and are not familiar with the nuances of rural practice. Thus, successful urban models lacking essential cultural components can be "transplanted" in small facilities or communities. Likewise, the act of creating something new is not necessarily the act of creating something successful, especially if the approach does not fit the local culture.

Historically, new rural nurses learned "to survive" in spite of what their leaders believed or did. Consequently, horizontal violence among employees coupled with the lack of administrative support challenged the novice to endure in a particular workplace. Supportive evidence proves that ignoring the learning and professional development needs of new employees contributes to high employee turnover, as well as impacting on the quality of care that is provided for patients. Motivated leaders can address these professional challenges with creativity, passion, and evidence-based principles. Thus, there is a need for information from experts about successful nurse transition-to-practice (TTP) models to guide future leaders in supporting and motivating employees, and thereby improving retention rates and addressing the quality of rendered care.

The text compiles the insights and experience of early transition-to-practice program adopters for the benefit of others who realize the importance of not needing to reinvent the wheel. By using principles of quality and safety, rural-based nurse administrators can improve on the work of the text contributors and increase patient care quality and thus the nursing profession. Rural nursing as a specialty area of practice emphasizes identification and efficient use of scarce resources, collaborative interprofessional relationships, autonomy, and accountability. These characteristics also are the core of successful TTP programs. The book includes chapters that describe both small and larger complex programs. Most involve partnerships that were supported by national and state governments, private enterprises, professional organizations, advocacy groups, health care facilities, or academic institutions.

Learning theories and educational principles such as learning through interactive experiences, building on existing knowledge, and measuring competence are noted throughout the book. Strategies for changing education and rural nursing practice are described. Creative approaches from national as well as international experts demonstrate that there is more than one way to increasing nurse knowledge, skills, or attitude. However, there are several common elements among the models presented that address the rural context among others, identifying a specific TTP need, asking why there is a status quo, and dreaming of more successful strategies are common themes. Program creators tend to first examine patients' and organizational needs and then proceed to develop and refine programs to address those priorities. This form of program development begins with the end in mind. Outcomes are delineated; goals and objectives are identified and strategies are refined that take into consideration system strength and resources. In determining effectiveness, cost and benefit analyses are undertaken, and findings are disseminated to target audiences. In other words, nurses apply a nursing process in an effort to design a program that nurtures and supports nurses, and can ultimately improve the patient quality of care. The book provides the rationale for transition-to-practice, recent research about rural nursing, examples of TTP, and suggestions for creating and maintaining programs. The authors of the various chapters present studies describing novice and expert rural nurses. Others highlight educational challenges and continuing education requirements for successful rural practice and workforce retention. The book features new-employee needs and offers insights into the practice and development of rural nurse generalists. This information can be useful to students, nurse educators, researchers, scholars, clinicians, administrators, and policy developers. Professional organizations such as the Rural Nurse Organization, academic and clinical educators, and researchers are poised to advocate for nurses in rural health care. Each of these entities is in a position to disseminate relevant evidence, as well as promote nursing standards and competencies.

In even the smallest community, a health care institution can become a center for excellence by nourishing its nurses. History provides examples of outcomes associated with doing little for the profession, as evidenced by an expectation that new nurses will learn naturally with time. Some refer to this as the "sink or swim" mentality for retaining survivors. Novice nurses are dared to succeed by learning the "hard way" what it is they need to know for practice and then by seeking out their own learning resources. This costly approach to nursing education leads to a high turnover rate among new employees. Agencies struggle to recruit and retain new nurses, and yet without changing transition-to-practice strategies, few agencies develop the loyalty needed for retention.

The need for overcoming the rural nurse shortage through improved recruitment and retention strategies is another theme running through the text. Several chapters address issues such as the global nurse shortage, turnover, job satisfaction, and personal practice perceptions. Research and program development reforms impact on administrators' interviewing and new-employee support strategies (Allen, Fiorini, & Dickey, 2010). Most rural administrators support residencies for two reasons: Retention and patient care (Holloway, Baker, & Lumby, 2009). The chapters indicate administrators need to do more than develop good reasons to create successful nursing organizations. Research indicates transition-to-practice requires administrators to create supportive staff cultures, design education delivery methods, provide preceptor and resident support, reserve participation time, and recognize educational accomplishments. Authors posit administrators' leadership impacts job satisfaction, personal practice perceptions, and patient safety (Baernholdt, Jennings, Merwin, & Thornlow, 2010; Molinari & Monserud, 2008; Wieck, Dols, & Landrum, 2010). Although the transition-to-practice challenge is colossal, the cost of ignoring new nurses is greater. Rural nurses can serve communities by collaborating on new TTP programming. Future rural nurse leaders will change the profession by producing new models of nurse support based on disseminated best practices.

Usually publishing a text indicates a culmination of topic knowledge. This book's purpose is to call rural nurses to the transition-to-practice debate, to encourage future studies, and to disseminate findings from dedicated rural nurses around the world. Experiment with the innovations described in the text, and share findings in professional venues. The future of rural nursing is in our focus—the care for rural populations is in our hands.

ACKNOWLEDGMENTS

A textbook requires the dedication and innovation of many people. We are deeply grateful to contributors for their rural nurse research and program development. Rural nurses' scholarly work improves health care. This text would be impossible without their daily efforts.

The most intense support, patience, and encouragement came from our fabulous spouses: Byron Molinari, and Jack Bushy. Their efforts kept us fed and healthy while we were tied to the computer. Our families' endurance permitted our persistence.

Many reviewers, editors, research assistants, and friends increased the project's quality. Special thanks are extended for the work of Debra Cassady, Lori Chovanak, Ashvin Jaiswal, Marla Jones, June Nilsson, Robin Raptosh, and Shilpa Siddhanti.

We also wish to thank the Springer staff, especially Allan Graubard, for their skills and patience. Allan's vision, faith, and feedback germinated, weeded, and fertilized our ideas.

I

Foundations of Rural Nursing Transition to Practice

The information in Section One presents an overview of nursing practice and its rural context. The first chapter by Bushy highlights characteristics of life in a small community where most people are familiar with one another. Rural is defined and features of rural nursing practice are examined. Chapter two, by Molinari, discusses current trends and the benefits and challenges of implementing new employee support programs. This is followed with a chapter by Spector and Silvestre who review evidence for the need to transition new graduates into competent and safe nurses.

Crooks offers an international perspective by presenting findings from a Canadian qualitative study exploring the phenomenon of dual interconnecting relationships in a small rural community. Another study by Molinari, Jaiswal and Peterson discusses nurses' perceptions of rural organizational cultures and the intent to leave. Since nursing is a predominately female profession, research focusing on women may provide insights about nurses and nursing practice. The section concludes with a chapter by Leipert examining the meaning of being both female and a nurse in a rural context.

1

The Rural Context and Nursing Practice

Angeline Bushy

---

*Although nursing is probably similar across settings and popu-
lations, there are some unusual features associated with practice
in a geographically remote area and small towns where most people are
familiar with one another. This chapter establishes a foundation for the
information provided in this textbook; beginning an historic overview
of "formal" rural nursing; followed by common definitions for rural.
An overview of rural populations' health status is presented along
with barriers experienced in obtaining a continuum of health care services. Given the rural context and the health status of people who live
there, nursing practice issues are examined that should be addressed in
rural nurse transition-to-practice programs.*
— Bigbee & Crowder, 1985; Bushy, 2011

HISTORICAL PERSPECTIVES

Formal rural nursing originated with the Red Cross Rural Nursing
Service, which was organized in November 1912. The Committee on
Rural Nursing was under the direction of Mabel Boardman (chair),
Jane Delano (vice-chair), and Annie Goodrich along with other Red
Cross leaders and philanthropists (Bigbee & Crowder, 1985). Before
the formation of the Red Cross Rural Nursing Service, care of the sick
in a small community was provided by informal social support systems. When self-care and family care were not effective in bringing
about healing, this task was assigned to healers, who often were
women who lived in the local community. Historically, the health
needs of rural Americans have been numerous, and although not
necessarily unique, they are different from those of urban populations.
Consistent problems of maldistribution of health professionals, poverty,
limited access to services, ignorance, and social isolation have plagued

some rural communities for generations. Overtime, the Red Cross Rural Nursing Service shows a consistent movement away from its initial rural focus, as demonstrated by its frequent name changes. Unfortunately, concern for rural health is similarly often temporary and replaced by other areas of greater need.

Defining Rural

Everyone has an idea as to what constitutes rural as opposed to urban residence. However, the two cannot be viewed as opposing entities. Moreover, with the increased degree of urban influence on rural communities, the differences are no longer as distinct as they may have been even a decade ago (Bureau of the Census Bureau, 2009; Gamm et al., 2003; U.S. Department of Agriculture [USDA], 2005, 2006, 2008a, 2008b). In general, rural is defined in terms of the geographic location and population density, or it may be described in terms of the distance from (e.g., 20 miles) or the time (e.g., 30 min) needed to commute to an urban center.

Both urban and rural communities are highly diverse and vary in terms of their demographic, environmental, economic, and social characteristics. In turn, these characteristics influence the magnitude and types of health problems that communities face. Urban counties, however, tend to have a greater supply of health care providers in relation to population, and residents of more rural counties often live farther from health care resources (CDC, 2010; Cromartie, 2008; Mead et al., 2008).

Some equate "rural" with farm residency and urban with nonfarm residency while others consider rural to be a "state of mind." For the more affluent, rural may bring to mind a recreational, retirement, or resort community located in the mountains or in lake country, where one can relax and participate in outdoor activities such as skiing, fishing, hiking, or hunting. For the less affluent, the term can impose grim scenes. For example, some people may think of an impoverished Indian reservation as comparable to an underdeveloped country, or it may bring to mind images of a migrant labor camp with several families living in a one-room shanty with no access to safe drinking water or adequate sanitation. Just as each city has its own unique features, it is also difficult to describe a "typical rural town" because of the wide population and geographic diversity. Furthermore, there can be vast differences between rural areas within one state. Still, descriptions and definitions for rural tend to be more subjective and relative in nature than those for urban. For example, "small" communities with populations of more than 20,000 have some features that one may expect to find in a city. Then again, residents who live in a community with a population of less than 2,000 may consider a community with a population of 5,000 or 10,000 to be a city. Although some communities may seem geographically remote on a map, the residents who live there may not feel isolated. Those residents believe they are within easy reach of services through telecommunication and dependable transportation; although extensive shopping facilities may be 50–100 miles from the family home, and obstetric care may be 150 miles away.

Often-used definitions to describe rural and urban are offered by several federal agencies. The definitions, which in many cases are dichotomous in nature, fail to take into account the relative nature of ruralness. Rural and urban residencies are not opposing lifestyles. Rather, they must be seen as a rural–urban continuum ranging from living on a remote farm, to a village or small town, to a larger town or city, to a large metropolitan area (Exhibit 1.1).

Several federal agencies classify counties according to population density, specifically, metropolitan area (1,090 U.S. counties), micropolitan area (674 U.S. counties), and noncore area (1,378 U.S. counties) (USDA, 2006). The terms metropolitan and micropolitan statistical

---

EXHIBIT 1.1   Terms and definitions

Farm residency: Residency outside area zoned as "city limits"; usually infers involvement in agriculture

Frontier: Regions having fewer than six persons per square mile

Large central: Counties in large (1 million or more population) metro areas that contain all or part of the largest central city

Large fringe: Remaining counties in large (1 million or more population) metro areas

Metropolitan county: Regions with a central city of at least 50,000 residents

Nonfarm residency: Residence within area zoned as "city limits"

Micropolitan county: Counties that do not meet SMSA criteria

Rural: Communities having less than 20,000 residents or fewer than 99 persons per square mile

Small: Counties in metro areas with less than 1 million people

Suburban: Area adjacent to a highly populated city

Urban: Geographic areas described as nonrural and having a higher population density; more than 99 persons per square mile; cities contain an urban core of at least 10,000 (but less than 50,000) population

areas (metro and micro areas) refers to geographic entities primarily used for collecting, tabulating, and publishing Federal statistics. Core-Based Statistical Area (CBSA) is a collective term for both metro and micro areas. A metro area contains a core urban area of 50,000 or more population. A micro area contains an urban core of at least 10,000 (but less than 50,000) population. Each metro or micro area consists of one or more counties containing the core urban area. Likewise, adjacent counties have a high degree of social and economic integration (as measured by commuting to work) with their urban core (Cromartie, 2008). Demographically, micro areas contain about 60% of the total nonmetro population. According to Bureau of the Census estimates (2009) about 25% of all U.S. residents live in rural settings.

In general, lack of an urban core and low overall population density may place these counties at a disadvantage in efforts to expand and diversify their economic base. The designation of micro areas is an important step in recognizing nonmetro diversity. The term also provides a framework to understand population growth and economic restructuring in small towns and cities that have received less attention than metro areas. Nationally and regionally, many measures of health, health care use, and health care resources among rural populations vary by the level of urban influence in a particular region. Micro areas embody a widely shared residential preference for a small-town lifestyle—an ideal compromise between large highly populated urban cities and sparsely populated rural settings.

Population Characteristics

Adding to the confusion about what constitutes rural versus urban residency are the special needs of the numerous underrepresented groups (minorities, subgroups) who reside in the United States. In general, there are a higher proportion of whites in rural areas than in urban areas. There are, however, regional variations, and some rural counties have a significant number of minorities. Little is documented on the needs and health status of special rural populations (Meade et al., 2008; USDHHS, 2010b, 2010c). Anthropologists are quick to report that, within a group, there often exists a wide range of lifestyles. Consequently, even in the smallest or most remote town or village, a subgroup may behave differently and have different values regarding health, illness, and patterns of accessing health care. Also, their lifestyle may be associated with health problems that are different from those of the predominant cultural group in a given community.

Demographically, rural communities include a higher proportion of younger and older residents. Consequently, a nurse who works in a rural health care facility can expect to encounter more residents under the age of 18 and over 65 years of age. Rural residents 18 years of age and older are more likely to be, or to have been, married than urban counterparts. As a group, rural adults are more likely to be widowed and have fewer years of formal education than do urban adults (Cromartie, 2008; USDA, 2008a, 2008b).

Although there are regional variations, rural families in general tend to be poorer than their urban counterparts. Comparing annual incomes with the standardized index established, more than one fourth of rural Americans live in or near poverty and nearly 40% of all rural children are impoverished (Gamm et al., 2003; Rand Corporation, 2010a, 2010b). Consequently, rural families are less likely to have private insurance and more likely to have public assistance or to be uninsured. Working poor in rural areas are particularly at risk for being underinsured or uninsured. In working poor families, one or more of the adults are employed but still cannot afford private health insurance. Furthermore, their annual income is such that it disqualifies the family from obtaining public insurance. A number of reasons are cited to explain why this phenomenon occurs more often in rural settings.

For example, a high proportion of residents are self-employed in a family business, such as ranching or farming, or they work in small enterprises, such as a service station, restaurant, or grocery store. Also, an individual may be employed in part-time or in seasonal occupations, such as farm laborer and construction, in which health insurance often is not an employee benefit. In other situations, a family member may have a preexisting health condition that makes the cost of insurance prohibitive, if it is even available to them. A few rural families fall through the cracks and are unable to access any type of public assistance because of other deterrents, such as language barriers, compromised physical status, the geographic location of an agency, lack of transportation, or undocumented-worker status. Insurance, or the lack of it, has serious implications for the overall health status of rural residents and the nurses who provide services to them (Agency for Health Care Policy and Research [AHCPR], 2009; Bennett, Olatosi, & Probst, 2008; Nelson & Stover-Gingerich, 2010; USDHHS, 2010c).

Health Status of Rural Residents

Even though rural communities constitute about one-fourth of the total population, the health problems and the health behaviors of the residents in them are not fully understood. Based on data from national health surveys, the overall health status of rural adults leaves much to be desired. This is attributed to a number of factors, including impaired access to health care providers and services, coupled with other rural factors. Thus, nurses in rural practice settings have an important role in coordinating a continuum of care to clients living in these underserved areas (Nelson et al., 2009). (Exhibit 1.2).

When the use of health care services is measured, the evidence shows that more than three-fourths of adults in rural areas received medical care on at least one occasion during a year. Despite their overall poorer health status and higher incidence of chronic health conditions, rural adults seek medical care less often than urban adults. In part, this discrepancy can be attributed to scarce resources and lack of providers in rural areas. Also, recruiting and retaining qualified health professionals in general and nurses in particular can be a challenge in rural communities, especially in more sparsely populated regions (AHCPR, 2009; BHPR, 2007; Cromartie, 2008; IOM, 2004; NACRHHS, 2008).

The ability of a person to identify a usual source of care is considered a favorable indicator of access to health care and a person's overall health status. Essentially, a person who has a usual source of care is more likely to seek care when ill and adhere to prescribed regimens. Having the same provider of care can enhance continuity of care, as well as a client's perceived perception of the quality of that

---

EXHIBIT 1.2   Characteristics of rural life

- More space; greater distances between residents and services
- Cyclic/seasonal work and leisure activities
- Informal social and professional interactions
- Access to extended kinship systems
- Residents who are related or acquainted
- Lack of anonymity
- Challenges in maintaining confidentiality stemming from familiarity among residents
- Small (often family) enterprises; fewer large industries
- Economic orientation to land and nature with industries that are extractive in nature (e.g., agriculture, mining, lumbering, marine-related, outdoor recreational activities)
- More high-risk occupations
- Town as the center of trade
- Churches and schools as socialization centers
- Preference for interacting with locals (insiders)
- Mistrust of newcomers to the community (outsiders)

care. Rural adults are more likely than urban adults to identify a particular medical provider as their usual source of care. As for the type of provider who delivers the care, general practitioners and advanced practice registered nurses (APRNs) increasingly are seen by rural adults, whereas urban adults are more likely to seek care from a medical specialist. However, this trend may be changing with health care reform, which emphasizes the importance of primary care (Bureau of Health Professions [BHRP], 2007, 2009; USDHHS, 2010a, 2010c).

Another measure of access to care is traveling time and/or distance to ambulatory care services. Rural persons who seek ambulatory care are more likely to travel more than 30 minutes to reach their usual source of care. Extended commuting time may also be a factor for residents in highly populated urban areas and those who must rely on public transportation. On arriving at the clinic or physician's office, however, no differences between rural and urban residents have been found in the waiting time to see the provider.

Measures of usual place and usual provider suggest that rural residents are at least as well-off as urban residents with regard to access to care (Woolston, 2010). However, caution must be used when making this generalization, because one out of 17 rural counties is reported to have no physician. Among rural respondents on national surveys, the ability to identify a usual site of care or a particular provider often stems from a community or county having only one or two physicians or nurse practitioners (Gamm et al., 2003; IOM, 2004). This finding may be attributable to the reality that it is not unusual for a rural health professional to live and practice in a particular community for decades.

Moreover, in a health professional shortage area (HPSA), a physician, a nurse practitioner, or a nurse often provides services to residents who live in several counties. Consequently, rural physicians and nurses frequently report, "I provide care to individuals and families with all kinds of conditions, in all stages of life, and across several generations" (J. A. Yost, personal communication); thus, it is no surprise that rural respondents who participate in national surveys are able to identify a usual source and a usual provider of health care (BHPR, 2009; NCHS, 2010).

Essentially, one cannot generalize about the health status of rural Americans associated with the diversity coupled with conflicting definitions of what differentiates rural from urban residences. Many vulnerable individuals and families live in rural communities across the United States, but little is known about most of them. This information deficit therefore is a potential area of research for nurses who practice in rural environments.

Barriers to Health Care

Although each rural community is unique, the experience of living in a rural area has several common characteristics (AHCPR, 2009; Bushy, 2008; USDA, 2008a, 2008b). Barriers to health care may include whether or not services and professionals are available, affordable, accessible, or acceptable to the rural consumer (Exhibit 1.3).

Availability implies the existence of health services as well as the necessary personnel to provide essential services. Sparseness of population limits the number and array of health care services in a given geographic region. Lacking a critical mass, the cost of providing special services to a few people often is prohibitive, particularly in frontier states where there are an insufficient number of physicians, nurses, and other types of health care providers. Consequently, where services and personnel are scarce, these must be wisely allocated. Accessibility implies that a person has logistical access to, as well as the ability to purchase, needed services. Affordability is associated with both availability and accessibility of care. It infers that services are of reasonable cost and that a family has sufficient resources to purchase these when needed. Acceptability of care means that a particular service is appropriate and offered in a manner that is congruent with the values of a target population, and unhampered by a client's cultural preference or the urban orientation of health professions (NACRHHS, 2008).

EXHIBIT 1.3   Barriers to health care in rural areas

- Lack of health care providers and services
- Great distances to obtain services
- Lack of personal transportation
- Unavailable public transportation
- Lack of telephone services
- Unavailable outreach services
- Inequitable reimbursement policies for providers
- Unpredictable weather and/or travel conditions
- Inability to pay for care/lack of health insurance
- Lack of "know-how" to procure publicly funded entitlements and services
- Inadequate provider attitudes and understanding about rural populations
- Language barriers (caregivers not linguistically competent)
- Care and services not culturally and linguistically appropriate

The past decade has seen the closure of many small hospitals over two decades. Of those that remain, many report financial problems that could lead to closure (NACRHHS, 2008; USDA, 2006). A shortage or the absence of even one provider, most often a physician or nurse, could mean that a small hospital must close its doors. Closure of the hospital has a ripple effect on the health of local residents, other health care services, and recruiting and retaining health professionals, as well as on economic development efforts in a small community (USDA, 2008a, 2008b).

Likewise, health care providers', in particular nurses', attitudes, insights, and knowledge about rural populations also are important. A patronizing or demeaning attitude, lack of accurate knowledge about rural populations, or insensitivity about the rural lifestyle on the part of a nurse can perpetuate difficulties in relating to those clients. Moreover, insensitivity perpetuates mistrust, resulting in rural clients' perceiving professionals as outsiders to the community. Some nurses in rural practice settings express feelings of professional isolation and community nonacceptance. To address disparate views, nursing faculty members should expose students to the rural environment and the people who live there. Clinical experiences must include opportunities to provide care to clients in their natural (e.g., rural) setting to gain accurate insight about a particular community and the local health care facilities.

Nursing Theory, Research, and Practice

Over the past two decades, the body of literature about nursing practice in small towns and rural environments has grown, and several themes have been noted (Exhibit 1.4).

The work of researchers from the University of Montana is widely accepted. They contend that existing theories do not fully explain rural nursing practice (Long & Weinert, 1989; Winters & Lee, 2009) (Exhibit 1.5).

Montana researchers examined the four concepts pertinent to a nursing theory (health, person, environment, and nursing/caring) and proposed relational statements that are relevant to clients and nurses in rural environments. Since the focus of their research was populations living in the Rocky Mountain area, care must be taken about generalizing those findings to other geographic regions and minorities. They propose that rural residents often judge their health by their ability to work. They consider themselves healthy, even though they may suffer from several chronic illnesses, as long as they are able to continue working. For them, being healthy is the ability to be productive.

EXHIBIT 1.4   Characteristics of nursing practice in rural environments

- Variety/diversity in clinical experiences
- Broader/expanding scope of practice
- Generalist skills with specialty knowledge of crises assessment and management across disciplines/specialties
- Flexibility/creativity in delivering care
- Sparse resources (e.g., materials, professionals, equipment, fiscal)
- Professional/personal isolation
- Greater independence/autonomy
- Role overlap with other disciplines
- Slower pace
- Lack of anonymity
- Increased opportunity for informal interactions with clients/coworkers
- Opportunity for client follow-up on discharge in informal community settings
- Discharge planning allowing for integration of formal and informal resources
- Care for clients across the lifespan
- Exposure to clients with a full range of conditions/diagnoses
- Status in the community (viewed as prestigious)
- Viewed as a professional role model
- Opportunity for community involvement and informal health education

Source: Bushy (2008), Hurme (2009), Nelson (2009), and Winters and Lee (2010).

Chronically ill people emphasize emotional and spiritual well-being rather than physical wellness.

Distance, isolation, and sparse resources characterize rural life and are seen in residents' independent and innovative coping strategies. Self-reliance and independence are demonstrated through their self-care practices and preference for family and community support. Community networks provide support but still allow for each person's and family's independence. Ruralites prefer and usually seek help through their informal networks, such as neighbors, extended family, church, and civic clubs, rather than seeking a professional's care in the formal system of health care, including services such as those provided by a mental health clinic, social service agency, or

EXHIBIT 1.5   Emerging conceptual framework for rural nursing

Nurse researchers at Montana State University proposed the following theoretical concepts and dimensions of rural nursing (Long & Weinert, 1999; Winters & Lee, 2010):

- **Health:** Defined by rural residents as the ability to work. Work and health beliefs are closely related.
- **Environment:** Distance and isolation are particularly important for rural dwellers. Those who live long distances from health care providers neither perceive themselves as isolated nor perceive health care services as inaccessible. Often there is suspicion of outsiders and "government" authorities who the community perceives as historically providing short-term resources without an understanding of the rural way of life.
- **Nursing:** Lack of anonymity, outsider versus insider, old-timer versus newcomer. Lack of anonymity is a common theme among rural nurses who report knowing most people for whom they care, not only in the nurse–client relationship but also in a variety of social roles, such as family member, friend, or neighbor. Acceptance as a health care provider in the community is closely linked to the outsider/insider and newcomer/old-timer phenomena. Gaining trust and acceptance of local people is identified as a unique challenge that must be successfully negotiated by nurses before they can begin to function as effective health care providers. Nurses often feel increased accountability for friends and neighbors.
- **Person:** Self-reliance and independence in relationship to health care are strong characteristics of rural individuals. They prefer to have people they know care for them (informal services) as opposed to an outsider in a formal agency.

health department. Although nursing is generally similar across settings and populations, there are some unique features associated with practice in a geographically remote area or in small towns where most people are familiar with one another. The next few paragraphs highlight a few of the variations that nurses in rural practice report (Hurme, 2009; Molinari & Monserud, 2008; Nelson, 2009; Skillman, Palazzo, Hart, & Butterfield, 2007).

A nurse's professional and personal boundaries often overlap and are diffuse. It is not unusual for a nurse to have more than one work-related role in the community. For example, a nurse may work at the local hospital or in a physician's office and may also be actively involved in managing the family farm, a local grocery store, or the pharmacy. For nurses, this means that many patients they encounter are personally known as neighbors, as friends of an immediate family member, or perhaps as part of one's extended family. Associated with social informality is a corresponding lack of anonymity in a small town. Some rural nurses say, "I never really feel like I am off duty because everybody in the county knows me through my work" (L. King, personal communication). In part, this report can be attributed to nurses being highly esteemed in their community and viewed by local people as experts on health and illness. It is not unusual for residents to informally ask a nurse's advice before seeing a physician for a health problem. Moreover, health-related questions are asked by residents when they encounter a local nurse in a grocery store, at a service station, during a basketball game, or at church functions.

Nurses in rural practice must make decisions about the care of individuals of all ages and with a variety of health conditions. They assume many roles because of the range of services that must be provided in a rural health care facility, given the scarcity of nursing and other health professionals. Stemming from rural residents' expectations of the health care delivery system, need to display nurses in rural practice technical and clinical competency, self-confidence, leadership, adaptability, flexibility, sound decision making, and interest in continuing education, together with skills in handling emergencies, teaching, and public relations. The nurse administrator, too, may be expected to be a jack-of-all-trades (i.e., a generalist) and to demonstrate competence in several clinical specialties in addition to managing and organizing staff within the facility for which he or she is responsible. Administrators often perform patient care in addition to their leadership and management responsibilities.

There are challenges, opportunities, and rewards in rural nursing practice. The manner in which each factor is perceived depends on individual preferences and the situation in a given community. Challenges of rural practice sometimes are listed as professional isolation, limited opportunities for continuing education, lack of other kinds of health personnel or professionals with whom one can interact, heavy workloads, an ability to function well in several clinical areas, lack of anonymity, and, for some, a restricted social life (Nelson, 2009; Roberge, 2009).

Of the many opportunities and rewards in rural nursing practice, those most commonly cited include close relationships with clients and coworkers, diverse clinical experiences that evolve from caring for clients of all ages who have a variety of health problems, caring for clients for long periods of time (in some cases, across several generations), opportunities for professional development, and greater autonomy. Many nurses value the solitude and quality of life found in a rural community, both personally and for their families. Others thrive on the outdoor recreational activities. Still others thoroughly enjoy the informal, face-to-face interactions coupled with the public recognition and status associated with living and working as a nurse in a small community.

Nursing in the Community

Although most of the publications about rural health care and nursing focus on hospital practice, much of that information is applicable to both community-oriented agencies and community-focused nursing (Davis & Droes, 1993; Molinari & Monserud, 2008; Skillman et al., 2007). The work-related stressors of community-focused nursing have received some attention in the literature. Early on, Case (1991) identified stressful experiences of nurses working in rural Oklahoma health departments including the following: political or bureaucratic problems, and interprofessional collaborations and interpersonal conflicts associated with inadequate communication; unsatisfactory work environment and understaffing; difficult or unpleasant nurse–client encounters, such as with relatives who refuse to deliver needed care to clients, and with clients who are hostile, apathetic, dependent, or of low intelligence; fear for personal safety; difficulty locating clients, and clients falling through the cracks of the health care system. (Decades later, similar stressors are cited by nurses who work in urban as well as rural public health agencies.) Anecdotal reports describe specific stressors associated with geographic distance, isolation, sparse resources, and other environmental factors that characterize rurality. Nursing in rural practice settings is characterized by physical isolation that may lend itself to any one of the following: professional isolation; scarce financial, human, and health care resources; and a broad scope of practice.

Anecdotally, this author has heard reports from nurses describing the lack of civility among nurses and other staff members in small health care facilities. Such behaviors may be related to low staff numbers who are employed in the facility who have day-to-day encounters. Sometimes the interpersonal conflicts that exist in the hospital or long-term care facility become common knowledge among community residents, and the targeted individuals are unable to "get away from it." Subsequently, the individuals may leave the facility or the community, and sometimes the profession. This dimension of retention of nurses in rural settings needs further study to identify risk factors and potential interventions to prevent the described outcomes (K. L., L. U., S. S. et al., personal communication).

Associated with personal familiarity with local residents, nurses often possess in-depth knowledge about clients and their families. Along with the acknowledged benefits, informal (face-to-face) interactions can significantly reduce a nurse's anonymity in the community and at times be a barrier to completing an objective assessment on a client. Like urban practice, rural community nursing takes place in a variety of locations, including homes, clinics, schools, occupational settings, and correctional facilities, and at community events such as county fairs, rodeos, civic and church-sponsored functions, and school athletic events.

Nursing Practice

Nurses in rural practice must have broad knowledge about nursing theory. Topics important in this practice environment include health promotion, primary prevention, rehabilitation, obstetrics, medical–surgical specialties, pediatrics, planning and implementing community assessments, and understanding the public health risks and needs for emergency preparedness in a particular state. A community's demographic profile and its principal industry(ies) can provide a snapshot of some of its social, political, and health risks. From this kind of information, a nurse can anticipate the particular nursing skills that will be needed to care for clients in a catchment area (U.S.A. Center for Rural Health Preparedness, n.d.).

Refer to Exhibit 1.6 for the health-related priorities for rural communities.

EXHIBIT 1.6   Health service priorities of rural communities

Access to care
Cancer (screening, early intervention, oncology services)
Diabetes (prevention, screening, tertiary care)
Maternal/Infant and children services
Mental Illness and behavioral health services
Nutrition/obesity
Drugs, Alcohol, and Substance abuse
Use of tobacco products
Education and an array of community-based programs

Public health infrastructures
Immunizations and infectious diseases
Injury and violence prevention
Family planning
Environmental and occupational health
Emergency medical services infrastructures
Long-term care/assistive living facilities
Other—that will vary by community based on predominate
  industry(ies) and age cohorts

Source: Bennett et al. (2008) and Gamm et al. (2003).

Nursing Research

Empirical data about rural family systems are sparse in terms of their health beliefs, values, perceptions of illness, and health care-seeking behaviors, as well as what is deemed to be appropriate nursing care. Therefore, nurse scholars must assume a more active role in implementing research on the needs of rural populations for nursing services to expand the profession's theoretical base and subsequently implement community-sensitive, evidence-based clinical interventions (Bushy, 2009; Graves, 2009; Merwin, 2008). Specific research topics that are of importance to nursing practice in rural environments include the following, among others.

- Most nurses indicate that they enjoy practicing in rural areas and are proud of what they do. They believe, however, that their work deserves more recognition by professional nursing organizations. Furthermore, the retention rate of nurses in some practice settings is poor. The perspective of nurses who are dissatisfied with rural nursing is necessary to provide a more complete picture of the rural experience. This information can be useful to a variety of people: Other nurses who are considering rural practice; nurse managers in need of better screening tools to assess the fit between the nurse and the environment when interviewing applicants; planners of continuing nursing education programs; and faculty members who teach undergraduate and graduate students.
- More information is needed about the stressors and rewards of rural practice. These data could lead to the development of stress management techniques to be used by nurses and their supervisors to retain nurses and improve the quality of their workplace environment.

■ With the increasing number of rural residents in all regions of the United States, empirical data are needed on the particular nursing needs of rural–client systems, especially underrepresented groups, minorities, and other at-risk populations that vary by region and state.

■ There also is a need for the international perspective on the health of rural populations, and on nursing practice within the rural community. Nurse scholars from Australian, New Zealand, and Canada have provided some insights into rural practice in these nations. Information is needed from less-industrialized nations as well as from those that are highly industrialized.

■ Technology increasingly is used in health care and seems to hold great potential in improving access to health care in rural and underserved areas. However, research is needed to determine the most efficient and effective way to meet the needs and preferences of rural clients, and to assure quality.

■ Communication technology increasingly is used by institutions of higher learning to deliver educational programs to nurses who live and work some distance from campus. Empirical studies are needed to measure the most effective modalities to achieve desired learning outcomes and the impact on recruitment and retention of nurses in rural settings.

■ Rural–urban disparities in health status and health behaviors need closer examination from the nursing perspective. Evidence-based practice nursing guidelines are needed that take into consideration the rural context and preferences of residents who obtain health care in these settings.

In summary, preparing nurses to practice in rural environments demands creative and innovative nursing educational opportunities, such as nurse transition to practice and extended residency programs. Communication technology and the internet hold great potential to link nurses in rural practice with nurse educators and researchers in urban-based academic settings. Collaboration and partnerships must be established to design and implement innovative learning experiences that include educators, rural nurses, and administrators of health care facilities in rural settings. To meet the demands and expectations of practice in that setting, nursing faculty members must expose students to the rural environment, facilitate the development and appreciation of generalist skills, and enhance the ability to function in several roles—that is, as expert generalists. The short supply and increasing demand for primary care providers in general, and nurses in particular, will continue for some time. In an effort to effectively respond to this opportunity, nurses must be creative to ensure delivery of appropriate and acceptable services to at-risk and vulnerable populations who live in rural and underserved regions. Nurses must be sensitive to the health beliefs of clients, and then plan and provide nursing interventions that mesh with the community's cultural values and preferences.

REFERENCES

Agency for Health Care Policy and Research (AHCPR). (2009). *Health care in urban and rural ar-eas combined years 2004–2006: Update of Content in MEPS Chartbook No. 13.* Retrieved 4/19/11 from http://www.ahrq.gov/data/meps/chbook13up.htm

Bennett, K., Olatosi, B., & Probst, J. (2008). *Health disparities: A rural—urban chart-book.* Retrieved 4/19/11 from http://rhr.sph.sc.edu/report/%287-3%29%20Health%20Disparities%20A%20Rural%20Urban%20Chartbook%20-%20Distribution%20Copy.pdf

Bigbee, J. L., & Crowder, E. L. (1985). The Red Cross Rural Nursing Service: An innovative model of public health nursing delivery. *Public Health Nursing, 2*(2), 109–121.

Bureau of the Census. (2009). *Annual esti-mates of the resident population for incorporated places.* Retrieved 4/19/11 from http://www.census.gov/compendia/statab/2008/tables/08s0028.pdf

Bureau of Health Professions (BHPR). (2007). *Nurse shortage counties.* Washington, DC: U.S. Department of Health and Human Services. Retrieved 4/19/11 from http://bhpr.hrsa.gov/healthworkforce/nursingshortage/issues.htm#f8

Bureau of Health Professions (BHPR). (2009). *Shortage designation: HPSAs, MUAs, MUPs.* Washington, DC: U.S. Department of Health and Human Services. Retrieved 4/19/11 from http://bhpr.hrsa.gov/shortage

Bushy, A. (2008). Conducting culturally compe-tent rural nursing research. *Annual Review of Nursing Research, 26,* 221–236.

Bushy, A. (2009). American nurses credentialing center (ANCC) pathway to excellence program: Addressing and meeting the needs of small and rural hospitals. *Online Journal of Rural Nursing and Health Care, 9*(1), 6–10. Retrieved 4/12/11 from http://www.rno.org/journal/index.php/online-journal/article/viewFile/171/221

Bushy, A. (2011). *Rural nursing: practice and issues—American Nurses Association On-line Continuing Education Program.* Retrieved 4/12/11 from http://www.nursingworld.org/mods/mod700/rurlfull.htm

Case, T. (1991). *Work stresses of community health nurses in Oklahoma.* In A. Bushy (Ed.), *Rural nursing* (Vol. 2). Newbury Park, CA: Sage.

Centers for Disease Control (CDC). (2010). *Healthy communities program: An overview.* Retrieved 4/12/11 from http://www.cdc.gov/healthycommunitiesprogram

Cromartie, J. (2008). Defining the "rural" in rural America. *Amber Waves, 6*(3), 28–35. Retrieved from http://www.ers.usda.gov/AmberWaves/June08/Features/RuralAmerica.htm

Davis, D. J., & Droes, N. S. (1993). Com-munity health nursing in rural and frontier counties. *The Nursing Clinics of North America, 28*(1), 159–169.

Gamm, L., Hutchison, L., Dabney, B. et al. (2003). *Rural Healthy People 2010: A companion document to Healthy People 2010,* Vols I, II, III. College Sta-tion, TX: Texas A&M University System Health Sci-ence Center, School of Rural Health, Southwest Rural Health Research Center. Retrieved 4/12/11 from http://www.srph.tamhsc.edu/centers/rhp2010/publications.htm

Graves, B. (2009). Community-based participa-tory research: Toward eliminating rural health dis parities. *Online Journal of Rural Nursing and Health Care, 9*(1), 12–14. Retrieved 4/12/11 from http://www.rno.org/journal/index.php/online-journal/article/viewFile/173/223

Hurme, E. (2009). Competencies for nursing practice in a rural critical access hospital. *Online Journal of Rural Nursing and Health Care, 9*(2), 67–81. Retrieved 4/12/11 from http://www.rno.org/journal/index.php/online-journal/article/viewFile/198/256

Institute of Medicine (IOM). (2004). *Quality Through Collaboration: The Future of Rural Health.* Washington, DC: IOM author. Retrieved 4/12/11 from http://www.iom.edu/report.asp?id=23359

Long, K. A., & Weinert, C. (1989). Rural nursing: Developing the theory base. *Scholarly In-quiry for Nursing Practice, 3*(2), 113–127.

Mead, H., Cartwright-Smith, L., Jones, K., Ramos, C., Woods, K., & Siegel, B. (2008). *Racial and Ethnic Disparities in U.S. Health Care: A Chartbook.* Retrieved 4/19/11 from http://www.commonwealthfund.org/~/media/Files/Publica tions/Chartbook/2008/Mar/Racial%20and%20Ethnic%20Disparities%20in%20U%20S%20%20Health%20Care%20%20A%20Chartbook/Mead_racialethnic disparities_chartbook_1111%20pdf.pdf

Merwin, B. (Eds.). (2008). *Annual review of nursing research: Focus on rural health, 26.* New York: Springer.

Molinari, D. L., & Monserud, M. A. (2008). Rural nurse job satisfaction. *Rural and Remote Health: The International Electronic Journal of Rural Re-mote Health, Research, Education, Practice and Pol-icy.* Retrieved 4/19/11 from http://www.rrh.org.au/articles/subviewnew.asp?ArticleID=1055

National Advisory Committee on Rural Health and Human Services (NACRHHS). (2008). *The 2008 Report to the Secretary: Rural Health and Human Services Issues.* Retrieved 4/19/11 from ftp://ftp.hrsa.gov/ruralhealth/committee/NACreport2008.pdf

National Center for Health Statistics (NCHS). (2010). *Health Behaviors of Adults United States -2005–2007.* Retrieved 4/19/11 from http://www.cdc.gov/nchs/data/series/sr_10/sr10_245.pdf

Nelson, J., & Stover-Gingerich, B. (2010). Rural health: Access to care and services. *Home Health Care Management Practice Online.* Retrieved 4/12/11 from http://hhc.sagepub.com/cgi/rapidpdf/1084822309353552v1

Nelson, W. (Ed.). (2009). *Handbook for rural health care ethics: A practical guide for professionals.* Lebanon, NH: Dartmouth. Retrieved 4/19/11 from http://dms.dartmouth.edu/cfm/resources/ethics/

Rand Corporation. (2010a). *U.S. Health Care Today: Coverage.* Retrieved 4/19/11 from http://www.randcompare.org/us-health-care-today/coverage

Rand Corporation. (2010b). *U.S. Health Care Today: Health*. Retrieved 4/12/11 from http://www.randcompare.org/us-health-care-today/health

Roberge, C. (2009). Who stays in rural nursing practice? An international review of the literature on factors influencing rural nurse retention. *Online Journal of Rural Nursing and Health Care, 9*(12), 82–93. Retrieved 4/19/11 from http://www.rno.org/journal/index.php/online-journal/article/viewFile/180/230

Skillman, S., Palazzo, L., Hart, G., & Butterfield, P. (2007). *Changes in the rural Registered Nurse workforce from 1980 to 2004*. Seatle, WA: WWAMI Rural Health Research Center. Retrieved 4/12/11 from http://depts.washington.edu/uwrhrc/uploads/RHRC%20FR115%20Skillman.pdf

U.S.A. Center for Rural Health Preparedness. (n.d.) Rural emergency preparedness toolkit (CDRom.). Retrieved 4/12/11 from http://www.rural-preparedness.org/index.aspx?page=3f3872b2-72dd-499f-8079-523bfd06d61f

U.S. Department of Agriculture (USDA). (2005). Measuring rurality: 2004 County typology codes. Retrieved 4/19/11 from http://www.ers.usda.gov/Briefing/rurality/Typology/

U.S. Department of Agriculture (USDA). (2006). *Measuring rurality: What is a micropolitan area?* Retrieved 4/12/11 from http://www.ers.usda.gov/Briefing/Rurality/MicropolitanAreas/

U.S. Department of Agriculture (USDA). (2008a). *Rural America at a glance: 2009 edi-tion*. Retrieved 4/12/11 from http://www.ers.usda.gov/Publications/EIB59/EIB59.pdf

U.S. Department of Agriculture (USDA). (2008b). *What is rural?* Retrieved 4/12/11 from http://www.nal.usda.gov/ric/ricpubs/what_is_rural.shtml#character

U.S. Department of Health and Human Services (USDHHS). (2010a). *More choices, better coverage: Health insurance reform and rural America*. Retrieved 4/12/11 from http://www.healthreform.gov/reports/ruralamerica/index.html

U.S. Department of Health and Human Services (USDHHS). (2010b). *Healthy People 2020*. Retrieved 4/12/11 from http://www.healthypeople.gov/hp2020/Comments/default.asp

U.S. Department of Health and Human Services (USDHHS). (2010c). *Health, United States, 2009: With special feature on technology*. Retrieved 4/12/11 from http://www.cdc.gov/nchs/data/hus/hus09.pdf

Winters, C., & Lee, H. (2009). *Rural nursing: Concepts, theory and practice* (3rd ed.). New York, NY: Springer Publishing Co.

Woolston, C. (2010, June 10). Lonesome doc: Medicine in a small town. *AARP Bulletin*. Retrieved 4/12/11 from http://www.aarp.org/health/doctors-hospitals/info-06-2010/medicine_in_a_small_town.html

2

Rural Nurse Transition-to-Practice Programs

Deana L. Molinari

The Institute of Medicine recommends offering transition-to-practice residencies for all recent nurse graduates as well as employees transitioning to new specialties. The discussion in this chapter highlights national and global trends; and examines the benefits and challenges of implementing such programs in small rural health care facilities.

The rural nurse transition-to-practice (TTP) discourse is a dialog about redesigning change. Transformation permeates a nurses' career development process. An individual alters him or herself through the sting of reflection, growth, and development, as well as the agony of testing and achievement. The nursing profession undergoes a similar redesigning process through discussions, initiatives, plans, and programs, as well as with transforming research and evaluation (Heinrich, 2011). The more transition is debated, the more the occupation is altered.

Florence Nightingale began professional redesigning 1855 by developing a new type of nursing school (Bloy, 2010). Yet, strangely, the more the discussion about altering nursing, the greater the realization of how little evidence is known about creating quality nurses (Baernholdt, Jennings, Merwin, & Thornlow, 2010; Lenz & Barnard, 2009). Current leaders debate the links between workforce performance management and patient care outcomes (Campbell, Roland, & Buetow, 2000). The nursing TTP discussion is related to several concepts such as: Professional education, patient care, performance measurement, job satisfaction, recruitment, and retention. Chapters in this text discuss each of these topics while calling for more information about rurally specific issues.

TTP is part of a larger nursing curriculum reformation which, in turn, is part of a larger health care professional curriculum initiative, and one aspect of the national demand for more accessible and affordable health care. In 2009, a collaborative initiative, *The Future of Nursing*, was implemented to transform nursing education. This initiative was undertaken by the Institute of Medicine (IOM) and the Robert Wood Johnson Foundation (RWJ) in an effort to identify the concepts that should be taught, how to instruct students to achieve competence, and when to teach the necessary content (Institute of Medicine [IOM], 2010a, 2010b).

The purpose of the initiative was to improve new graduates' competence in an expanding knowledge discipline. The literature indicates newly licensed nurses are not adequately prepared for the transition to professional practice (Billings, 2008). To survive in the health care system as it currently exists, a nurse must have the ability to practice in fast-paced change settings, lead teams of health care providers, and work under the pressure of a decreasing nurse supply. In addition, the gap between education and professional practice needs to be crossed by the nurse (Allen, 2008).

Basic education reforms are detailed in the collaborative initiative report titled, *The Future of Nursing: Leading Change, Advancing Health* (IOM, 2010a). The alterations under discussion include: Introducing youth to the profession, revising the academic curriculum, standardizing professional entry degrees, forming TTP collaborations, and requiring periodic performance competency measurements. Specific proposals highlighted are:

- Encouraging nurses to practice to the full extent of their education and training.
- Assisting nurses in achieving higher levels of education and training through an improved education system that promotes seamless academic progression.
- Partnering nurses with physicians and other health care professionals, to redesign health care in the United States.
- Collecting data and improving the information structure to develop effective nurse workforce plans and policies.

The IOM report essentially urges the nursing profession to move from a supportive to a leadership role within the health care system. Achieving a leadership role will require the active involvement of all health care layers: Individual nurses, health care organizations, third-party payers, professional organizations, business enterprises, health care organizations, as well as state and federal governments. Leadership in designing accessible and safe patient care with improved health outcomes requires nurses to exert the power of numbers and knowledge. The more-than-three-million nurses will need to work together and with other health care professionals to define the new leadership role. The IOM report also urges nursing to identify professional needs and develop creative solutions. So, what does the information in the IOM report mean for rural TTP?

Although a study by the National Council of State Boards of Nursing (NCSBN) conducted in 2006 found a majority of newly licensed nurses participate in some type of orientation program, about 41% experienced a comprehensive transition program that included a hospital orientation and a clinical supervision component. Most of the two-pronged orientation programs are offered in larger urban-based hospitals with a staff development department and perhaps collaborating with academic institutions. Currently, there are no national standards for nurse TTP programs that list specified content, outcomes, or the length of time for the course. Still, studies indicate nurse TTP programs improve individuals' competencies, lower stress levels, enhance self-confidence, reduce the time required for orientation, and improve retention rates within the facility (Beyea, Von Reyn, & Slattery, 2007).

The *Future of Nursing* initiative recommends offering TTP residencies that are designed for recent graduates as well as employees moving to specialty positions. Academic curricula do not prepare graduates with the skills for situational decision making or the professional attitudes needed to manage highly stressful workplaces. Likewise, new employees require mentoring along with on-the-job supervision, whether they are employed by community agencies or hospitals (Stokowski, 2011).

Providing a nurse residency program indicates an institution is moving beyond the goal of increasing the number of available bedside nurses to a goal of providing accessible, safe, and affordable patient care (Stokowski, 2011). Health care organizations consider a number of other issues as well. Consumers increasingly demand competent care based on evidence. Subsequently, health care institutions are changing organizational structures and the manner in which nurses provide care in order to meet consumer demands. Organizations are reshaping employment practices to accommodate a growing influx of aging individuals with diverse backgrounds and multiple chronic health conditions, and a decreasing number of nurses entering the profession. Organizations are learning to provide more health promotion, illness prevention, self-care, and diversity sensitivity services. In order to "reduce" the cost of health care, payers intend to spend less on acute care and more on preventative care. All these organizational changes affect the manner in which nurses are educated and their relationship with other health professionals.

The Institute of Medicine (IOM, 2010b) addressed another issue in *Redesigning Continuing Education for the Health Professions.* The report recommends five major changes for postlicensure education. Continuing education (CE) must change the way it is conducted, financed, regulated, and evaluated. The following issues are addressed:

- The science underpinning CE is insufficient, fragmented, and must be developed.
- Interprofessional CE requires constructing tailored learning environments so that teamwork and collaboration can be fostered.
- A comprehensive vision of professional development is needed to replace the present CE culture.
- Establishing a national interprofessional CE institute is a recommended way to foster these goals.

CE IMPROVEMENTS

The IOM's report expands the work accomplished by several other groups. The Josiah Macy Jr. Foundation Report (Hager, Russell, & Fletcher, 2008) found that the existing system of CE is flawed and does not support the development of health care professionals. The report states that the absence of a comprehensive national vision and regulatory body contributes to the lack of professional knowledge production and the number of performance deficiencies. The authors contend that systematic CE concerns are further complicated by instructional design failures. CE instructors need educational design methods that support performance-based competency validation.

The American Nurses Association defined CE as staff development and in-service education until 2010. The revised *Scope and Standards of Practice* (American Nurses Association, 2011) expanded the professional development model to include the following components: Continuing nursing education (CNE), in-service education, staff development, academic education, clinical skill competencies, and professional development. This document significantly impacts on organizations providing educational services as well as nurses who purchase educational products. The document also alters the way information (content) is delivered, designed, and measured. Ultimately, this reform may reduce the number of formal conferences and lectures while increasing the number of simulation experiences and bedside learning opportunities.

Traditionally, CE contact hours were awarded based on the time the learner spent on the offering rather than what the learner gained from the session. The revised goals are meant to improve nurse performance. Educational products will be developed differently. There will be a focus on measuring participants' competencies. Teachers will be required to teach strategies based on evidence and identified standards. The American Nurses Association recommends nurses design personal professional development plans based on learning preferences, needs, environments, and expectations. In other words, the educational environment will shift from the desk and chair to the point of care (DeSilets, 2010). The new approaches to CE provide a researcher's playground.

The scarcity of research about professional development and its impact on patient care is alarming according to the IOM (2010). The discipline lacks a data-based infrastructure to guide practice. There is insufficient information to support present practices or project future trends. The IOM's call to change professional development offers a venue for providers to market new products. Providers without knowledge of best practices and a supporting culture of data collection are likely to create products that waste time and money and can ultimately harm patients. The initiative calling for more research will impact on nurse residency program design (Allen et al., 2010). Transitioning nurses to professional practice requires evidence about how nurse practice impacts patient care outcomes. Data collection will need to expand from participant satisfaction surveys to performance achievement validation. Since the purpose of educational products are changing from knowledge transfer to performance improvement, designing the courses is also changing.

Instructional designers are challenged to develop interprofessional learning in patient care settings. The current literature provides little information as to the best way to teach numerous professionals representing various disciplines in one classroom setting. Some disciplines focus on diagnosis, others on treatment interventions, while still others translate data-based evidence into care, support, education, and communication, which facilitate progressing through a complex health care system. Collaborative education programs address the various roles while improving shared skills such as assessment, care management, outcomes evaluation, teaching, quality improvement, policy development, leadership, collaboration, and communication.

Interprofessional staff development can occur in nurse residencies. Physicians and pharmacists, for example, can be included in a "rural community hospital" exercise. Recently, professional nurses performed various nursing roles (certified nurse assistant, licensed practical nurses, registered nurses, and an advanced practice nurse) while caring for simulated patients (standardized patients and high-fidelity simulators) in a virtual (online hospital). In one simulated experience, a patient "crashed" every 20 minutes. Participants collaborated in a team to develop solutions. In this cyber hospital, a drug reaction, an end-of-life decision, a fall, and a myocardial infarction encouraged the participants' problem solving. The exercise focused on teamwork communication using the TeamSTEPPS® competencies. Combining professionals from several disciplines in one learning environment teaches more than exercise solution. Learning how other professionals think and communicate can break down barriers and diffuse professional "silo thinking." National professional organizations, such as the American Nurses Association and the American Medical Association encourage CE reformation that will bring various disciplines together and address similar patient care topics.

RURAL AND URBAN INEQUITIES

CE in rural facilities requires even more restructuring than in urban settings, for several reasons. First and foremost, there are few nurses, fewer (if any) staff developers, and even less knowledge about the educational and learning needs of the rural nurse, as well as scarce professional development resources (Molinari & Monserud, 2009). These realities contribute to reduced educational opportunity. Small facilities in remote settings can collaborate with nursing schools and professional organizations to increase professional development frequency, appropriateness, and quality. Since so much diversity exists in rural communities, there is little likelihood for one approach to appeal or be suitable for all agencies.

The World Health Organization (WHO) reports an inequality of nurse distribution in the world, with 60% of nurses practicing in urban centers (Roberge, 2009). In the United States, the urban to rural distribution of nurses is 80% to 20%. Economic declines in small communities may result in an inadequate population base to support full-time nurses. Another outcome of declining fiscal resources is that local nurses may choose to commute to urban centers for full-time employment, further complicating the rural employment issue. (Other recruitment, and retention issues are discussed in other chapters of this volume.)

Recruitment and retention issues found in rural communities often relate to nurse education. More specifically, a study conducted in Colorado indicates nurse recruitment in small rural facilities takes 60% longer than in a more populated setting, causing greater expense (Roberge, 2009) and reducing available funds for new employee educational support.

Rural nurses experience inequitable access to education, training, and professional development for a number of reasons (Francis, Bowman, & Redgrave, 2001). There are few staff developers in rural facilities. Professional development is delivered by a nurse who also has patient care and/or management responsibilities. Local educational offerings are often limited to state and hospital accreditation requirements. Moreover, part-time nurses receive less education than do their full-time counterparts. Some education topics require nurses to travel, limiting frequency due to related expenses. Including registration, travel, accommodation, childcare, and a relief nurse. Likewise, professional development record maintenance is often lax, thus impairing proof of accomplishment. Urban facilities are better able to match a nurse's skills with patient acuity on a particular unit. However, this practice is rare in small hospitals due to low staffing numbers along with the lack of technological infrastructure (Holloway, Lumby, & Baker, 2009).

Although staff development programs promote both the confidence and competence demanded of rural nurses (Keahey, 2008), and the literature indicates that rural practice requires nurses with advanced practice skills, there is little to indicate how nurses attain this level of competence. There is a paucity of data addressing the question: Should rural nursing skills be taught prelicensure or postemployment? Finding an answer to the question may be difficult due to infrequent academic courses and few staff development courses covering rural specialty skills.

Theoretical Foundation

Most education theories were developed in urban settings, resulting in possible rural inequity or even inappropriate application. Theoretical frameworks are needed to enlarge the body of knowledge unique to rural nursing. Theories that provide systematic approaches to studying rural nurses, consumers, and patients are needed (Alligood & Tomey, 2010). In addition, evidence-based information about rural CE associated with staff development patterns and impact on patient care outcomes are needed.

There is a critical need to study rural nurse TTP needs and develop programs designed to address those needs. Few articles discuss the theoretical and practice issues. At present, several theories support TTP but these are insufficient for rural skill development. Theories such as Benner's *Novice to Expert* theory of professional development, adult learning theory, and rural nursing theory are often mentioned in the nursing literature. Benner posits that employees need time, experience, and increasing knowledge to blend practical knowledge with academic studies. "Expertise develops as the clinician tests and modifies principle based expectations in the actual situation" (Alligood & Tomey, 2010, p. 141). These theoretical foundations fail to address many of the issues described in this text, such as "place," practice setting variations, and the lack of recognition for rural nursing as a specialty. More information is needed about differences among urban and rural residency outcomes. Since rural nurses describe practice in different terms, does CE differ? Rural nurses practice differently from urban nurses, as explained in chapter one; however, there is little information about how rural competencies are taught or measured. For example, nurses often enter the profession as midlevel managers without the needed knowledge resources.

The topic of developing rural TTP is widely discussed at this time. Globally, national governments, professional organizations, and individual facilities are making an effort to develop new graduates for professional responsibilities. While numerous methodologies are employed to achieve the goal, few studies measure the strengths and weaknesses of the initiatives. The lack of consistency in defining new employee support complicates the restructuring of education discussion. For example, some support programs begin before licensure. The N2K program sponsored by the Oregon Office of Rural Health and housed in the Oregon Health Careers Center was designed to reduce rural nurse shortage (Helseth, 2010). Rural hospitals enroll promising employees, assist them to obtain a degree, and then ask for a contracted service period postlicensure. The Washington Rural Outreach in Nursing Education program possesses a similar philosophy. Facilities can "grow their own" nurses rather than hire strangers. (Both programs are described in this text.) Retention outcomes of this type of program should be compared with various internships, residencies, and preceptorships.

Some residency programs are developed by "expert" urban nurses and offered as "outreach" to rural facilities. Other programs are task oriented, and do not address role skills such as crisis assessment and management, rural nursing theory, rural collaborative practice, rural community accountability, use of formal and informal rural resources, population-focused health issues, or communication patterns in small communities. Some rural transition curricula address pertinent topics such as local rural morbidity and mortality patterns, along with local patterns of chronic disease including diabetes, stroke, heart and vascular disease, and mental and behavioral health problems (Australian Institute of Health and Welfare, 2010).

Not all nurse transition programs meet rural-specific learning needs, which is due to the shortage of rural research. The lack of information creates an educational bias for urban practice. Educator rural bias is evident when an educator states there is no difference in treating patients in urban or rural settings; or when large tertiary care facilities provide "outreach" education to rural facilities without involving rural "expert" nurses. Even the term "outreach" can be considered biased, suggesting a charitable act to improve patient care in a needy environment.

Rural professionals possess their own expertise. For instance, rural nurses differentiate roles according to unique small community needs. Rural communication patterns and interprofessional relationships occur differently than in large urban hospitals (Williams, 2001). Sharing tasks, collaboration, and making-do with less are rural proficiencies. Nurses often perform tasks not executed in urban settings, such as blood gas analysis and discharge planning. Therefore, rural nurses can address their own TTP issues, study rural practice patterns, and disseminate research.

The chapters in this book describe other transition strategies as well.

- Orientation: Or the transfer of knowledge about specific skills, tasks, policies, and procedures provided by facilities and corporations. Orientations last for a short time and enable nurses to function in specific locations.
- Internships are defined as programs offered either before or shortly after graduation that teach a variety of practice skills such as career management, communication, and delegation, although orientation programs are still required to develop specific tasks. The word internship is often used as a substitute for residency.
- Residencies occur shortly after graduation and when changing career focus. The difference between an internship and a residency is that the latter is specialty specific rather than time period specific. The idea is to provide specialty role knowledge, socialization, and competency measurement when it is needed. Many topics are included in the curriculum such as leadership, communication, professional practices, clinical reasoning, assessment, and management.
- Preceptorships focus on developing cultures where experts share with newcomers. One benefit of educating experienced nurses and providing them processes to educate novices is improvement of the whole staff. The culture of nourishing all nurses is established. A disadvantage of providing only preceptors is the reliance on older teachers with established bad habits and a tendency to teach the way they were taught before competency education.
- Competency measurement programs seek to define nursing practice as skills that must be demonstrated. The behavioral method of

teaching, demonstration, and regurgitation can also have negative consequences. The competencies can become protocols for tasks and lack nursing-role emphasis. Role performance is harder to measure. The advantage of competency programs is that the institution speaks a common expectation language (Bassendowski & Petrucka, 2009).

- Staff development programs are courses often associated with nurse contact hours and focus on a specific topic. The certificates indicate achievement in special skills like trauma assessment and reading EKGs. There are larger content programs that prepare nurses to take national certification courses like informatics, case management, or staff development. The Rural Nurse Organization (rno.org) and academic institutions provide education programs to support rural staff development in specific practice matters.
- A combination of approaches is supported by most TTP programs. There is not enough evidence yet to suggest best practices. Although the evidence is strong that baccalaureate preparation for nursing is associated with lower mortality rates, no one has yet compared internships with residencies for effectiveness. Although competencies are growing in popularity, the types that produce safe patient care are not yet identified. More study is needed.

In summary, the IOM recommends TTP programs for novice nurses and those seeking to function in another specialty area. Rural programs are needed. The benefits and challenges of implementing such programs in rural health care institutions are extensive.

REFERENCES

Allen, L. (2008). The nursing shortage continues as faculty shortage grows. *Nursing Economics, 26*(1), 35–40.

Allen, S. R., Fiorini, P., & Dickey, M. (2010). A Streamlined clinical advancement program improves RN participation and retention. *The Journal of Nursing Administration, 40*(7/8), 316.

Alligood, M. R., & Tomey, A. M. (2010). *Nursing theorists and their work* (7th ed.) Maryland Heights, MO: Mosby/Elsevier. ISBN: 978-0-323-05641-0.

American Nurses Association. (2011). *Nursing professional development: Scope and standards of practice.* Silver Spring, MD: American Nurses Association.

Australian Institute of Health and Welfare. (2010). Risk factors disease and death. Retrieved March 24, 2011 from http://aihw.gov.au/

Bassendowski, S., & Petrucka, P. (2009). Continuing competence program of the Saskatchewan Registered Nurses' Association. *Journal of Continuing Education in Nursing, 40*(12), 553–559.

Baernholdt, M., Jennings, B., Merwin, E., & Thornlow, D. (2010). What does quality care mean to nurses in rural hospitals? *Journal of Advanced Nursing, 6*(6), 1346–1355.

Beyea, S. C., von Reyn, L., & Slattery, M. J. (2007). A nurse residency program for competency development using human patient simulation. *Journal for Nurses in Staff Development, 23*(2), 77–82.

Billings, D. M. (2008). Quality care, patient safety, and the focus on technology. *Journal of Nursing Education, 47*(2), 51–52.

Bloy, M. (2010). Florence Nightingale. Retrieved March 24, 2011 from http://www.victorianweb.org/history/crimea/florrie.html

Campbell, S., Roland, M., & Buetow, S. (2000). Defining quality of care. *Social Science & Medicine, 51*, 1611–1625.

DeSilets, L. D. (2010). The Institute of Medicine's Redesigning Continuing Education in the Health Professions. *The Journal of Continuing Education in Nursing, 41*(8), 340–341. doi: 10.3928/00220124-20100726-02

Francis, K., Bowman, S., & Redgrave, M. (2001). Rural nurses: Knowledge and skills required by to meet the challenges of a changing work environment in the 21st century: A review of the literature. *National Review of Nursing Education*. Retrieved March 18, 2011 from http://www.dest.gov.au/archive/HIGHERED/nursing/pubs/rural_nurses/1.htm#contents

Hager, M., Russell, S., & Fletcher, S. (2008). *Continuing education in the health professions*. New York, NY: Josiah Macy, Jr. Foundation.

Helseth, C. (2010). Education partnerships enhance nurses' skills, encourage retention. *The Rural Monitor*. Retrieved from http://www.raconline.org/newsletter/spring10/feature.php#story1

Heinrich, C. J. (2011). A behavioral model of innovative search: Evidence from public hospital services. *Journal of Public Administration Research and Theory, 21*, 181–210.

Holloway, K., Lumby, J., & Baker, J. (2009). Specialist nursing framework for New Zealand: A missing link in workforce planning. *Policy, Politics and Nursing Practice, 10*(4), 269–75.

Institute of Medicine. (2010a). *The future of nursing: Leading change, advancing health*. Washington, DC: The National Academies Press.

Institute of Medicine. (2010b). *Redesigning continuing education in the health professions*. Washington, DC: The National Academies Press.

Keahey, S. (2008). Against the odds: Orienting and retaining rural nurses. *Journal for Nurses in Staff Development, 24*(2), E15–E20. doi: 10.1097/01.NND.0000300875.10684.be

Lee, S. M., Coakley, E. E., Dahlin, C., & Carleton, P. F. (2008). An evidence-based nurse residency program in geropalliative care. *Journal of Continuing Education in Nursing, 40*(12), 536–542. doi: 10.3928/00220124-20091119-01

Lenz, B. K., & Barnard, P. (2009). Advancing evidence-based practice in rural nursing. *Journal for Nurses in Staff Development, 25*(1), E14–E19. doi: 10.1097/NND.0b013e318194b6d0

Molinari, D. L., & Monserud, M. (2009). Rural nurse cultural self-efficacy and job satisfaction. *Journal of Transcultural Nursing 20*(2), 211–218.

National Council of State Boards of Nursing. (2006). *A national survey on elements of nursing education*. Chicago: Author.

Roberge, C. M. (2009). Who stays in rural nursing practice? An international review of the literature on factors influencing rural nurse retention. *Online Journal of Rural Nursing and Health Care*, 9(1). Retrieved from http://www.rno.org/journal/index.php/online-journal/article/view/180

Stokowski, L. A. (2011). *Overhauling nursing education. Medscape nursing.* Retrieved March 18, 2011 from http://www.medscape.com/viewarticle/736236 Medscape Nursing>Nursing Perspectives

Williams, L. A. (2001). Imogene King's interacting systems theory: Application in emergency and rural nursing. *Online Journal of Rural Nursing and Health Care*, 2(1), 25–30.

3

Quality of Care and Patient Safety: The Evidence for Transition-to-Practice Programs

Nancy Spector and Josephine H. Silvestre

This chapter reviews the literature on the topic of nurses' transition to practice; challenges and outcomes. Much has been written about effective models in large urban-based health care institutions. However, little has been documented about approaches that fit nursing practice in small rural-based facilities. The discussion herein lays the groundwork for developing and evaluating rural-focused nurse transition-to-practice programs and ascertaining associated outcomes.

Nurses first became aware of the employment-related challenges confronting recent graduates' transition to practice (TTP) when Marlene Kramer (1974) published her seminal work on "reality shock." Several decades later, Patricia Benner (2004) expanded on Kramer's work as she described competence characteristics of nurses as they progressed from novice, to advanced beginner, to proficient, and finally to expert. Within the last decade there has been a proliferation of studies that focused on recent graduates when entering the workforce as Registered Nurses (RN) relative to outcomes of patient safety, retention rates, along with individual competency and confidence levels. This chapter presents an overview of the literature on novice nurses' TTP challenges and outcomes within the health care system; strategies and models that can enhance TTP are highlighted. Of note is the paucity of information addressing novice nurses' experiences in a rural context, thus reinforcing the need for the information provided by the contributing authors in this volume.

PATIENT SAFETY AND NEW GRADUATE ISSUES

Nursing practice requires more education than in the past. Health care grows increasingly complex with a patient population that is diverse, older, and sicker with multiple diagnoses. Technology, too, is becoming ever more sophisticated. Nurses work at a "staccato" pace to survive (Wiggins, 2006). In turn, patients are discharged "quicker and sicker" from the hospital, going home with complex medical, social, and economic issues. Patient safety and health care outcomes become ever more important.

Michael Berens (2000), an investigative reporter for the *Chicago Tribune*, analyzed three million governmental computer records to quantify RN's role in medical errors. Because of incomplete and inconsistent reporting, these numbers just hint at the national scope of the nurse's role in medical errors. Berens included poignant stories such as the following: In Chicago, a 2-year-old child received a deadly overdose of sedatives by a new graduate nurse who was left alone to perform a delicate medical procedure without training (Berens, 2000, p. 20). Consumers also are concerned about safety when seeking health care. Adults ($N = 2,012$) over the age of 18 responded to a national survey supported by the Kaiser Family Foundation, the Agency for Healthcare Research and Quality, and the Harvard School of Public Health (Kaiser Family Foundation, 2004). About one-third of the respondents (34%) stated that a family member experienced a medical error at some point in life. About one-fifth (21%) stated the medical error caused "serious health consequences," including death (8%), long-term disability (11%), and/or severe pain (16%). Nearly half (48%) reported concerns about the safety of the health care that they and their families receive.

Safety questions arise regarding newly licensed nurses. A reliable analysis of patient care errors does not seem possible when using self-reported errors. The health care industry attempts to promote a culture of "not blaming" the individual in order to improve systems, but this makes data collection difficult. In a survey by NCSBN (2007) of 560 newly licensed nurses (average of 11.4 months in practice), 55.2% reported charting on the wrong record, 43.2% reported making medication errors, 39.3% reported contributing to treatment delays, 38.5% reported missing physicians' orders, 34.9% were involved with patient falls, and 28.2% made errors in performing skills.

The NCSBN surveyed employers (Budden, 2011) who reported that new nurses were slightly more likely to make errors than more experienced nurses. The trend held across hospitals, home health agencies, and nursing homes settings. These two preliminary studies reveal a need for additional research related to new nurses and patterns of medical errors. A number of other reports link new nurses to patient safety issues, such as near misses, adverse events, and practice errors (Berens, 2000; Bjørk & Kirkevold, 1999; Board of Registration in Nursing, 2007; del Bueno, 2005; Ebright, Urden, Patterson, & Chalko, 2004; Johnstone & Kanitsaki, 2006; Johnstone & Kanitsaki, 2008; Orsolini-Hain & Malone, 2007). Berens' (2000) news reporting found that temporary nurses in Illinois were increasingly the focus of disciplinary action. The reasons for their errors most often were linked to lack of knowledge of hospital procedure and unfamiliarity with patients. Also, unfamiliarity with patients and units were cited by the Massachusetts Board of Nursing (Board of Registration in Nursing, 2007) and Ebright et al. (2004) as reasons for near misses or errors.

Other researchers report that newly licensed nurses experience significant job stressors (Elfering, Semmer, & Grebner, 2006; Fink, Krugman, Casey, & Goode, 2008; NCSBN, 2007; Williams, Goode, Krsek, Bednash, & Lynn, 2007) linked to patient errors (NCSBN, 2007; Elfering et al., 2006). Investigators in Sweden studied 23 novice nurses from 19 hospitals for 2 weeks and found job stressors and low job control to be risk factors for patient safety (Elfering et al., 2006). The most frequently occurring safety issues associated with nurses' stress included incorrect documentation, medication errors or near misses, delays in patient care delivery, and violence among patients or toward nurses. Another study found that newly licensed nurses reporting higher stress made significantly more errors than new nurses reporting lower stress levels (NCSBN, 2007). Interestingly, in the NCSBN national study (2007) of newly licensed nurses, stress levels of new nurses were found to be highest during their 3–6 month period of practice. This is most likely the time frame when the nurse no longer participates in a transition or orientation program. A study by American Association of Colleges of Nursing/University Healthsystem Consortium (AACN/UHC) of a yearlong residency program found that stress gradually decreases (Williams et al., 2007). These findings suggest that a comprehensive yearlong transition program is linked to decreased stress, which, in turn, is related to safe patient care.

The NCSBN Nursys® data on discipline in the boards of nursing (NCSBN, 2009a) found that 4.1% of disciplinary actions were with novice nurses. Data also should that there was an increased disciplinary action trend in 1996–2006, supporting the IOM's report of an increase in practice errors. An Australian study (Johnstone & Kanitsaki, 2008) found that incident reporting increased during the novice nurse's first year in a supportive transition program. This finding was attributable to nurses being taught the importance of reporting errors and near misses and of focusing on root cause analyses. Nurses were able to integrate patient safety into the system within 3–4 months of this 12-month program. Key indicators measured included new graduates' familiarity with the following (Board of Registration in Nursing, 2007; Ebright et al., 2004; Johnstone & Kanitsaki, 2008):

- Hospital layout
- Hospital policies regarding risk assessment tools
- Processes of evidence-based practice
- Incident reporting

New nurses tend to engage in concrete thinking, focusing on technology and skills (Benner, 2004; Orsolini-Hain & Malone, 2007), but missing the broader context of quality, patient-centered care. This approach can be devastating in a complex health care system (Benner, Sutphen, Leonard, & Day, 2010; del Bueno, 2005; Ebright et al., 2004). Inexperienced nurses without support can impact on patient safety stemming from missed nursing care. Kalisch (2006), in a qualitative study focused on missed nursing care, identified nine themes, including the lack of patient surveillance. Members in the focus group reported that there were too many inexperienced nurses with inadequate orientations and inconsistent assignments. In other words, novice nurses without an opportunity to understand their patients lacked the ability to recognize changes in their patients' health conditions. When nursing care is omitted, patient outcomes can be adversely affected, thus contributing to falls, failure to rescue, pressure ulcers, etc.

Benner et al. (2010) recommend a yearlong transition program for new nurses, in part because students do not have the opportunity to follow up with patients in academic programs. Therefore, novice nurses do not have the opportunity to detect subtle changes, which quickly lead to patients' deterioration. For example, Ashcraft (2004) discusses how crucial pattern recognition is when patients are in pre-arrest states. In presenting three cases, she notes that novice nurses take longer to "put the pieces together" and would benefit from consulting with an experienced nurse in critical situations. A supportive transition program can assist new nurses to identify subtle changes and avoid practice errors.

The NCSBN's (2007) national study found that when transition programs in hospitals focused on specialty care, new nurses reported making significantly fewer practice errors. Similarly, when nurses perceived being more competent, they also reported fewer errors; in particular, they reported greater competence in clinical reasoning abilities, communication, and interpersonal relationships.

Johnstone and Kanitsaki (2006, 2008) studied the impact of integrating new nurses into clinical risk management systems in Australia and emphasized the importance of not reeducating new nurses on what they have already learned in their nursing programs. Rather, novice nurses should learn by experience with support from experienced nurses how to prevent and manage risks in practice. When new graduates were introduced to clinical risk management in these studies, none were involved in a preventable adverse patient event. The researchers, however, did not have a comparison group without risk management knowledge.

COMPETENCE AND NEW NURSES

Keller, Meekins, and Summers (2006) provide insight as to why new nurses need continued support for the first year, even after graduating from an approved nursing program and passing the National Council Licensure Examination for Nursing (NCLEX®). The authors suggest that basic nursing education programs cannot prepare graduates for workplace acculturation and correct language use. Keller asserts that new graduates are expected to become skilled in a wide range of absolutely necessary skills and gain a broad sense of their organization and health care. Some of the necessary skills include self-awareness and learning about team dynamics, leading teams, coordinating care, managing conflict, understanding the psychological effects of change and transition, communication, evidence-based practice, systems thinking, and financial pressures. Neophyte nurses can become overwhelmed and stressed with all these expectations (Elfering et al., 2006; NCSBN, 2007; Williams et al., 2007), supporting other findings that stress in the first year of practice is significantly related to practice errors.

Some employer studies reported that new graduates are not ready to practice like experienced nurses. Two studies by the NCSBN (2002, 2004a) found fewer than 50% of employers reported new graduates are ready to provide safe and effective care. Similarly, Berkow, Virkstis, Stewart, and Conway (2008) surveyed more than 5,700 frontline nurse leaders, about new graduates' competencies. Improvement was needed across education program levels (ADN and BSN). For example, 53% of employers were satisfied with the top-rated competence, while only 10% were satisfied with the lowest-rated competency. Competencies where the nurse leaders reported the most improvement was needed included:

- Understanding of quality improvement
- Completion of tasks within the expected time frame

- Ability to track multiple responsibilities
- Conflict resolution
- Ability to prioritize
- Ability to anticipate risk
- Delegation of tasks

Berkow et al. (2008) noted that the bottom-rated competencies would be better taught in an experiential environment, such as a TTP program.

A recent NCSBN study (Budden, 2011) of employers found more optimistic results. This study found that 17% of employers disagreed that new nurses were prepared to deliver safe and effective care to their patients, while 67% agreed. There is more evidence linking competence to the need for effective transition programs (Benner et al., 2010; Beyea, Slattery & von Reyn, 2010; Bjørk & Kirkevold, 1999; del Bueno, 2005; NCSBN, 2007, 2009b; Orsolini-Hain & Malone, 2007; Williams et al., 2007). NCSBN (2007) reported that new graduates are more likely to self-report practice errors when reporting decreased competence and increased stress.

In the Bjørk and Kirkevold (1999) study, investigators videotaped new nurses in practice for 1 year. As there were no opportunities for feedback or reflective practice, researchers that found the nurses made the same errors (such as contaminating wounds or unsafely removing wound drains) at the end of their first year in practice. In the Dartmouth–Hitchcock transition program (Beyea et al., 2010), investigators measured confidence, competence, self-efficacy, and readiness to practice, all of which increased after participation in the TTP program. This program uses simulation vignettes, with debriefing strategies, that highlight high-risk and low-frequency events, as well as commonly occurring clinical situations. Reflection is a highly effective way of developing competency and confidence in new graduates.

RETENTION RATES OF NEWLY LICENSED NURSES

Some authors question if job retention is a fair measure of quality and safety in patient care. Turnover is described as nurses leaving the job during the first year. The literature reports moderate-to-high turnover rates during novice nurses' first year of practice. Findings vary, but nurse turnover rates have been reported to be between 35% and 60% during the first year on the job (Advisory Board Company, 2006; Halfer, Graf, & Sullivan, 2008; Pine & Tart, 2007; Williams et al., 2007). There are inconsistent reports in the literature and Kovner and Djukic (2009) discuss problems with turnover statistics for the newly licensed nurse. For example, some studies include turnover within the institution, while others report turnover after completion of a comprehensive transition program. Using unpublished raw data from the RN Work Project, Kovner and Djukic (2009) report a 26% nurse turnover rate within 2 years.

Other variables affecting nurse turnover rates are economic factors. Budden (2011) found 61% of hospital employers reported that new nurse turnover was not a problem. However, it was unclear as to whether or not the finding was related to the nation's economic decline. On the other hand, Randolph (2010) reports nurses across the nation are not leaving their positions until the economic climate improves.

Several authors state that comprehensive transition programs decrease turnover rates (Beecroft, Kunzman, & Krozek, 2001; Halfer et al., 2008; Pine & Tart, 2007; Williams et al., 2007). While some novice nurse turnover is expected in the first year of practice associated with life events, the literature reports that a turnover rate over 7–10% most likely is related to job-related factors.

The turnover of newly licensed nurses is more often analyzed in acute care settings than in long-term care settings. The American Health Care Association (2008) study focusing on vacancy and turnover in long-term care settings found overall high nurse turnover among RNs (41%) and LPNs (49.9%). This study, however, did not specifically target novice nurse turnover rates. One can speculate that these findings probably are true for recent nurse graduates as well. The authors conclude that high-quality care is highly dependent on a stable, well-trained workforce and the development of sound fiscal policies designed to strengthen the workforce should be a top national priority.

Do novice nurses who quit their first jobs leave the profession of nursing? Orsolini-Hain and Malone (2007) found a trend of nurses leaving the nursing profession. In 2007, about 4.5% of nurses were employed outside of nursing compared to 2004, when 16.8% of nurses were employed outside of health care settings. However, this trend may not hold true for recent graduates. Kovner & Djukic (2009) report that 98% of new graduates passing the NCLEX were employed as nurses 2 years later.

OVERVIEW OF NURSE TRANSITION-TO-PRACTICE PROGRAMS

One solution to improve patient safety and healthcare outcomes is to provide all novice nurses with a TTP (Spector & Echternacht, 2010). Medicine, pharmacy, and pastoral services have transition programs funded by the Center for Medicare and Medicaid Services (CMS).

Other professions also promote TTP. More than 30 states mandate mentor induction programs for novice teachers and 17 states fund the mentoring that generally is 2 years in length (The American Association of State Colleges and Universities, 2006).

National organizations and research findings support post-basic education. The Joint Commission (2002), the Carnegie study of nursing education report (Benner et al., 2010), the American Association of Colleges of Nursing, and the University Health System Consortium (Goode, Lynn, Krsek, & Bednash, 2009) call for nursing TTP initiatives. The Carnegie study recommends lower entry-level salaries as one approach to funding. Very recently, the Institute of Medicine (Committee, 2011) landmark report on the *Future of Nursing* recommends a year-long residency program for novice nurses.

INTERNATIONAL PERSPECTIVES

Several countries support TTP. Portugal developed a national regulatory model termed Nurse Professional Development Program in which a new graduate is given a provisional license and participates in a 9-month supervised practice. At the end of the 9 months, the new nurse writes a "reflective report" and his or her supervisor writes an evaluative report. Both reports are reviewed by a committee (body) that is separate from the Board of Nursing. The committee, in turn, makes a recommendation to the Board regarding issuing permanent licensure. If the committee recommends not awarding permanent licensure, the new nurse is given a second opportunity to learn these skills that extends for three additional months. The federal government funds this TTP model and there are about 59 thousand nurses in Portugal.

Scotland has a web-based voluntary transition model (Roxburgh et al., 2010), termed as "Flying Start," which incorporates an online mentorship. Elements of this model include communication, teamwork, clinical skills, safe practice, research for practice, equality and diversity, policy, reflective practice, professional development, and career pathways. The model was evaluated with a convenience sample of 97 graduates who completed the program for future job intentions, knowledge and skill dimensions (self-perception), self-reported competency, self-efficacy, and job demands. The evaluation did not address quality and safety outcomes and there was no comparison control group (Roxburgh et al., 2010).

Canada, too, supports nurse preceptorship and mentorship programs for new graduates (http://www.cna-nurses.ca/CNA/default_e.aspx). The Canadian Nurses Association sent a representative to the

NCSBN TTP Committee meetings to learn about the U.S. initiative. Ireland took a different approach and mandated a transition program that is a component in the student's last year of school. This consists of a 36-week internship prior to graduation (http://www.nursingboard.ie/en/education.aspx). Employers pay students' salaries during the internship period. Australia implemented national licensure in July 2010 and incorporated a yearlong graduate mentorship program for new graduates (http://tinyurl.com/y99mqf3).

UNITED STATES PERSPECTIVES

RN transition programs vary widely across the United States in structure, length, experiences, and outcomes; some are more successful than others. NCSBN (2006b) investigated transition experiences in a geographically representative sample of newly licensed registered nurse graduates ($N = 628$). The findings indicate that a majority of the graduates participate in some sort of orientation or transition program that averages 11.4 weeks. About 41% of new graduates working in hospitals participated in comprehensive transition programs that included hospital orientation, and an internship, preceptorship, or mentorship experience. All RNs reporting no type of transition program came from ADN programs. Other studies reported similar findings (NCSBN, 2004b 2006a; Scott, Keehner Engelke, & Swanson, 2008).

A recent NCSBN study (Budden, 2011) confirmed this variability in a survey of 1,733 employers. While 84–97% reported providing a new hire orientation (i.e., introduction to the organization's policies, procedures, and other site-specific information), about 31% reported hosting a TTP program (i.e., a formal, time-limited program that incorporates active learning to support the new nurse's progression into practice). The National Council of State Boards of Nursing campaigns for a national, standardized transition program. Associated with faculty shortages nurse educators are working harder, and smarter, to educate sufficient and qualified nurses to meet the demands of the health care industry. A mandated transition model is not needed because practice settings are expecting new nurses to "hit the ground running." A number of institutions have developed such programs associated with challenges of transitioning new graduates to nursing practice. However, the caliber and outcomes of programs are highly variable (NCSBN, 2006a, 2006b; Scott et al., 2008).

In summary, TTP programs can help the novice nurse to successfully progress from a student role to a professional nursing role. Nationally and internationally, innovative models have been developed with notable improvements in patient safety, quality of care, and nurse retention rates. While there is extensive information focusing on TTP models in large health care facilities, little is known about the fit of these approaches for nurses who work in small health care facilities located in rural settings. There is a critical need for information about effective rural nurse TTP models and the associated outcomes. The various chapters in this volume go a long way to fill the information void on rural nursing practice issues and challenges.

REFERENCES

Advisory Board Company. (2006). *Transitioning new graduates to hospital practice: Profiles of nurse residency program exemplars.* Washington, DC: Author.

American Association of State Colleges and Universities. (2006). Teacher induction programs: Trends and opportunities. *Policy Matters, 3*(10).

American Health Care Association (2008). *Report of findings: 2007 AHCA survey nursing staff vacancy and turnover in nursing facilities.* Retrieved from http://www.ahcancal.org/research_data/staffing/Documents/Vacancy_Turnover_Survey2007.pdf

Ashcraft, A. S. (2004). Differentiating between pre-arrest and failure-to-rescue. *MEDSURG Nursing, 13*(4), 211–215.

Beecroft, P. C., Kunzman, L., & Krozek, C. (2001). RN internship: Outcomes of a one-year pilot program. *Journal of Nursing Administration, 31*(12), 575–582.

Benner, P. (2004). Using the dreyfus model of skill acquisition to describe and interpret skill acquisition and clinical judgment in nursing practice and education. *Bulletin of Science, Technology & Society, 24*(3), 188–199. doi: 10.1177/0270467604265061

Benner, P., Sutphen, M., Leonard, V., & Day, L. (2010). *Educating nurses: A call for radical transformation.* San Francisco, CA: Jossey-Bass.

Berens, M. J. (2000, September 10). Nursing mistakes kill, injure thousands: Cost-cutting exacts toll on patients, hospital staffs series: Dangerous care: Nurses' hidden role in medical error. First of three parts. *The Chicago Tribune,* p. 20.

Berkow, S., Virkstis, K., Stewart, J., & Conway, L. (2008). Assessing new graduate nurse performance. *Journal of Nursing Administration, 38*(11), 468–474.

Beyea, S. C., Slattery, M. J., & von Reyn, J. (2010). Outcomes of a simulation-based nurse residency program. *Clinical Simulation in Nursing, 6*(5), e169–e175. doi: 10.1016/j.ecns.2010.01.005

Bjørk, I. T., & Kirkevold, M. (1999). Issues in nurses' practical skill development in the clinical setting. *Journal of Nursing Care Quality, 14*(1), 72–84.

Board of Registration in Nursing, Division of Health Professions Licensure, Massachusetts Department of Public Health. (2007). *A study to identify evidence-based strategies for the prevention of nursing errors.* Massachusetts: Author.

Budden, J. S. (2011). A survey of nurse employers on professional and practice issues affecting nursing. *Journal of Nursing Regulation, 1*(4), 17–25. Retrieved from http://www.journalofnursingregulation.com/content/F3RVR1L8074VM710

Committee on the Robert Wood Johnson Foundation Initiative on the Future of Nursing at the Institute of Medicine. (2011). *The future of nursing: Leading change, advancing health.* Washington, DC: National Academies Press.

Del Bueno, D. (2005). A CRISIS in critical thinking. *Nursing Education Perspectives, 26*(5), 278–282.

Ebright, P. R., Urden, L., Patterson, E., & Chalko, B. (2004). Themes surrounding novice nurse near-miss and adverse-event situations. *Journal of Nursing Administration, 34*(11), 531–538.

Elfering, A., Semmer, N. K., & Grebner, S. (2006). Work stress and patient safety: Observer-rated work stressors as predictors of characteristics of safety-related events reported by young nurses. *Ergonomics, 49*(5/6), 457–469. doi: 10.1080/00140130600568451

Fink, R., Krugman, M., Casey, K., & Goode, C. (2008). The graduate nurse experience: Qualitative residency program outcomes. *Journal of Nursing Administration, 38*(7–8), 341–348.

Goode, C. J., Lynn, M. R., Krsek, C., & Bednash, G. D. (2009). Nurse residency programs: An essential requirement for nursing. *Nursing Economics, 27*(3), 142–159.

Halfer, D., Graf, E., & Sullivan, C. (2008). The organizational impact of a new graduate pediatric nurse mentoring program. (Cover story). *Nursing Economics, 26*(4), 243–249.

Johnstone, M.-J., & Kanitsaki, O. (2006). Processes influencing the development of graduate nurse capabilities in clinical risk management: An Australian study. *Quality Management in Health Care, 15*(4), 268–278.

Johnstone, M.-J., & Kanitsaki, O. (2008). Patient safety and the integration of graduate nurses into effective organizational clinical risk management systems and processes: An Australian study. *Quality Management in Health Care, 17*(2), 162–173.

Joint Commission White Paper. (2002). *Health care at the crossroads: Strategies for addressing the evolving nursing crisis.* Retrieved November 15, 2009, from http://www.jointcommission.org/NR/rdonlyres/5C138711-ED76-4D6F-909F-B06E0309F36D/0/health_care_at_the_crossroads.pdf

Kaiser Family Foundation. (2004). *Five years after IOM report on medical errors, nearly half of all consumers worry about the safety of their health care.* Retrieved from http://www.kff.org/kaiserpolls/pomr111704nr.cfm

Kalisch, B. J. (2006). Missed nursing care: A qualitative study. *Journal of Nursing Care Quality, 21*(4), 306–315.

Keller, J. L., Meekins, K., & Summers, B. L. (2006). Pearls and pitfalls of a new graduate academic residency program. *Journal of Nursing Administration, 36*(12), 589–598.

Kovner, C. T., & Djukic, M. (2009). The nursing career process from application through the first 2 years of employment. *Journal of Professional Nursing, 25*(4), 197–203.

Kramer, M. (1974). *Reality shock: Why nurses leave nursing.* Saint Louis: CV Mosby.

National Council of State Boards of Nursing (NCSBN). (2002). *Report of findings from the 2001 employers survey.* Chicago: Author.

National Council of State Boards of Nursing (NCSBN). (2004a). *Report of findings from the 2003 employers survey.* Chicago: Author.

National Council of State Boards of Nursing (NCSBN). (2004b). *Report of findings from the 2003 practice and professional issues survey: Spring 2003.* Chicago: Author.

National Council of State Boards of Nursing (NCSBN). (2006a). *A national survey on elements of nursing education.* Chicago: Author.

National Council of State Boards of Nursing (NCSBN). (2006b). *Transition to practice: Newly licensed registered nurse (RN) and licensed/vocational nurse (LPN/VN) activities.* Chicago: Author.

National Council of State Boards of Nursing (NCSBN). (2007). *The impact of transition experience on practice of newly licensed registered nurse.* Data presented on February, 2007, Transition Forum, Chicago, IL.

National Council of State Boards of Nursing (NCSBN) (2009a). *An analysis of NURSYS® disciplinary data from 1996–2006.* Retrieved from https://www.ncsbn.org/09_AnalysisofNursysData_Vol39_WEB.pdf

National Council of State Boards of Nursing (NCSBN). (2009b). *Post-entry competence study.* Retrieved from https://www.ncsbn.org/09_PostEntryCompetence Study_Vol38_WEB_final_081909.pdf

Orsolini-Hain, L., & Malone, R. E. (2007). Examining the impending gap in clinical nursing expertise. *Policy, Politics & Nursing Practice, 8*(3), 158–169. doi: 10.1177/1527154407309050

Pine, R., & Tart, K. (2007). Return on investment: Benefits and challenges of a baccalaureate nurse residency program. *Nursing Economics, 25*(1), 13–39.

Randolph, P. K. (2010). What happened to the nursing shortage? *Leader to Leader,* Spring. Retrieved from https://www.ncsbn.org/L2L_Spring2010.pdf

Roxburgh, M., Lauder, W., Topping, K., Holland, K., Johnson, M., & Watson, R. (2010). Early findings from an evaluation of a post-registration staff development programme: The Flying Start NHS initiative in Scotland, UK. *Nurse Education in Practice, 10*(2), 76–81. doi: 10.1016/j.nepr.2009.03.015

Scott, E. S., Keehner Engelke, M., & Swanson, M. (2008). New graduate nurse transitioning: Necessary or nice? *Applied Nursing Research: ANR, 21*(2), 75–83.

Spector, N., & Echternacht, M. (2010). A regulatory model for transitioning newly licensed nurses to practice. *Journal of Nursing Regulation, 1*(2), 18–25.

Wiggins, M. (2006). Clinical nurse leader, evolution of a revolution: The partnership care delivery model. *Journal of Nursing Administration, 36*(7/8), 1–5.

Williams, C. A., Goode, C. J., Krsek, C., Bednash, G. D., & Lynn, M. R. (2007). Postbaccalaureate nurse residency 1-year outcomes. *Journal of Nursing Administration, 37*(7–8), 357–365.

4

Dual Relationships and Rural Nurse's Transition to Practice: A Canadian Ethnographic Study

Kathryn H. Crooks

This chapter highlights background information and discusses select findings from a qualitative study conducted in Canada that explored nurses' experiences in a small rural community, specifically the phenomenon of dual relationships. Three major themes are discussed herein: rural nursing—living where you work, rural nursing—working where you live, and rural nursing practice—more than just tasks. *While this study occurred in Canada, the findings are congruent with anecdotal stories by U.S.-based rural nurses' practice experiences, and highly relevant for transition to practice programs.*

While the study occurred in a rural western Canadian setting, the findings reflect the dynamics of nursing practice in rural settings within the United States; more specifically, the phenomenon of dual interconnecting relationships. Interest in the topic originated thus:

> Shortly after graduating from my basic nursing education and procuring a position at a small rural hospital, I married a farmer. One of the most difficult lessons I learned following my marriage related to being able to integrate into my new community while trying to learn the "ropes" in my new position as a rural acute care nurse. Having grown up and being educated in a mid-size urban Canadian location, I had little understanding that the environment that I was entering, would present me with a large measure of learning about the multidimensional features of rural nursing but more importantly the unique nature of the rural health care relationship.

Early exposure to rural health care paved the way for a career that has spanned decades. From front line nursing care to academia, my entire career has focused on the health and well-being of the rural population of Canada. My early difficulties integrating into a rural community led me to pursue research regarding the rural health care relationship.

Essentially, nursing practice is similar, be it a rural or an urban area. However, the context as well as the surroundings in which nursing care is delivered influences the experiences of the nurse, both as an individual and as a professional. For example, nurses who work in rural health care facilities report that they provide care to patients across the life span, with a variety of diagnoses and health conditions. In turn, the competency expectation for rural nurses is to be an "expert generalist," possessing a wide range of nursing skills, having a broad understanding of nursing knowledge along with an innate ability to be "flexible" (Scharff, 2006). Context may also influence job satisfaction and whether or not a nurse chooses to remain in a particular community to work as a professional nurse (Kulig et al., 2009).

Associated with informal social dynamics in small communities, a nurse's professional and personal boundaries are often blurred and diffuse. For instance, it is not unusual for a rural nurse to care for friends, neighbors, and even relatives while in the professional role. Likewise, local residents are often acquainted with the nurse stemming from interactions at community functions. In turn, such interactions influence community members' perceptions of the nurse, both as a member of the community and as a nurse. Ultimately, rural context-driven dynamics can impact on the recruitment and retention of nurses in local health care settings; therefore, these elements must be addressed in all "transition to professional practice programs" in a rural setting. Essentially, experiences that merge with and support or detract from the nurse's life ultimately influence nursing practice. Rural contextual dynamics, as described, became the focus of this ethnographic study addressing the following question. *What is it like for a nurse to care for people with whom there is an ongoing relationship* (Crooks, 2007)?

NURSING AND DUAL RELATIONSHIPS

Many aspects of the nurse–patient relationship have been studied in the past. Considered as fundamental to all dimensions of nursing, the nurse–patient relationship stimulates particular questions for nurses who live and work with a concentrated population within the same locale. Frequently, these individuals find themselves in relationships that create a blurring of the lines that separate the personal and professional life. For nurses in the rural environment, when there is a marked possibility of a preexisting relationship, it may be difficult to move the relationship from its position as friend, neighbor, or even acquaintance, to one that is professional in nature (Crooks, 2007). This circumstance, commonly referred to as a dual or multiple relationship, happens repeatedly to rural residents regardless of the community or practice environment.

Various sources agree that a dual relationship exists when another meaningful association occurs simultaneously between a professional and the person for whom they are caring (Gottlieb, 1996; Kagle & Giebelhausen, 1994; Pope, 1988; Reamer, 2003). Kagle and Giebelhausen point out that the dual relationship is present regardless of which connection is the initial source of the bond. Reamer (2003) noted that dual relationships include a spectrum of affiliations ranging from sexual to social to business or religious attachments provided they occur simultaneously with the professional association. This would include the nurse–patient relationship and any other association that the nurse may have with the patient or other health care professionals outside the health care environment.

It has been suggested that dual relationships frequently occur in rural practice merely because of the limited choice of associations available to the professional (Jennings, 1992). A dual relationship is often the result of the extreme visibility of the professional within the rural community (Lee, 1998; McNeely & Shreffler, 1998). Because extreme visibility is an essential requirement of acceptance in many rural areas, it is also the catalyst for conflict between the professional and personal role (Schank & Skovholt, 1997). Gottlieb (1996) suggests that all the concerns that emerge as a result of the existence of the dual relationship are actually related to the disparate expectations between the professional and social roles.

Researchers discovered, while engaging in the study, that the term "dual relationship" was less than descriptive of what was observed or spoken about by the key participants. The term "dual relationship" gives the false sense that the two affiliations that occur are disconnected even though they occur simultaneously. Observations and the spoken words of the participants demonstrated a fusion of various complex experiences that thread the community and the working environment inextricably together. Further, it is not the frequency of exposure or the reciprocal nature but the depth and duration of the relationship that create a sense of permanence or attachment. Consequently, the term interconnecting bond provides a more realistic description of the nature of the rural health care relationships in this study.

METHODS

Focused ethnography was chosen as the most appropriate method for the study because of its essentially holistic and contextual character. In addition, focused ethnography allowed the research to occur in a time-limited way with a small group of participants, while providing additional questions to emerge as the research progressed (Muecke, 1994). Permission to conduct research was received from the University of Calgary Conjoint Health Research Ethics Board and from the Health Region Ethics Committee. The study included nurses living and working in towns and municipalities outside the commuting zone of urban centers with 10,000 or more population (du Plessis, Beshiri, Bollman, & Clemnson, 2001). The inclusion criteria required the nurses to be individuals engaged in the practice of professional nursing requiring the designation of Registered Nurse; participants had to live and work in the same area for a period of 5 years or more; participants could work in home care, acute care, or public health, and must work a minimum of 50% or more of a full-time schedule. Eventually, 10 key participants met the established criteria and consented to be included in the research. All key participants were located at three separate and distinct locations within a large rural health region in western Canada.

Data generation took place over a 1-year time period and consisted of becoming familiar with the areas through windshield survey techniques; participant observation, observer as participant; semistructured tape-recorded interviews utilizing an open-ended questioning technique, and informal conversations with key participants and others (Burnard, 1991; LeCompte & Schensul, 1999). Sampling continued until recurring patterns of data resulted. Credibility and trustworthiness were established through triangulation and participant verification of data. Transferability was determined by anecdotal comments during various presentations of the material. The comments reflected a sense of recognition by rural registered nurses and a broadened understanding on the part of administrators.

Ferdinand Tönnies's 1888 mental construct of *Gemeinschaft und Gesellschaft*, which theoretically describes the difference between and among groups of people, provided support for the demarcation of the major dimensions of the interconnecting bond. *Gemeinschaft* includes the social bonds that individuals within a community have with each other (Kornbeck, 2001); relationships within the concept are thought to be based on "sentiment, friendship, kinship and neighborliness" (Mellow, 2005, p. 52) resulting in intimate interpersonal relationships (McNeely & Shreffler, 1998). The notion of *Gesellschaft* on the other hand is epitomized by impersonal relationships often bounded by legal codes and contracts. Professional work has often been identified as an expression of *Gesellschaft* (Mellow, 2005).

In this research, rather than singular elements, *Gemeinschaft* is conceptualized as the notion of living where you work, whereas *Gesellschaft* is conceptualized as working where you live. These two elements are further conceptualized as two threads made up of separate personal behaviors spiraling around each other. The two separate threads are linked at various points by the notion of individual and community evaluation. The result is a double helix that is intended to demonstrate the influence one dimension has on the other. Neither aspect is exclusive but relies on the existence of the other to create the rural relational phenomenon known as the interconnecting bond (Crooks, 2007).

DISCUSSION OF FINDINGS

Content analysis procedures of the interviews revealed several major themes. Of these, select themes highlighted in this chapter include *rural nursing—living where you work, rural nursing—working where you live,* and *rural nursing practice—more than just tasks.* Each of these themes is examined in greater detail in the next few paragraphs.

Rural Nursing: Living Where You Work

Being recognized as a professional in the community, while a feature of the interconnecting bond, does not mean the nurse is better known within the community than any other individual. Frequently in rural communities, individuals are powerless to remain unidentified, regardless of their role, simply because chance encounters with others occur while going about the activities of daily living. As individuals within the community are frequently seen in an array of settings and functioning in an assortment of roles, there is a great deal of cross-referencing of individuals and functions taking place at all times (Bonner, 1997). Consequently, sometimes the nurse is a nurse, at other times she is the "hockey mom," at still other times she is the church group leader (Long, Scharff, & Weinert, 1998). For the long-term resident, the diversity of features that craft the individual has become woven into the substance of a community in such a way that the nursing identity is only one piece of the fabric (Crooks, 2007).

In the study, how the nurse's professional persona became known in the community was not an essential element of the interconnecting bond. That is, it did not matter if the nurse grew up in a particular area, or arrived there as a newly graduated nurse or young bride. However, being known as a nurse was an essential element of developing an interconnected relationship with the community.

The phenomenon of being acknowledged as a professional is not unique to nursing, as the rural lawyer, physician, social worker, and minister, to name a few, are usually linked to their professional role as well (Mellow, 2005). Just as the nurse is often asked to provide health information outside the professional realm, the lawyer/neighbor may be asked for legal advice, or the teacher/neighbor may provide information regarding a child's learning problems. Being recognized in a professional role, however, is only one of the elements that secure a connection to the community (Crooks, 2007).

For nurses just entering the community, the role of professional may provide the starting point for the relationship; however, it is vital for the recent rural resident to integrate into the community (Crooks, 2007). Caniparoli (1998) suggests that to become accepted within a community requires the individual to establish relationships within the community. This means being present for the variety of activities that help create the unique character of the community. For some it means joining a volleyball league or volunteering for the grounds crew at a baseball tournament; for others it means joining the local drama club, or chairing the yearly fashion show. In the study, key participants demonstrated connection to the community in several ways; the most relevant, however, was being present in the role of the nurse when needed. One of the participants pointed out "... you have to be able to be there as they want you there." Making a connection means taking part in the day-to-day activities that form the fabric of the community so that the nurse then becomes known in a variety of roles (Crooks, 2007).

Making a community connection can mean acceptance by the overall population in all the aspects of day-to-day life. Some of the participants, because of their professional role, talked of feeling a sense of responsibility or even "ownership" related to the health and well-being of the community. This belief or feeling caused the participants to be present as a nurse even when not in the professional role. One participant pointed out

> ... they always see me as a nurse first ... I'm a Lions member and if I'm working down at the playground cleaning it up and um well we're okay we have a nurse here so if they twist an ankle or you know that type of thing so they always see me as a nurse ... maybe I just slip into it when I need to ...

Being available as a nurse even when off-duty may also enhance the participant's acceptance by the larger community while working in the professional role (Waltman, 1986). In a Canada-wide study of rural and remote nursing, MacLeod et al. (2004) stress the importance of community involvement as a means of securing acceptance in the working environment. Indeed, while this often means being present in the role of the nurse at times outside the working environment it is an essential element of the interconnecting bond of rural health care. A participant related the following:

> I was at choir practice a week ago and a lady came up to me after choir and said you know I hurt my arm. So she shows me ... she wanted to clean it with what I wouldn't have recommended ... so we talked about it and then in the end [right after choir practice] I had her come over here [homecare office] and I cleaned it and I did a dressing on it ... she was perfectly capable of dealing with it herself with just a bit of guidance.

Rural Nursing: Working Where You Live

Making a connection with the community provides momentum for the experiences that take place within the working environment. However, this may lead the new rural nurse into features of the interconnecting bond that create additional concerns. The informality of day-to-day activities that take place in the community often trickles into the rural health care environment in ways that the nurse may be unprepared for. For example, nurses are educated to rely on policies, rules, and regulations to guide function while in the working environment. While this is essential for safe, competent health care to occur, functioning in this prescribed manner may require a different approach to working with patients when there is the likelihood of prior or future contact. On this note, one participant suggests "you have to be able to be there as they want you there . . . ."

Interestingly, the seemingly relaxed character of many rural health care settings is ripe for the development of unclear expectations particularly for the new nurse. That is, the natural commitments of friendship or kinship may conflict with the role the nurse has been educated and socialized to assume in professional life. For example, when learning about the traditional therapeutic relationship, nurses are urged to avoid self-disclosure unless there is proven therapeutic benefit to the patient (Balzer-Riley, 2000; College and Association of Registered Nurses of Alberta, 2005). Because of the necessity to integrate into the community, as well as the condensed nature of many rural sites, it may be difficult for the nurse to prevent private information from becoming public knowledge, increasing the potential for role strain.

Knowing intimate information and context about the patient is acknowledged to enhance care. For a variety of reasons, however, this aspect of rurality may result in additional personal distress to the nurse. For the nurse, coping with personal distress is a feature of the health care relationship that is pivotal to maintaining a successful connection to the community. One participant suggests "... you know volumes of information about people and they know you know, so it's better just to blank it out." Another nurse suggests that she is "the secret keeper" for her community.

When functioning in the role of the professional, it is often essential for the nurse to disconnect from any form of emotional engagement to be able to function safely, competently, or ethically. One participant referred to this element as "nurse face ... [versus] private face ... you gotta know when to use them." Another participant suggested that during emotionally stressful events "... you put it aside and worry about it later ... later you can fall apart." While some authors suggest that connection with the patient is essential to providing appropriate care (Morse, 1991), in this study, it is essential to unlock from the previously established connection, and move toward a less involved stance.

Achieving balance between engagement and detachment when providing patient care is a feature of all aspects of nursing. When there is a preexisting connection, achieving balance is made more difficult. "... there's a lot of emotional investment and I think when you're looking at the emotional involvement it goes on at all sorts of different levels ... [but] they [patients] come to the hospital expecting you to perform at your normal level". Fortunately, during stressful patient care events, being able to detach and place the patient into a category becomes a necessity that has at least two positive outcomes: (1) the patient has the expectation of receiving optimum health care from a professional educated to do so and (2) the ability to categorize or compartmentalize may also serve as an emotional shield for nurses who must work with those known from another relationship (Crooks, 2007). By being able to rely on habit when providing care, the rural nurse is able to safeguard against an emotional assault that could prove overwhelming and render the nurse useless to the patient during a time of great need (Crooks, 2007). Indeed, for the rural nurse, achieving the balance between engagement and detachment is particularly demanding work and requires ability that when done well goes largely unrecognized (James, 1992).

While at work or out in the greater community, the participants in the study were aware of being assessed and subsequently analyzed by others. Each stressed in one way or another, the necessity of learning and knowing "the rules." Immersion in the area was essential because each location had subtle differences that necessitated exposure to the site to be able to "learn the rules." One of the participants referred to this as "... kind of like an osmosis thing you kind of learn it overtime."

While learning rules is essential, all the participants in the study felt that self-awareness was a key attribute and was the prime reason each had worked successfully in their particular rural setting for many years. In the study, self-awareness allowed the nurses to navigate the often subtle yet treacherous aspects of the interconnecting bond. A participant shared her beliefs about this: "You have to be very mature ... you have to have some life skills ... the high maintenance girls are going to get burnt."

RURAL NURSING PRACTICE: MORE THAN JUST TASKS

For the nurse, the professional aspect of living and working in the same rural environment takes on special meaning. The nurse–patient dyad is an interactive process in which each member of the dyad negotiates the best possible position in the relationship to facilitate optimum health care (Crooks, 2007). It is up to the nurse with an interconnecting bond to assess which relationship is the most appropriate at the time. That is, the nurse must be able to decide what type of relationship to have with the patient or prospective patient depending on the circumstances. Indeed, a cultural standard is being used to calculate the nurse's acceptability not only in the workplace but also in the community. Consequently, the rural nurse must learn about and integrate into the elements of the community to function at the best possible level regardless of the circumstances or context. Further, the nurse must be intuitive enough to be able to assess the expectations of others so that potential missteps are avoided. The very nature of the work that nurses do calls for an emotional investment that is far greater when there is an interconnecting bond with the community. The nurse must be prepared to face difficult and emotionally troubling situations and to have a depth of self-knowledge to realize when events are beyond their capacity. The relational components inherent in a rural setting, which are integral in the creation of an interconnecting bond, actually assist the nurse in developing a therapeutic association with the patient (Crooks, 2007). Taking particular note of the interconnecting bond in a rural health care setting would make discussions of the nurse–patient relationship more than an academic exercise and would provide real-world information to the phenomenon of the therapeutic relationship (Crooks, 2007).

Ongoing Concerns

The idea of caring for people known from another relationship appears often in rural literature, particularly when nurses try to describe the various dimensions of rurality (Bushy, 2002; Kulig et al., 2008). What is not mentioned, however, is what the nurse must do to successfully navigate the subtle elements of the interconnecting bond.

Because the interconnecting bond is generally unavoidable in the rural setting it is essential to inform the body of literature. Further, it would be interesting to find out if distance from various cultural and recreational activities makes a significant difference in the way the nurse perceives the interconnecting bond? Likewise, modulation of emotion when the nurse categorizes the patient requires additional investigation. Indeed, because the nurse is known from an existing professional relationship, it is likely necessary to temper emotion from time to time in a social setting as well. In turn, what does this mean for the nurse personally and professionally?

In a recent study examining job satisfaction, Hunsberger, Baumann, Blythe and Crea (2009) identify the need for "extensive orientation and mentoring" (p. 23) as a means of improving retention of novice nurses in the rural setting. Further, experienced nurses suggested that patient care was being compromised when novice nurses were unprepared for the rigors of rural health care. Several authors recognize the necessity of preparing nurses at the undergraduate level to seek opportunities for employment in the rural sector (Andrews et al., 2005; Bushy, 2002; Van Hofwegen, Kirkham, & Harwood, 2005). In addition, nurses who have had contact to all aspects of life in rural and remote areas during undergraduate education tend to value the unique qualities inherent in this type of nursing simply because of exposure. Therefore, providing government financing to expedite practicum placements for nursing students is essential. Those that tend to choose rural nursing as a career, however, usually have significant relationships in the community (Bushy & Leipert, 2005). Consequently, creative methods of recruiting individuals with preexisting rural relationships into nursing education are essential, as is providing rural communities with professional nursing education. Orpin and Gabriel (2005) point out when attempting to recruit students into rural practice, it is less a matter of persuading them to accept rural as a practice area and more a matter of keeping up the interest of those who already have the connections.

Policy makers appreciate the value that a nurse with an interconnecting bond provides to a community. Ultimately, for the nurse, having established relationships provides social capital to the area. That is, a patient who is able to relinquish vigilance during a health care experience is more likely to have an optimum environment in which to heal (Morse, 1991), resulting in cost saving to the health care system. In due course, providing incentives to those with a bond with a community will create the means to sustain the community.

While there are commonalities among rural areas, each community has distinct differences, which give the area a unique quality (Thomlinson, McDonagh, Baird Crooks, & Lees, 2004). Regardless of the setting, however, the climate of the professional relationship between the nurse and the patient in a rural venue is frequently the result of a prior association. The mood of the relationship between the nurse and the prospective patient that takes place in the community often spills over into the professional realm, creating a phenomenon unique to rural nursing. The reality of the relationship is the element that makes rural nursing different from its urban counterpart (Crooks, 2007).

In summary, the rural health care relationship is a reciprocal entity that weaves its way through all aspects of the nurse's life. Each relational element merges inextricably with the other and is bonded together by the multiplicity of connections experienced daily by the nurse participants. The relationship experienced by the nurses in the study was not a straightforward element, but the fusion of various complex experiences that thread the community and the working environment together. A key participant expressed this best by sharing her feelings thus:

> It's probably the best decision I ever made. I got to come here and work here and belong here . . . it just feels right.

REFERENCES

Andrews, M. E., Stewart, N. J., Pitblado, R., Morgan, D. G., Forbes, D., & D'Arcy, C. (2005). Registered nurses working alone in rural and remote Canada. *Canadian Journal of Nursing Research, 37*(1), 14–33.

Balzer-Riley, J. (2000). *Communication in nursing* (4th ed.). Toronto: Mosby.

Bonner, K. (1997). *A great place to raise kids: Interpretation, science, and the urban-rural debate.* Montreal: McGill-Queen's University Press.

Burnard, P. (1991). A method of analyzing interview transcripts in qualitative research. *Nurse Education Today, 11,* 461–466. doi: 10.1016/0260-6917(91)90009-Y

Bushy, A. (2002). International perspectives on rural nursing: Australia, Canada, USA. *Australian Journal of Rural Health, 10*(2), 104–111. doi: 10.1046/j.1440-1584.2002.00457.x

Bushy, A., & Leipert, B. (2005, April 19). Factors that influence students in choosing rural nursing practice: A pilot study. *Rural and Remote Health 5*: Article 387 (Online). Retrieved August 10, 2006 from http://rrh.deakin.edu.au

Caniparoli, C. D. (1998). Old-timer. In H. J. Lee (Ed.), *Conceptual basis for rural nursing* (pp. 102–112). New York, NY: Springer Publishing Company.

Christenson, J. A. (1984). Gemeinschaft and gesellschaft: Testing the spatial and communal hypothesis. *Social Forces, 63*(1), 160–168.

College & Association of Registered Nurses of Alberta. (2005). *Professional boundaries for registered nurses: Guidelines for nurse-client relationship.* Retrieved June, 2006 from www.nurses.ab.ca/documents

Crooks, K. H. (2007). *Where everyone knows your name: An ethnographic exploration of rural nursing* (Unpublished doctoral dissertation). University of Calgary, Calgary, AB. Canada.

Du Plessis, V., Beshiri, R., Bollman, R. D., & Clemenson, H. (2001). Definitions of "rural". *Rural and Small Town Canada Analysis Bulletin 3,* 1–16. Retrieved January 28, 2002, from http://www.statcan.gc.ca/pub/21-006-x/21-006-x2001003-eng.pdf

Gottlieb, M. C. (1996). Avoiding exploitative dual relationships: A decision-making model. *Psychotherapy, 30*(1), 41–48. doi: 10.1037/0033-3204.30.1.41

Hunsberger, M., Baumann, A., Blythe, J., & Crea, M. (2009). Sustaining the rural workforce: Nursing perspectives on worklife. *The Journal of Rural Health, 25*(1), 17–25. doi: 10.1111/j.1748-0361.2009.00194.x

James, N. (1992). Care = organisation + physical labour + emotional labour. *Sociology of Health & Illness, 14*(4), 488–509. doi: 10.1111/1467-9566.ep10493127

Jennings, F. L. (1992). Ethics of rural practice. *Psychotherapy in Private Practice, 10*(3), 85–104.

Kagle, J. D., & Giebelhausen, P. N. (1994). Dual relationships and professional boundaries. *Social Work, 39*(2), 213–220.

Kornbeck, J. (2001). 'Gemeinschaft' skills versus 'gesellschaft' skills in social work education and practice. Applying Tonnies' dichotomy for a model of intercultural communication. *Social Work Education, 20*(2), 247–261.

Kulig, J. C., Andrews, M. E., Stewart, N. L., Pitblado, R., MacLeod, M. L. P., Bentham, D., & Smith, B. (2008). How do registered nurses define rurality? *Australian Journal of Rural Health, 16,* 28–32. doi: 10.1111/j.1440-1584.2007.00947.x

Kulig, J. C., Stewart, N., Penz, K., Forbes, D., Morgan, D., & Emerson, P. (2009). Work setting, community attachment, and satisfaction among rural and remote nurses. *Public Health Nursing, 26*(5), 430–439. doi: 10-1111/j.1525-1446.2009.00801.x

LeCompte, M. D., & Schensul, J. J. (1999). *Designing & conducting ethnographic research.* Lanham, MD: Alta Mira Press Rowman & Littlefield Pub Inc.

Lee, H. J. (1998). *Conceptual basis for rural nursing.* New York, NY: Springer Publishing Company.

Long, K. A., Scharff, J. E., & Weinert, C. (1998). Rural nursing: Developing the theory base. In H. J. Lee (Ed.), *Conceptual basis for rural nursing* (pp. 3–17). New York, NY: Springer Publishing Company.

MacLeod, M., Kulig, J., Stewart, N., Pitblado, R., Banks, K., D'Arcy, C., & Bentham, D. (2004). *The nature of nursing practice in rural and remote Canada.* Canadian Health Services Research Foundation. Retrieved from http://www.chrsf.ca

McNeely, A. G., & Shreffler, M. J. (1998). Familiarity. In H. J. Lee (Ed.), *Conceptual basis for rural nursing.* New York, NY: Springer Publishing Company.

Mellow, M. (2005). The work of rural professionals: Doing the gemeinschaft-gesellschaft gavotte. *Rural Sociology, 70*(1), 50–69. doi: 10.1526/0036011053294637

Morse, J. M. (1991). Negotiating commitment and involvement in the nurse-patient relationship. *Journal of Advanced Nursing, 16*(4), 455–468. doi: 10.1111/1365-2648.ep8531749

Muecke, M. (1994). On the evaluation of ethnographies. In J. M. Morse (Ed.), *Critical issues in qualitative research methods* (pp. 186–209). Thousand Oaks, CA: Sage Publishing.

Orpin, P., & Gabriel, M. (2005, October 4). Recruiting undergraduates to rural practice: What the students can tell us. *Rural & Remote Health, 5*(4), 412 (Online). Retrieved August 10, 2006 from http://rrh,deakin.edu.au/

Pope, K. S. (1988). Dual relationships: A source of ethical, legal, and clinical problems. *The Independent Practitioner: Bulletin of the Division of Independent Practice, Division 42 of the American Psychological Association, 8*(1), 17–25.

Reamer, F. G. (2003). Boundary issues in social work: Managing dual relationships. *Social Work, 48*(1), 121–133.

Schank, J. A., & Skovholt, T. M. (1997). Dual-relationship dilemmas of rural and small-community psychologists. *Professional Psychology: Research & Practice, 28*(1), 44.

Scharff, J. E. (2006). The distinctive nature and scope of rural nursing practice: Philosophical bases. In H. J. Lee, & C. A. Winters (Eds.), *Rural nursing: Concepts, theory, and practice* (2nd ed.) (pp. 179–196). New York, NY: Springer Publishing Company.

Thomlinson, E., McDonagh, M. K., Crooks, K. B., & Lees, M. (2004). Health beliefs of rural Canadians: Implications for practice. *Australian Journal of Rural Health, 12*(6), 258–263. doi: 10.1111/j.1440-1854.2004.00627.x

Van Hofwegen, L., Kirkham, S., & Harwood, C. (2005). The strength of rural nursing: Implications for undergraduate nursing education. *International Journal of Nursing Education Scholarship, 2*(1), 1–13.

Waltman, G. H. (1986). Main Street revisited: Social work practice in rural areas. *Social Casework, 67*(8), 466–474.

5

Rural Nurse Perceptions of Organizational Culture and the Intent to Move

Deana L. Molinari, Ashvin R. Jaiswal, and Teri Peterson

This chapter highlights select findings from a study addressing the question: How are personal and organizational factors related to rural nurses' feelings of support and their intent to move? The sample of rural nurses (N = 106) responded to a survey about determinants influencing initial employment decisions (lifestyle, cost of living, close to family, social relationships, spousal employment opportunity) and organizational characteristics associated with nurses' intent to leave (intra/interprofessional dynamics, vulnerability for violence, and the workplace environment). Findings could be useful for designing, implementing, and evaluating rural nurse transition-to-practice programs.

About 20% of the U.S. population lives in rural and frontier communities and registered nurses (RN) are central to a rural hospital's ability to provide health care to local residents. Thus, recruiting and retaining nurses in rural communities is of major concern (Palumbo, McIntosh, Rambur, & Naud, 2009). Retention of nurses is important to the economic sustainability of a small community since health care is one of the predominate industries in rural areas (Tourangeau, Cummings, Cranley, Ferron, & Harvey, 2010). Thus, the departure of a nurse who works at the local hospital indirectly impacts on the entire community, that is, the loss of nursing expertise, which is a much-valued health care resource (Skillman, Palazzo, Keepnews, & Hart, 2006).

Recruiting nurses to a rural area can be costly. For example, when a nurse leaves a small hospital, the replacement cost can be as much as $388,000 (Jones & Gates, 2007). The challenges are compounded by a small applicant pool of qualified individuals for the vacancy (American

Association of Colleges of Nursing, 2011; Winters & Lee, 2008). Other often-cited rural nurse recruitment barriers to rural recruitment are lower salaries, limited spousal employment opportunities, and limited health care resources along with the exodus of working age young adults to urban centers for education and employment opportunities (Bushy & Leipert, 2005; Kenny, 2009; Lindsey & Kleiner, 2005; Molinari & Monserud, 2008). Consequently, rural hospitals are more likely to recruit and hire employees who are older, established in the community, and do not require spousal employment.

A popular strategy to recruit nurses in rural settings is for the community to "grow their own." More precisely, the hospital seeks individuals with the potential of completing the educational requirements for becoming a health professional, most often a physician or nurse. Generally, the employee is an adolescent or young adult who is provided financial support to pursue an academic degree, with a contractual commitment to return and practice in the community (Chapter 17). While this strategy can have drawbacks, many underserved rural communities find the strategy effective for recruiting and retaining nurses (Pine & Tart, 2007).

Retaining nurses who are not from a rural community is a concern because they may not be familiar with the rural culture and lifestyle (Kenny, 2009; Newhouse, Morlock, Pronovost, Colantuoni, & Johantgen, 2009). Of all nonfederal, short-term, general, and specialty hospitals, rural facilities make up ~41%. Annually, these small facilities have 7.5 million patient discharges. Consequently, an individual's knowledge of the rural lifestyle and culture is an important consideration for institutions' recruitment and retention strategies.

Adequate staffing levels are a critical dimension of patient outcomes (El-Jardali, Dimassi, Jamal, Jaafar, & Hemadeh, 2011). For example, California-elected officials introduced staffing regulations several years ago, and recent findings indicate that increased staffing reduced patient mortality rates (Horsham, 2010; Ross, 2010). Staffing patterns should not be a convenience or a budgetary concern, but rather a matter of assuring quality patient care (Aiken, Clarke, Sloan, Lake, & Cheney, 2008; Van den Heede et al., 2009).

Nursing administrators employ a variety of strategies to retain nurses (Coshow et al., 2008). Increasing job satisfaction through supportive environmental factors is one of the most common approaches (Cohen, Stuenkel, & Nguyen, 2009; DiMattio, Roe-Prior, & Carpenter, 2010; Hendren, 2009; Larrabee et al., 2010). Another common technique is to apply a "carrot or stick" approach. The carrot strategy serves to motivate recruitment and retention while sticks are designed to discourage termination.

Another recruitment and retention strategy is to improve the organizational culture that supports nurses and nursing practice. With that in mind, hospitals can even achieve recognition for nurse-supportive policies, in particular the American Nurses Credentialing Center (ANCC) Magnet Status and ANCC Pathway to Excellence (Allen, Fiorini, & Dickey, 2010; McCarthy & Kemnitz, 2010; Scott, Sochalski, & Aiken, 1999; Ulrich, Buerhaus, Donelan, Norman, & Dittus, 2007; Wood, 2009). However, small facilities designated as critical access hospitals (CAHs) rarely achieve such national recognition. CAHs lack the resources required for rewards, such as financial resources and the appropriate nurse academic preparation for credentialing.

Intent to move is a measure that has been used to determine job satisfaction (Beecroft, Dorey, Wenten, 2008; Bowles & Candela, 2005; Coomber & Barriball, 2007; DiMattio et al., 2010; Hayes, 2006). Organizational factors influence employee's job satisfaction; in turn, this impacts on nurses' intent to move and retention rates (Aiken et al., 2008; Beecroft et al., 2008; Lacey et al., 2008). While there are articles about the relationship of organizational climate and nurses' intent to leave (Shader et al., 2001), little is documented about rural health care organizational structures and recruitment and retention of nurses. The study described in this chapter was an effort to address the information deficit on rural nurses' perception of organizational support and intent to leave.

METHODOLOGY

A descriptive, correlational design was used to answer the following question: How are personal and organizational factors related to rural nurses' feelings of support and their intent to move? Concepts from the rural nurse theory were used to provide potential explanations for the findings (distance, isolation, social networks, self-reliance) (Lee & Winters, 2004; Long & Weinert, 1989; Winters & Lee, 2008). In this study, an employee's "intent to move" was defined as the desire to leave employment within the next 2 years and, "support" was defined as the employee's satisfaction with the administration's workforce strategy(ies). The "probability of turnover" measured nurses' anticipation of perceptions of staff stability. The variable "feeling supported" measured nurses' perceptions of organizational support strategies. Approval to conduct the study was obtained from the Idaho State University Institutional Review Board.

Data were obtained via an online survey from rural nurses ($N = 106$) located in 22 states. Subjects were enrolled in a residency program either as a nurse resident (novice) or a nurse preceptor (expert). The instrument included items related to demographic information, self-perceived adequacy of educational preparation, and perceptions of the employing organization's characteristics. Likert scales measured the following variables: the importance of select lifestyle characteristics when choosing a rural placement and perceived adverse and supportive workplace conditions. One item specifically asked whether or not the participant intended to move within the next 2 years. Another item asked how well supported the subject felt in his or her current position as a nurse. Data analysis included descriptive, correlational, and inferential statistics.

DISCUSSION OF FINDINGS

The next section discusses select findings from the study, including sample demographics, criteria nurses associated with feeling supported, feelings of violence vulnerability, and finally comments about the intent to leave and projected turnover. The discussion integrates concepts from rural nursing theory in an effort to describe the rural context.

Demographically, the sample was predominately Caucasian (95%). About one-third (35%) were over 40 years if age; a slightly higher proportion were under 30 years of age (41%). Most reported having rural birthplace (67%). The majority completed an associate degree (53%) as their highest level of education; were married (68%); and had children under the age of 18 in the home (51%). Nurses reported from 2 weeks to 36 years in their current positions, with the majority (69%) employed less than 1 year. A small, significant proportion (11%) indicated intent to move within the next 2 years.

The findings revealed that most nurses selected a rural community and a rural lifestyle rather than a rural generalist employment position. Individuals who were married with children at home were more likely to choose a rural lifestyle. Other influencing determinants in the nurses' employment decisions included: [reasonable] cost of living, close to [extended] family, [opportunities for] social relationships, and employment [opportunity] for a spouse.

Nurses specified that the most likely organizational culture deterrents for retention were insufficient staffing, [high] turnover rates, [heavy] workload, physical injury due to work requirements, [mandated] staff downsizing, and [risk] for patient accidents. Still of concern, but less likely to occur, were the use of temporary nurses, [mandated] overtime, patient turbulence, harassment [horizontal violence] by staff members, violence against nurses, and harassment by a physician. Overall, these rural nurses reported being satisfied with their workplace environment and the culture of the employing organization (Meraviglia et al., 2009). It is important to point out that these nurses were enrolled in a transition-to-practice program, either as a novice nurse or a supervising preceptor expert nurse. In and of itself, this fact demonstrates a certain degree of administrative support for nursing within the organization.

The survey further asked subjects about perceived reasons for nurse turnover. Answers included [nonsupportive] professional relationships; unwilling to ask for advice; perceived [threat] of violence; harassment by physician(s), patients, and staff; and [unsafe] staffing patterns, use of temporary [traveling] nurses, heavy workload, downsizing [number] of employee numbers, [mandated] overtime, and a risk of patient safety [errors].

Feeling Supported

Feeling supported by administrators (managers) was noted as a critical factor for employee retention. Nurses in the study generally felt supported by supervisors and physician colleagues, while those not feeling supported were more likely to leave. Only a few nurses indicated intent to move within 2 years, while a high proportion of the sample reported experiencing negative organizational culture factors. Possessing a rural background and a preference for the rural lifestyle was associated with a supportive work environment. Since the association of an employee's lifestyle preference with job satisfaction has not been examined in management models, particularly relative to nurses in rural contexts, the importance of the finding is unknown (Meraviglia et al., 2008).

Management models usually address the availability and management of resources. Nurses rated the lack of resources contributed to feeling less supported. Nurse administrators are in a position to modify policies and working conditions related to staffing patterns, communication style, educational progression, and interpersonal behaviors. Administrators assist in procuring biotechnology and providing the necessary education for using the equipment safely and appropriately. Continuing education was highly rated as important to feeling supported among all nurses in this study.

Participation in continuing education offerings is often associated with challenges that may not be present in larger urban facilities. For example, given the tenuous fiscal status of many small rural facilities, continuing education may not be a budgetary priority. Administrators may find continuing education too costly. That is to say, paying a nurse to commute the long distance to an event, and then funding the registration fee, room, and board during the conference, as well as the replacement nurse can cost more than a facility has. Then, there may be constraints associated with the low number of nursing staff. For instance, if one of the nurses goes out of town to attend a conference, there may be insufficient staff to provide nursing coverage during that time period. Telecommunication and the internet are increasingly employed as budgetary solutions. Rural nurse transition-to-practice models are examined in more detail in other chapters within this volume.

Interpersonal professional dynamics are a critical characteristic defining the culture of an organization (Van Bogaert, Meulemans, Clarke, Vermeyen, & Van de Heyning, 2009). In a hospital setting, interpersonal dynamics infers the comfort level that nurses have in asking another professional for advice. In addition, in rural settings, the problem may center on the nurse not having "immediate" geographical access to another professional who could be asked for advice. In this study, those who were most likely to ask for advice also reported having heavy workloads and were intent on moving. This dimension of job satisfaction has not been examined in the rural literature, but was identified as important by subjects. This begs the following questions: In a rural setting, could the inability of a nurse to ask for advice be related to feeling professionally or geographically isolated? Could advice seeking, or the lack of it, be a characteristic of the inexperienced nurse, given that the majority of nurses in this study had less than 12 months of experience? Further, is it feasible for professional inquiry behaviors to be taught in nursing education programs? If so, what are the best approaches to achieve this outcome among graduates of nursing programs and how can this characteristic be evaluated? Are variations needed when preparing nurses to practice in the rural context? These and other questions need further exploration given that individual inquiry and intraprofessional discussion preempt implementing evidence-based care.

Vulnerability for Violence

Feeling vulnerable to violence (the antithesis of feeling supported) emerged in this rural-focused study. In other words, not feeling supported at work could potentially be associated with the perceived threats of violence (Applebaum, Fowler, Fiedler, Osinubi, & Robson, 2010; Ferns, 2006; Health and Safety Administration, 2004). Violence and patient turbulence appear to be associated with unpredictability, loss of control, excessive responsibility, noise, problems with equipment and supplies, and workload (Jennings, 2008; Pawlin, 2008). Further, patient turbulence impacts on nursing care by distracting nurses, and disrupting schedules and communication (Jennings, 2008).

While reasons for vulnerability for violence were not specified, almost all the subjects (88%) indicated feeling "risks" or "threats" of violence. Among the sample, the frequency of reported violence was related to the intent to move. The relationship of staffing patterns and safety of nursing staff is not fully understood, particularly in rural facilities. More specifically, how are staff size and mix related to violent occurrences? How do "tight" homogenous social networks and dual relationships, which characterize the rural context, impact on the reporting by nurses of a violence act? Further, how does the insider/old timer—outsider/newcomer dynamic (identified in the rural literature) influence whether or not a newly hired nurse (not of the community) is accepted by employees who have worked in the facility for many years (Long & Weinert, 1989)? Horizontal violence among nurses in small health care facilities with low staff numbers, in particular, needs further exploration in light of the comments provided by nurses in this study (Fern, 2006; Shields & Wilkins, 2009; Stokowski, 2009).

Intent to Leave and Projected Retention Rates

Turnover and intent to leave are measures to assess probable retention rates and sometimes are associated with anticipation of an increased practice burden (Perrine, 2009; Teasley et al., 2007). For this sample, retention of employees was not dependent on the management's incentives and disincentives. Likewise, salary, an often-cited incentive in the literature, was not indicative of turnover or intent to move for nurses in this study (Meraviglia et al., 2008; Perrine, 2009). These rural nurses reported more concern for negative organizational elements, including insufficient staff, Licensed Vocational/Practical Nurses turnover, heavy workload, patient turbulence, staff downsizing, and violence. Having a supportive nurse manager during a conflict with the organization was noted to be a critical factor in feeling support, and thus decreased the potential for nurse turnover.

Concepts from rural nursing theory may be useful to explain some of the findings in this study. For instance, self-reliance among rural residents might be a reason for an individual to be reluctant to ask for advice or, perhaps, not feel supported. Then, too, geographical distances between resources could be a confounding factor for longevity by employees within a particular institution in spite of a nonsupportive organizational environment or adverse working conditions.

In summary, this chapter examined select findings from a study with rural nurses ($N = 106$) where participants were in a formal transition-to-practice program. Additional research is needed to replicate and expand these preliminary findings. A larger and more diverse sample of nurses in other rural contexts is suggested. As the national economy rebounds, nurse retention rates will probably be impacted in rural as well as urban settings. In anticipation of future trends, it would be prudent for administrators in rural health care facilities to consider these findings relative to rural nursing frameworks when proposing and evaluating nurse recruitment and retention strategies (Lee & Winters, 2004).

REFERENCES

American Association of Colleges of Nursing. (2011). *Nursing Shortage.* Accessed on October 7 at http://www.aacn.nche.edu/Media/FactSheets/NursingShortage.htm

Aiken, L. H., Clarke, S. P., Sloane, D. M., Lake, E. T., & Cheney, T. (2008). Effects of hospital care environment on patient mortality and nurse outcomes. *The Journal of Nursing Administration, 38*(5), 223–229.

Allen, S. R., Fiorini, P., & Dickey, M. (2010). A streamlined clinical advancement program improves RN participation and retention. *The Journal of Nursing Administration, 40*(7/8), 316.

Applebaum, D., Fowler, S., Fiedler, N., Osinubi, O., & Robson, M. (2010). The impact of environmental factors on nursing stress, job satisfaction, and turnover intent. *JONA: The Journal of Nursing Administration, 40*(7/8), 323–328.

Beecroft, P. C., Dorey, F., & Wenten, M. (2008). Turnover intent in new graduates: A multivariate analysis. *Journal of Advanced Nursing, 62*(1), 41.

Bowles, C., & Candela, L. (2005). First job experiences of recent RN graduates: Improving the work environment. *Journal of Nursing Administration, 35*(3), 130–137.

Bushy, A., & Leipert, B. D. (2005). Factors that influence students in choosing rural nursing practice: A pilot study. *Rural and Remote Health.* Retrieved January 2011 from http://www.rrh.org.au

Cohen, J., Stuenkel, D., & Nguyen, Q. (2009). Providing a healthy work environment for nurses: The influence on retention. *Journal of Nursing Care Quality, 24*(4), 308.

Coomber, B., & Barriball, K. L. (2007). Impact of job satisfaction components on intent to leave and turnover for hospital-based nurses: A review of research literature. *International Journal of Nursing Studies, 44*(2), 297.

Coshow, S., Davis, P., & Wolosin, R. J. (2008). The 'big dip': Mid-career nurses show decreased satisfaction. *Satisfaction Monitor, 2,* 21–23.

DiMattio, M. J., Roe-Prior, P., & Carpenter, D. R. (2010). Intent to stay: A pilot study of baccalaureate nurses and hospital nursing. *Journal of Professional Nursing, 26*(5), 278.

El-Jardali, F., Dimassi, H., Jamal, D., Jaafar, M., & Hemadeh, N. (2011). Predictors and outcomes of patient safety culture in hospitals. *BMC Health Services Research, 24,* 11(1), 45.

Ferns, T. (2006). Under-reporting of violent incidents against nursing staff. *Nursing Standards, 20*, 41–45.

Hayes, L. J. (2006). Nurse turnover: A literature review. *International Journal of Nursing Studies, 43*(2), 237–263.

Health and Safety Administration. (2004). *Guidelines for preventing workplace violence for health care & social workers.* Retrieved from http://www.osha.gov/Publications/OSHA3148/osha3148.html

Hendren, R. (2009). *Focus returns to nurse retention in 2010.* Retrieved from http://www.healthleadersmedia.com/content/NRS-244148/Focus-Returns-to-Nurse-Retention-in-2010

Horsham. (2010). California's mandated staff ratios reduce mortality. *Nursing, 40*(6), 21.

Jennings, B. M. (2008). *Patient safety and quality: An evidence-based handbook for nurses.* Rockville MD: Agency of Health Care Research and Quality. http://www.ncbi.nlm.nih.gov/bookshelf/br.fcgi?book=nursehb&part=ch29.

Jones, C., & Gates, M. (2007). The costs and benefits of nurse turnover: A business case for nurse retention. *OJIN: The Online Journal of Issues in Nursing, 12*(3), 4.

Kenny, A. (2009). Nursing shortages will cripple rural health care, ABC News. Retrieved from http://www.abc.net.au/news/stories/2009/02/02/2479976.htm

Lacey, S. R., Teasley, S. L., Henion, J. S., Cox, K. S., Bonura, A., & Brown, J. (2008). Enhancing the work environment of staff nurses using targeted interventions of support. *Journal of Nursing Administration, 38*, 336–340.

Larrabee, J. H., Wu, Y., Persily, C. A., Simoni, P. S., Johnston, P. A., Marcischak, T. L., Mott, C. L., & Gladden, S. D. (2010). Influence of stress resiliency on RN job satisfaction and intent to stay. *Western Journal of Nursing Research.* Beverly Hills, 32(1), 81.

Lee, H. J., & Winters, C. A. (2004). Testing rural nurse theory: Perceptions and needs of service providers. *Online Journal of Rural Nursing and Health Care, 4*(1).

Lindsey, G., & Kleiner, B. (2005). Nurse residency program: An effective tool for recruitment and retention. *Journal of Healthcare Finance, 31*(3), 25–32.

Long, K. A., & Weinert, C. (1989). Rural nursing: Developing the theory base. *Scholarly Inquiry for Nursing Practice, 3*, 113–127.

McCarthy, P., & Kemnitz, R. (2010). Avoiding a key employee exodus. *Broker World, 30*(9), 24–26.

Meraviglia, M., Grobe, S. J., Tabone, S., Wainwright, M., Shelton, S., Miner, H., & Jordan, C. (2009). Creating a positive work environment: Implementation of the nurse-friendly hospital criteria. *Journal of Nursing Administration, 39*(2), 64–70.

Meraviglia, M., Grobe, S. J., Tabone, S., Wainwright, M., Shelton, S., Yu, L., & Jordan, C. (2008). Nurse-Friendly Hospital Project: Enhancing nurse retention and quality of care. *Journal Nursing Care Quality, 23*(4), 305–313.

Molinari, D. L., & Monserud, M. (2008). Rural nurse job satisfaction. *Journal of Rural and Remote Health. 8*(1). Retrieved from http://www.rrh.org.au/articles/defaultnew.asp?IssueNo=8x

Newhouse, R. P., Morlock, L., Pronovost, P., Colantuoni, E., & Johantgen, M. (2009). Rural hospital nursing: Better environments=shared vision and quality/safety engagement. *Journal of Nursing Administration, 39*(4), 189–195.

Palumbo, M. V., McIntosh, B., Rambur, B., & Naud, S. (2009). Retaining an aging nurse workforce: Perceptions of human resource practices. *Nursing Economics, 2*(4), 221–227. 232.

Pawlin, S. (2008). Reporting violence. *Emergency Nurse, 16*(4), 16–21.

Perrine, J. L. (2009). Strategies to boost RN retention. *Nursing Management, 40*(4), 20.

Pine, R., & Tart, K. (2007). Return on investment: Benefits and challenges of a baccalaureate nurse residency program. *Nursing Economics, 21*(5), 13–18, 39. Retrieved from http://www.medscape.com/viewarticle/555120

Ross, J. (2010). Legislating nurse staffing: Understanding the issues and reviewing the evidence. *Journal of Perianesthia Nursing, 25*(5), 319–321.

Scott, J. G., Sochalski, J., & Aiken, L. (1999). Review of magnet hospital research: Findings and implications for professional nursing practice. *The Journal of Nursing Administration, 29*(1), 9–19.

Shader, K., Broome, M., Broome, C., West, M., & Nash, M. (2001). Factors influencing satisfaction and anticipated turnover for nurses in an academic medical center. *Journal of Nursing Administration, 31*, 210–216.

Shields, M., & Wilkins, K. (2009). *Factors related to on-the-job abuse of nurses by patients.* Health Reports, 20(2), 7–19. Retrieved from http://www.statcan.gc.ca/pub/82-003-x/2009002/article/10835-eng.pdf

Skillman, S. M., Palazzo, L., Keepnews, D., & Hart, G. (2006). Characteristics of registered nurses in rural versus urban areas: Implications for strategies to alleviate nursing shortages in the United States. *Journal of Rural Health, 22*(2), 151–157.

Stokowski, L. A. (2009). Nurse staffing for safety: Safe staffing legislation. Retrieved from http://www.medscape.com/viewarticle/711116_6

Teasley, S. L., Sexton, K. A., Carroll, C. A., Cox, K. S., Riley, M., & Ferriell, K. (2007). Improving work environment perceptions for nurses employed in a rural setting. *Journal of Rural Health, 23*(2), 179–182. DOI: 10.1111/j.1748-0361.2007.00087.x

Tourangeau, A. E., Cummings, G., Cranley, L. A., Ferron, E. M., & Harvey, S. (2010). Determinants of hospital intent to remain employed: Broadening our understanding. *Journal of Advanced Nursing, 66*(1), 22.

Ulrich, B. T., Buerhaus, P. I., Donelan, K., Norman, L., & Dittus, R. (2007). Magnet status and registered nurse views of the work environment and nursing as a career. *Journal of Nursing Administration, 37*(5), 212–220.

Van Bogaert, P., Meulemans, H., Clarke, H., Vermeyen, K., & Van de Heyning, P. (2009). Hospital nurse practice environment, burnout, job outcomes and quality of care: Test of a structural equation model. *Journal of Advanced Nursing, 65*(10), 2175.

Van den Heede, K., Lesaffre, E., Diya, L., Vleugels, A., Clarke, S. P., Aiken, L. H. et al. (2009). The relationship between inpatient cardiac surgery mortality and nurse numbers and educational level: Analysis of administrative data. *International Journal of Nursing Studies, 46*(6), 796–803.

Winters, C. A., & Lee, H. J. (2010). *Rural nursing: Concepts, theory and practice* (3rd ed.). New York: Springer.

Wood, D. (2009). *ANCC's Pathway to Excellence: Commitment to Good Nursing Environments.* Retrieved from http://www.nursezone.com/Nursing-News-Events/more-features/ANCC%E2%80%99s-Pathway-to-Excellence-Commitment-to-Good-Nursing-Environments_32216.aspx

6

Women's Health and Nursing Practice in Rural Canada

Beverly D. Leipert

There is a paucity of research on nursing in rural Canada and the literature presents conflicting information, paralleling U.S. findings. Nursing is a predominately female profession; thus, research focusing on women's issues offers general insights about nurses and nursing practice. In this chapter, the author justifies the case for further examination surrounding the dynamics of being both female and a nurse in rural contexts.

Canada's vast rural and remote lands are home to ~22% of its people (Canadian Institute for Health Information [CIHI], 2006). Six million people are scattered across 99.8% of the second-largest nation on earth (Health Canada, 2001; Kulig, 2010). Yet, in spite of the obvious needs of such a diverse and isolated population, little is known about the specific health needs or even the nature, such as the gender composition, of Canada's rural and remote population. In addition, although health care personnel shortages are reputed to be widespread throughout rural Canada (Romanow, 2002), little attention has been given to nursing, a profession dominated by females. This chapter discusses what is known about rural nursing in Canada and includes information about the health concerns of rural women. Recommendations are included for educators, clinicians, researchers, and policy developers that could impact on rural nursing practice in particular and the health of Canada's rural women in general.

Unfortunately, there is no agreed-upon definition for rural in Canada. One of the more frequently cited ones defines rural as communities with populations of <10,000 that are removed from urban services and resources (du Plessis, Beshiri, & Bollman, 2002). Other rural definitions include additional criteria such as source of income (e.g., agricultural, mining, and forestry) and social organization and representation (e.g., people living in an area consider themselves as rural) (Halfacree, 1993; Troughton, 1999). Varying definitions, while commendable in their attempts to accurately reflect the diverse nature of rural contexts in Canada, are also problematic in that a lack of a singular definition, together with limited political interest in rural health issues, allows governments to defer establishing policies that pertain to rural nursing practice and rural women's health.

Governmental support for the health of rural people, although minimal in these past few decades, has decreased even further in recent years (Senate Standing Committee on Agriculture and Forestry [SSCAF], 2006). Although national reports have been prepared that address rural people's health (CIHI, 2006; Health Canada, 2001; Romanow, 2002), and the health of segments of the population that have particular relevance to rural populations because of their increasing prevalence and needs in rural communities (Hodge, 2008; Keating, 2008), such as the elderly (Canadian Nurses Association [CNA], 2008) and women (CIHI, 2003), these reports minimally address rural nursing practice. The prevailing dialogue by governments and rural agencies such as The Rural Ontario Institute (see http://ruralontarioinstitute.ca) tends to narrowly focus on increasing treatment resources and personnel such as physicians rather than taking a more holistic approach to include health promotion, illness and injury prevention, and other initiatives that are also required to effectively support the recruitment and retention of diverse health care professionals, such as rural nurses, and the health of rural people.

RURAL NURSING IN CANADA

Minimal research has been conducted on rural nursing in Canada. What is known is that there were ~41,500 registered nurses (RNs) working in rural Canada in 2000, a 2% decline from 1994, even though the population of rural people had increased (Kulig, Macleod, Stewart, & Pitblado, 2008). Most nurses were female (95.6%) with just over 50% working full time, the average age was 42.9 years, and 18.5% held a baccalaureate degree. On average, in 2000, there were 62 nurses per 10,000 in rural Canada compared to 78 per 10,000 in urban Canada, 17.9% of all RNs employed in nursing in Canada worked in rural areas but served 21.7% of the population, and 169 rural communities were being served by only one RN (CIHI, 2002). In 54 of these communities, the nurse was below 30 years of age with limited experience in nursing; also, higher proportions of nurses worked in community settings (12.7%) compared to their urban counterparts (7.8%) (Kulig et al., 2008).

A national 3-year study of 3,933 rural nurses conducted in 2001–2005 (Macleod, Kulig, Stewart, Pitblado, & Knock, 2004) revealed similar findings. However, more rural RNs (27%) held the baccalaureate degree than in the 2000 reports, and 5% identified as First Nations or Metis ethnicity. The areas of nursing practice included acute care (39%), long-term care (17%), community health (14%), home care (8%), and primary care (7%). Other findings from the study include (a) the terms "rural" and "remote" require additional investigation to accurately depict rural RNs' experience, (b) more RNs are needed to meet demands in rural and remote areas, (c) rural RNs need more educational support and opportunities, (d) the complexity of rural nursing practice is poorly understood and acknowledged, and (e) out-migration has a very negative effect on the supply of rural RNs (Pitblado, Medves, & Stewart, 2005). Specific information about the practice of rural RNs regarding rural women's health was not sought in this study. Implications from these findings suggest that rural nursing requires enriched valuing, understanding, and support to enhance recruitment, retention, and high-quality practice, such as preceptor or mentoring programs for novice nurses to facilitate transition from the student role to practice competency in the workplace. In addition, it is vital that research be conducted that explores the practice of rural nurses regarding specific populations, such as rural women.

The Canadian Association for Rural and Remote Nurses (CARRN; see www.carrn.com), a voluntary organization that serves as a voice for and that represents and advances rural and remote nursing practice in Canada, and the CNA, the professional body to which almost all RNs in Canada belong, have illuminated several issues regarding rural and remote nursing practice in Canada (CAARN, 2008; CNA, 2005), including inadequate numbers of nurses coupled with geographic and sociocultural factors. These documents reveal that rural nurses carry tremendous responsibility in being the only or one of a few health care providers who must provide care to a diverse array of clients, and that rural nurses are often the only formal health care provider, and often the only female health care provider in their communities, whose mandate is to promote health (rather than to provide treatment). For many rural women, rural nurses are the major, if not the only, source of gender-sensitive health promotion care and information (Leipert & Reutter, 1998). Thus, the question must be asked: Who cares and provides support for the caretaker, in this case the nurse in the rural community?

Characteristics of rural nursing practice include significant autonomy and responsibility, the ability to be both a generalist and a specialist and to take on aspects of care that would normally be provided by others, such as physicians and social workers, having to perform complex tasks competently but infrequently, the ability to be culturally safe, able to use technology, flexibility, resilience, and excellent assessment, communication, advocacy, and leadership skills (CARRN, 2008; CNA, 2005; Leipert & Reutter, 1998; Scharff, 2006). However, in spite of these significant professional demands and expectations, rural nurses have lower levels of formal education and support compared to urban nurses (Pitblado, 2005), and require more support and resources to practice effectively (CNA, 2005).

Additional challenges that rural nurses in Canada face relate to several issues. Recruitment and retention of nurses in isolated settings are problematic due to financial, education and training, professional development, quality-of-life, and quality-of-work-life factors (CNA, 2005). Recent economic measures in Canada have resulted in health care restructuring whereby small rural hospitals have either been closed, and nursing jobs lost, or hospitals are converted into providing alternate types of health care, which changes the skill set that nurses in those communities need or can obtain. In addition, the rural education that is available to nursing students in most nursing programs in Canada is limited and requires enrichment to enable all nursing students to consider rural practice, to function competently in rural settings, and to remain in the independent generalist practices in which they will engage in rural locations. In addition, access to continuing education while working in rural communities must be made available, and accommodate distance, weather, and travel issues. Quality of life and quality of work life for nurses are often affected by the "living in a fish bowl" nature of life in small communities (Leipert, 1999, p. 287), where everyone knows everyone else and where one's privacy and anonymity may be compromised.

For some nurses, such as those who were raised in rural settings, these factors may be familiar and not pose particular problems; however, for others who may be considering rural nursing practice, these factors and issues may discourage them from applying for and remaining in rural nursing settings (Leipert, 1999). Particular challenges for Aboriginal nurses and Aboriginal communities, which are often located in rural and remote locations, include recruitment and retention issues, acceptance of the nurse within the community, recognition that the nurse is a professional meeting standards of competency, and the need for ethical practice guidelines and clear regulations for practice (Aboriginal Nurses Association of Canada, 1995). Formal pre-ceptorships, internships, and mentorship arrangements of adequate duration and substantive quality that include cultural knowledge development (contextual as well as ethnic) hold significant potential to effectively prepare nurses to enter the rural health system workforce.

RURAL NURSING AND RURAL WOMEN'S HEALTH

Some of the first research on rural nursing and rural women's health explored women's health and the practice of public health nurses in northern British Columbia (BC) (Leipert, 1999; Leipert & Reutter, 1998). Using a phenomenological approach, interviews with 10 female public health nurses in northern BC revealed rich data about rural women's health (needs, how women stay healthy in northern commu-nities, and conditions that affect northern women's health), rural public health nursing practice (activities, strengths, conditions, and ways to strengthen), and the rural context (definitions, and benefits and chal-lenges) (Leipert). The value of nurses in advancing women's health in northern communities was clearly evident; however, further acknowl-edgment, valuing, support, and research were strongly advised.

More recent research has explored aspects relevant to rural nursing and rural women's health related to a variety of topics including the determinants of rural women's health (Leipert & George, 2008), rural context and rural women's health promotion (Leipert et al., 2011), abuse and violence (Riddell & Leipert, 2009), various diseases such as cancer (Brophy et al., 2006), mental health issues such as those related to stress (Kubik & Moore, 2003a, 2003b), and health issues and resources, such as resilience, of women in various rural locations (the north, farms, fishing communities) (Leipert, 2010; Leipert & Reutter, 2005; Sutherns, McCallum, & Haworth-Brockman, 2007; Sutherns, McPhedran, & Haworth-Brockman, 2004). An emerging field of study is the practice of nurse practitioners (NPs) and rural women's health. NPs, who work with an expanded scope of practice and often in rural settings, are becoming integrated into the health care systems of many Canadian pro-vinces. The time, attention, and care that NPs devote to rural women's health and the information that they impart to rural women are highly valued by the women who have access to them (Wagner, 2007). More research that explores the nature and practice of rural NPs with respect to rural women's health in Canada, and ways to advance and tailor practice to fit the needs and preferences of women in these commu-nities, is needed.

Explicit research in Canada about the practice of rural nurses with respect to rural women's health is in its infancy. The *Canadian Journal of Nursing Research* [CJNR], a key nursing journal in Canada, has recently dedicated two issues to rural health research (CJNR, 2005, 2010). In the first Rural Health Research issue of the *Canadian Journal of Nursing Research* (CJNR, 2005), submissions focused primarily on rural nursing workforce issues. The 2010 CJNR Rural Health Research issue (CJNR, 2010) has focused more on clinical issues for rural nurses and perspectives of rural residents; two of the seven research articles in this issue focus on rural nursing and rural women's health. As rural nursing and rural women's health research is published in other nursing journals and in journals of other disciplines and in other countries, it is challenging to obtain a clear picture of the breadth and depth of knowledge about this topic. Nonetheless, it is obvious that more information is needed. The creation in 2003 of the first Research Chair in North America in Rural Women's Health at the University of Western Ontario will help to foster research, development, and advocacy in this area.

RECOMMENDATIONS

Delivering nursing care to anyone in rural Canada is challenging. Models for the delivery of rural health care are few and far between, they are not well researched or disseminated, and may not be suitable for every rural setting, rural population, or rural culture. No models for rural nursing practice or for the practice of rural nursing to address rural women's health have yet been proposed or implemented nationwide in Canada. Nonetheless, several initiatives have been undertaken to support rural nursing practice. These include refining the NP role and nurse-managed care systems; coordinating formal preceptorship, internship and mentorship arrangements; working with indigenous paraprofessionals especially in remote settings; integrating telehealth and communication technology to deliver health care across remote distances; and using incentives, such as retention bonuses, northern salary enhancements, bursaries, forgivable loans, and tax reductions to enhance recruitment and retention (CNA, 2005; Macleod, Browne, & Leipert, 1998).

Canadian health care planners and policy developers must learn about and consider the distinctive features and challenges of the rural context (Anderson, 2006). Program accessibility, affordability, acceptability, appropriateness, awareness, and sustainability are important considerations when planning and implementing rural health programs (Anderson, 2006). Other ways in which nurses may help to eliminate or reduce rural health problems include:

1. Address socioeconomic factors that contribute to rural Canadians having lower incomes and less secure employment than their urban counterparts.
2. Attend to rural occupational hazards, as rural workers tend to have higher occupational hazards.
3. Develop strategies to improve rural roads and address other transportation issues that affect the health of rural people.
4. Enhance rural health promotion and illness and disease prevention programs.
5. Address accessibility issues for rural people regarding services that provide early detection and secondary prevention of acute and chronic diseases (CIHI, 2006). Considering what works and the successes of rural health programs in Canada (Health Canada, 2001) and elsewhere could also help to provide usable rural-friendly health care resources. Nurses must have a voice and advocate meaningful strategies to address rural nursing practice. Recommendations to support rural nursing practice and promote the health of rural residents, women in particular, follow.

   ■ Enrich professional nurse education programs to include relevant topics about the rural context and the people who live there.
   ■ Coordinate student clinical experiences and formal mentorship arrangements in rural facilities to enhance recruitment, retention, and delivery of safe and effective nursing services in professionally underserved settings.
   ■ Employ more public health nurses and NPs in rural Canada; support nurses in these practices with formal orientation and mentorship programs; and provide the necessary resources, authority, and ability to implement their full scopes of nursing practice.
   ■ Disseminate information about successful rural nurse mentorship and preceptorship models. The Canadian Association of Rural and Remote Nurses and the Canadian Nurses Association could lead this initiative.
   ■ Invite nurses and other health professionals with diverse geographical and cultural backgrounds as guest speakers in nursing education and professional continuing education programs to expose students and clinicians to effective current rural practice.
   ■ Inform policy developers at local, regional, provincial, and national levels about current and potential rural nursing practices

to elicit support for innovative programs that enhance recruitment and retention of nurses in underserved areas.

■ Educate CNA, CARRN, and CIHR about the need to lobby government entities and philanthropic organizations to fund more research related to nursing, as a predominately female profession, in the rural context. Evidence-based studies could provide important insights and strategies that address the health of rural women and rural female nurses as well as rural nursing practice.

■ Establish and publish national and provincial databases, standards, and objectives for rural women's health; then review the data to develop effective policy and clinical practice guidelines.

■ Implement recommendations by the World Health Organization (WHO, 2010) for recruitment and retention of rural health care personnel:

■ Use targeted admission to enroll students with rural backgrounds to increase rural practitioners, nurses in particular.

■ Locate health professions schools outside urban areas.

■ Introduce and regulate enhanced scopes of practice in rural and remote areas to increase the potential for job satisfaction, thereby assisting recruitment and retention of nurses.

■ Develop and support career development programs and provide senior posts so that nurses can progress on the career trajectory as a result of experience and training, without leaving rural areas.

■ Conduct more studies on rural factors and situations to enhance further understanding of "why" and "how." For example, further research about the practice of nurses in diverse rural areas could assist understanding of practice characteristics and needs, such as why and how nursing practices are constructed, or could be constructed, to enhance the health of the nurse as well as rural residents.

In summary, information about nurses and nursing practice in rural Canada is sparse and often times conflicting. What is known is that women dominate the nursing profession. In rural settings, the nurses tend to be older and have more years of work experience, but with fewer years of formal nursing education than urban counterparts. Research on rural Canadian women's health is a relatively new initiative and findings, so far, indicate these women experience disparities in accessing care and in their health status. Finally, there is a need for closer examination of the dynamics associated with being female and a nurse in the rural context, and the impact this has on nursing practice in rural communities.

ACKNOWLEDGMENT

I thank Dr. Rebecca Sutherns and Dr. Judith Kulig for their reviews and recommendations regarding this work.

REFERENCES

Aboriginal Nurses Association of Canada. (1995). *Band nurse workshops summary report*. Ottawa: Author.

Anderson, A. (2006). *Delivering Rural Health and Social Services: An Environmental Scan*. Retrieved from http://www.alzheimerontario.org/local/files

Brophy, J. T., Keith, M. M., Gorey, K. M., Luginaah, I., Laukkanen, E., Hellyer, D. et al. (2006). Occupation and breast cancer: A Canadian case-control study. *Annals of the New York Academy of Sciences, 1076*, 765–777.

Canadian Association of Rural and Remote Nurses. (2008). *Rural and Remote Nursing Practice Parameters Discussion Document*. Retrieved from http://www. carrn.com/files/NursingPracticePararmeters.pdf

Canadian Institute for Health Information [CIHI]. (2002). *Supply and distribution of registered nurses in rural and small town Canada, 2000*. Ottawa: Author.

Canadian Institute for Health Information [CIHI]. (2003). *Women's health surveillance report: A multidimensional look at the health of Canadian women*. Ottawa: Author.

Canadian Institute for Health Information [CIHI]. (2006). *How healthy are rural Canadians? An assessment of their health status and health determinants*. Ottawa: Author.

Canadian Journal of Nursing Research. (2005). *37*(1).

Canadian Journal of Nursing Research. (2010). *42*(1).

Canadian Nurses Association. (2005). *Rural nursing practice in Canada: A discussion paper* (Draft 3). Retrieved from http://www.carrn.com/files/RUral-Nursing-discussion-paper_Draft3-Sept%2005-1.pdf

Canadian Nurses Association. (2008). *Healthy Aging*. Retrieved from www. cna-aiic.ca

Du Plessis, V., Beshiri, R., & Bollman, R. (2002). Definitions of rural. (Catalogu 21-006-XIE). *Rural and Small Town Canada Analysis Bulletin, 3*(3), 1–16. Ottawa, ON: Statistics Canada.

Halfacree, K. H. (1993). Locality and social representation: Space, discourse and alternative definitions of the rural. *Journal of Rural Studies, 9*(1), 23–37.

Health Canada. (2001). *Canada's rural health strategy: A one-year review*. Retrieved from http://www.hc-sc.gc.ca

Hodge, G. (2008). *The geography of aging: Preparing communities for the surge in seniors*. Montreal, QC: McGill-Queen's University Press.

Keating, N. (Ed.). (2008). *Rural ageing: A good place to grow old?* Bristol, UK: The Policy Press, University of Bristol.

Kubik, W., & Moore, R. (2003a). Changing roles of Saskatchewan farm women: Qualitative and quantitative perspectives. In R. Blake, & A. Nurse (Eds.), *The trajectories of rural life: New perspectives on rural Canada* (pp. 25–36). Regina, SASK: Saskatchewan Institute of Public Policy, University of Regina.

Kubik, W., & Moore, R. (2003b). Farming in Saskatchewan in the 1990s: Stress and coping. In H. Diaz, J. Jaffe, & R. Stirling (Eds.), *Farm communities at the crossroads: Challenge and resistance* (pp. 119–133). Regina, SASK: Canadian Plains Research Centre, University of Regina.

Kulig, J., Macleod, M., Stewart, N., & Pitblado, R. (2008). Clients in rural areas. In L. Stamler, & L. Yiu (Eds.), *Community health nursing: A Canadian perspective* (2nd ed.) (pp. 301–310). Toronto: Pearson Prentice Hall.

Kulig, J. C. (2010). Rural health research in Canada: Assessing our progress. *Canadian Journal of Nursing Research, 42*(1), 7–11.

Leipert, B. (1999). Women's health and the practice of public health nurses in Northern British Columbia. *Public Health Nursing, 16*(4), 280–289. doi: 10.1046/j.1525-1446.1999.00280.x

Leipert, B. (2010). Rural and remote women and resilience: Grounded theory and photovoice variations on a theme. In C. Winters, & H. Lee (Eds.), *Rural nursing: Concepts, theory, and practice* (3rd ed.) (pp. 105–129). New York: Springer.

Leipert, B., & George, J. (2008). The determinants of rural women's health: A case study in southwest Ontario. *Journal of Rural Health, 24*(2), 210–218.

Leipert, B., & Reutter, L. (1998). Women's health and community health nursing practice in geographically isolated settings: A Canadian perspective. *Health Care for Women International, 19*(6), 575–588. doi: 10.1080/073993398246133

Leipert, B., & Reutter, L. (2005). Women's health in northern British Columbia: The role of geography and gender. *Canadian Journal of Rural Medicine, 10*(4), 241.

Leipert, B., Plunkett, R., Meagher-Stewart, D., Scruby, L., Mair, H., & Wamsley, K. (2011). I couldn't imagine my life without it! Curling and health promotion: A photovoice study. *The Canadian Journal of Nursing Research, 43*(1), 60–78.

MacLeod, M., Browne, A. J., & Leipert, B. (1998). Issues for nurses in rural and remote Canada. *The Australian Journal of Rural Health, 6*(2), 72–78.

MacLeod, M. L. P., Kulig, J. C., Stewart, N. J., Pitblado, J. R., & Knock, M. (2004). The nature of nursing practice in rural and remote Canada. *Canadian Nurse, 100*(6), 27–31.

Pitblado, J. (2005). *How many registered nurses are there in rural and remote Canada?* Retrieved from www.carrn.com/files/RuralNsgFactSheet1.pdf

Pitblado, J., Medves, J., & Stewart, N. (2005). For work and for school: Internal migration of Canada's rural nurses. (2005). *CJNR (Canadian Journal of Nursing Research), 37*(1), 102–121.

Riddell, T., Ford-Gilboe, M., & Leipert, B. (2009). Strategies used by rural women to stop, avoid, or escape from intimate partner violence. *Health Care for Women International, 30*(1), 134–159.

Romanow, R. (2002). *Building on values: The future of health care in Canada.* Ottawa: The Romanow Commission Report.

Scharff, J. E. (2006). The distinctive nature and scope of rural nursing practice: Philosophical bases. In H. J. Lee, & C. A. Winters (Eds.), *Rural nursing: Concepts, theory, and practice* (2nd ed.) (pp. 179–196). New York, NY: Springer Publishing.

Senate Standing Committee on Agriculture and Forestry [SSCAF]. (2006). *Understanding freefall: The challenge of the rural poor.* Retrieved from www.parl.gc.ca

Sutherns, R., McCallum, M., & Haworth-Brockman, M. (2007). A thematic bibliography and literature review of rural, remote, and northern women's health in Canada 2003–2006. *Resources for Feminist Research, 32*(3/4), 142–178.

Sutherns, R., McPhedran, M., & Haworth-Brockman, M. (2004). *Rural, remote, and northern women's health: Policy and research directions.* Winnipeg, MA: Prairie Center of Excellence for Women's Health.

Troughton, M. J. (1999). Redefining "rural" for the twenty-first century. In W. Ramp, J. Kulig, I. Townshend, & V. McGowan (Eds.), *Health in rural settings: Contexts for action* (pp. 21–38). Lethbridge, AB: University of Lethbridge.

Wagner, J. (2007). *Rural women's experiences with primary health care nurse practitioners.* (Unpublished Master's thesis). University of Western Ontario, London, Ontario, Canada.

World Health Organization. (2010, October). *WHO Guidelines on Rural Recruitment and Retention.* Retrieved from http://www.rrh.org.au/news/shownewsnew.asp?NewsID=222

II

Transition to Practice: Exemplar Models

Section Two focuses on transition-to-practice exemplar models. Models authored by both national and international authors present different approaches to the question, "How can providers assist new graduates or nurses changing career focus become both confident and competent in the new roles?" This section begins with two international exemplars. Chapter Seven, by Ross, elaborates on a "place based" practice model (PBPM), designed to facilitate transition of a student to professional nursing practice in rural New Zealand. Chapter Eight, by Francis and Jacob, provides an overview of Australia and its nursing workforce. They offer a case study describing the decision-making process of one nurse choosing a rural practice environment.

Two larger models delivered in both rural and urban settings are described next. McElroy and McGuinn focus on the University Health-System Consortium's (UHC) & the American Association of Colleges of Nursing's (AACN) Nurse Residency Program (UHC/AACN Nurse Residency Program™). The transition-to-practice model consists of a series of learning and work experiences for increasing the clinical and leadership skills necessary for an advanced beginner nurse to become a successful healthcare team partner. In Chapter 10, Silvestre and Spector offer details about the National Council of State Boards of Nursing's (NCSBN's)—Transition to Practice (TTP) Regulatory Model. This exemplar is appropriate for health care agencies that hire newly licensed nurses at many educational levels; including practical nurses, associate degree, diploma, baccalaureate and other entry-level graduates.

Molinari, in Chapter 11 presents another national exemplar designed for small rural facilities. In Chapter 12 Boyer highlights the Vermont Nurses In Partnership (VNIP) Model. This exemplar integrates an internship framework that supports safe, effective transitions for new graduate nurses who successfully complete the NCLEX. State programs from North Carolina are featured in Chapter 13. Johnson, Hall, and Roth provide details about Regionally Increasing Baccalaureate Nurses (RIBN) & Evidence-based Transition-to-Practice Program. The programs were created to increase the number of Baccalaureate prepared nurses in the state and to retain new graduates in rural settings.

Kuebel and Joiner contributed a chapter that elaborates on a Washington state program educating nurses in their rural hospitals called the Rural Outreach Nursing Education (RONE) Program. The program increases the number of individuals who can complete nursing education as well as retains the new graduates because they are longtime rural community residents.

Chapter 15 features an Alaskan competency measurement exemplar. The program, entitled Alaska Frontier: Statewide Competency Development Initiative, was contributed by Roleff, McNulty, and Montague. The authors describe the statewide collaboration process on a required competency measurement tool and the outcomes of standardizing preceptor competencies.

In Chapter 16, von Dielingen describes the outcomes of another statewide collaboration, New Mexico: Nurse Residence Program. Hosted by the state Center for Nursing Excellence, the process created new partnerships, generated innovative ideas, and facilitated insights regarding RNs transition into the state's nursing workforce. Wappes, in Chapter 17, describes a different type of support program designed in Oregon for small hospital employees wanting to become nurses. Hospitals create cohorts at nearby schools in exchange for work guarantees.

Chapter 18 offers an international perspective from Canada, by Yonge, Myrick, Ferguson, and Grundy, about preceptor evaluation issues. The grounded theory study addresses the difficulties preceptors experience when evaluating visiting students.

7

Place-Based Practice: A New Zealand Nursing Education Model

Jean Ross

This chapter describes New Zealand, the land and its people; examines features of nursing in rural New Zealand; and presents an overview of a Bachelor of Nursing program at the School of Nursing, Otago Polytechnic, Dunedin, New Zealand. For this model, the concept of place provides meaning and experience in reference to "location," "locale," and "sense of place." The aim of this Place-Based Practice Model was to facilitate transition of a student to professional nursing practice in rural New Zealand.

The Bachelor of Nursing (BN) program at the School of Nursing, Otago Polytechnic developed the *Place-Based Practice Model (PBPM)* in an effort to address distinct, diverse, and challenging nature of New Zealand (NZ) nursing practice. The PBPM focuses on the concept of rural as "place," in reference to *location, locale,* and *sense of place.* The first component of place introduces nursing students to geographical "locations." "Locale" addresses social relationships that a nurse develops within and external to a rural setting. While "sense of place" refers to attachment and belonging, which are important dimensions of positive learning experiences that can facilitate transition of a student to professional nursing practice in a rural area.

OVERVIEW OF NEW ZEALAND'S HEALTH CARE SYSTEM

New Zealand consists of three main islands, the North Island, the South Island, and the Stewart Island, and two smaller islands, the Chatham and Great Barrier Islands. Geographically, NZ is very diverse with glaciers, fjords, mountains, plains, subtropical forest, a volcanic plateau, and miles of coastline. The total population of NZ is about 4.5 million, of which about 30% live on the South Island; a third live on the North Islands. The population density of NZ is relatively low with 15 people per square kilometer. Of the total NZ land mass, rural areas account for 97% of land having about 15% of the total population (Jones, 2007). Rural is defined as a town with a population of 1,000 people or less (Statistics New Zealand, 2006). The terrain of NZ is conducive to numerous sporting activities (winter and summer sports). Thus, tourism has become a dominant industry for international visitors along with seasonal workers supporting the industry. In some small towns, the population may double in size during certain times of the year associated with recreational events.

Politically, the changing focus of the provision of health care in the community was a strategic direction of the NZ Labor government in the early 2000s. The Primary Health Care Strategy (2001), an initiative of this government, was designed to promote and maintain health of the populations through District Health Boards, Primary Care Organizations, and rural communities in the form of community trusts to promote accessible, affordable, approachable, available, and appropriate health care to the people of NZ (Primary Health Care Strategy, 2001). Equitable access and appropriate, affordable, health care for all New Zealanders is a fundamental principle set out in the *Primary Health Care Strategy* (2001) and *Implementing the Primary Health Care Strategy in Rural New Zealand* (2002). In turn, appropriate access and acknowledging social networks that provide formal and informal rural care become the focus of rural nursing practice.

RURAL NURSING PRACTICE

Successful rural practice requires that nurses offer health services that are innovative, autonomous, and collaborative (New Zealand's Ministry of Health Primary Health Care Strategy, 2001). To achieve competence, rural nurses are expected to adapt their knowledge and clinical skills to meet the needs of individuals in the community in which they practice (Howie, 2008; Jones & Ross, 2000; O'Malley & Fearnley, 2007; Ross, 1996).

Understanding the political background along with the nuances of the geographical or physical environment is essential for the nursing practice. Population trends as described above can pose challenges for a local health care system, placing additional strain on nurses and the institution's financial resource (Fitzwater, 2008; Health Workforce Information Programme, 2009). In NZ, rural nursing practice is shaped by the context or "place," as illustrated in the following statement:

> Rural is not a scope of practice, it is a context of practice. Rural nursing practice is shaped by its situatedness. Distinctive settings determine nursing roles and responses—which differ according to the health needs and health service provision in particular rural communities.
>
> —*Jones & Ross, 2003, p. 18*

In NZ, rural nursing occurs in many settings, among others, homes, schools, long-term care facilities, health centers, local shops, and sporting events. Nurses also work in very small and tertiary hospitals as well as mobile [surgical] buses/service (Jamison, 2008). Understanding rural peoples' culture will ultimately decrease inequalities for access to health care and assist in developing a collaborative nurse–client relationship. These federal health policies were instrumental in revising the BN curriculum at School of Nursing, Otago Polytechnic, Dunedin, New Zealand and development of the PBPM.

PHILOSOPHY OF PBPM

The philosophical underpinnings of PBPM for nursing education emphasize physical environment (context), distance from regional and local health services, and local amenities when planning health care. Knowledge about the context is important for nurses who work in urban as well as rural facilities. However, the PBPM curriculum integrates *distinctive rural competencies* (Jones & Ross, 2003) that are based on the following NZ definition of rural nursing:

> A distinctive way to nurse: rural nurses are specialist-generalists who use insider knowledge of the communities they live/work/study in, combined with advanced clinical skills to provide a nursing service, particular to the unique health needs of their community. Professional and personal roles are interwoven so managing professional/personal boundary issues along this continuum are critical to achieving success in the role
>
> —*Adapted by O'Malley, Lawry, Barber, & Fearnley, 2009, p. 17*

This definition highlights the complexity of rural nursing in New Zealand. First, it emphasizes an understanding of location relative to the rural nurse's practice. Second, the definition alludes to relationships developed and maintained by the rural nurse. Third, the definition highlights an interface of the personal and professional self that occurs within a rural community.

The three aspects of rural nursing practice relative to "place" ("location," "locale," and "sense of place") are based on the work of Agnew (1987) and are examined in more detail relative to the PBPM nursing curriculum. Place, as a physical site indicated on a map marked to scale, with the purpose of specifying a place or location. However, place takes on far greater meaning than simply being a physical location relative to a student successfully transitioning to rural nursing practice (Agnew, 1987; Cresswell, 2004; Massey, 2005; Vanclay, Higgins, & Blackshaw, 2008). Within the PBPM place, "location" (Agnew, 1987) is used in reference to environment, or more specifically, the rural context in which the nurse works. Here the competent nurse must be able to adapt nursing practice to meet the needs and preferences of the people who live there (Primary Health Care Strategy, 2001).

The concept of "locale" is used in reference to a setting in which everyday life takes place, to include development and maintenance of relationships both internal and external to the community. For a nurse, relationships within a community include local residents, health professionals, and social networks. Those relationships that are external to a rural community often support a nurses' professional and personal development. Building and sustaining effective relationships by a nurse with local residents is a unique feature of rural nursing (O'Malley et al., 2009; Ross, 1998). According to Agnew (1987), social relationships are more complex than simply an interaction between humans; rather, these include dynamic political movements among those who are in the relationship (Massey, 2005). For the rural nurse, it is important that he or she learn to understand the political tensions (local, regional, and national) as this ability facilitates the transition from student to professional practice.

Agnew (1987) describes "sense of place" as the location in which meaning emerges for an individual, through emotion and attachments to the location. For the novice nurse, sense of place is established when he or she develops an emotional attachment and a sense of physical belonging to a particular rural place. Attachment, subsequently, strengthens an individual's commitment to the rural (place) community (Vanclay, et al., 2008). Attachments are accompanied by a willingness of local residents, including the nurse, to contribute to the community.

According to Vanclay et al. (2008), sense of place, or homogeneity, includes the notion of belonging and cohesion. A person's awareness of self is linked to the location in which a sense of belonging evolves, evidenced by behavior and actions that construct a community member's performance. For nurses in rural practice, this concept connotes differentiation of personal and professional boundaries of relationships that occur within the community.

Tertiary education in New Zealand is generally focused on a traditional model of delivering programs in main urban educational centers. While clinical placements are provided outside of the main urban centers, students return to the main educational center for ongoing theoretical study. There is a mix of student nurses from both urban and rural backgrounds who attend the program. Small groups of students (cohorts) from rural locations form local groups while receiving all their clinical placements in their local rural location and travel to the main urban center for their ongoing theoretical study. However, recent advances in technology and internet connections have aided these students with blended learning styles. Positive experiences and faculty support of rural clinical practice are associated with student success in their transition to practice (Sedgwick & Yonge, 2008). Research demonstrates that students who experience rural practice as a positive learning encounter are more likely to practice rural nursing following graduation (Smith, Edwards, Courtney, & Finlayson 2001).

PBPM: BN CURRICULUM

The PBPM curriculum incorporates a rural thread to aid the successful transition of student nurse into rural nursing practice. This thread includes knowledge and clinical experience relating to the study of rural culture, society, and the practice of nursing, rural people/whanau (related to as families) and iwi (tribes or groups) through the delivery of primary and secondary health care contexts. Preparation of nurses for the workplace either within a rural setting or nursing rural people in the urban setting also drives the rural thread (see Table 7.1 for detailed content).

The placed-based practice model rural content offers the student nurse essential knowledge and skills to blend in professionally with the community and achieve clinical competency. The knowledge generated to adapt rural nursing practice to meet the demands and specific features of the rural community within a flexible environment enables the nurse to deliver a health service that is based on defined community need. This is specific to local rural people within the appropriate social and geographical context, that is, locally rather than regionally and nationally driven. The rural content is built on

TABLE 7.1
PBPM Curriculum Overview: Objectives and Rural Content

YEAR	LEARNING OBJECTIVES	CLINICAL OBJECTIVE/EXPERIENCE
Year 1	Overview of "place" as "location," a geographical position on the earth's surface and sites of practice	Exposure to rural society/economics and culture, including Maori the indigenous people of New Zealand Exposure to rural health services Introduction to rural online resources, journals, textbooks and workbook/tools and online activities Introduction to rural organizations, local, regional, national, and international
Year 2 Builds on year 1 content	Overview of "place" as "locale," where social relations occur both within and external to "location"	Exposure to rural people accessing and receiving health care in urban and rural contexts Exposure to various rural population groups Understanding physical environment, distance and access from regional and local health services Accessing rural organizations, local, regional, and national
Year 3 Builds on year 1 and year 2 content	Overview of "place" as "sense of belonging," to blend professionally into rural society and culture	Preparation for transition to rural practice Incorporation of community profile and assessment and health needs Reflection of rural community life and shared values Providing effective and responsive health care dedicated to rural context Contributing to rural organizations, local, regional, and national

the foundation research studies undertaken within New Zealand in the early 2000s and the development of relevant educational resources, including distinctive rural competencies, orientation to rural practice tool, a rural nursing textbook, web-based resources, and a documentary film.

DISTINCTIVE RURAL COMPETENCIES

Distinctive Rural Competencies (Exhibit 7.1) developed by Jones and Ross (2003) comprise four main themes with a number of corresponding subthemes.. These competencies guide student learning for clinical placements in Years 2 and 3. These competencies are measured student learning and practice with course objectives that align with the three aspects of "place."

EXHIBIT 7.1 PBPM: Overview of Distinctive Rural Competencies

Related to isolation and distance, availability of backup

- Assessment and triage as **first-response** to trauma and other life-threatening or serious emergency
- **Mobilizing and coordinating** local and distant resources in emergencies and nonemergencies
- **Planning care** (self, family, nursing, and others) that is appropriate to the patient's situation and resources (care anticipates, supplements, involves those resources)
- **Telephone consultation**, including advising, counseling, and triage
- **Accessing internet-based resources** for clinical management, service, and community development, and own professional development and networks as a rural nurse

Related to managing the professional and personal self in a smaller community

- Gaining entree and **trust**, and establishing **credibility** in a community
- Establishing both **boundaries** for self and with others as a professional and community member; negotiating a changing role; dealing with breaches and breakdowns
- Establishing and utilizing appropriate/safe/discreet sources of **personal and professional support**
- Selecting **community involvements** and roles to align/amplify professional responsibilities

Related to nurse/patient relationships

- Moving into and out of (establishing/negotiating/disengaging from) **effective nurse/patient relationships** with fellow community members/persons known to oneself
- Establishing an effective relationship with the visitor/tourist/stranger/foreigner
- Engaging with or entering parts of the community where one is not of the dominant **culture** *in ways that are safe, appropriate, and effective*

Related to independence and interdependence with other health professionals and anticipating resolution of unsatisfactory legal provisions

- Practising within current legal provisions and/or **managing cover or accountability** for breaches and difficulties

■ Building respectful and productive **collegial relationships** with doctors, other health personnel, and other "officers of the community"
■ Managing **timely and appropriate responses and treatment orders** from other health professionals

Source: From Jones & Ross, 2003. Reprinted with permission.

ORIENTATION TO RURAL PRACTICE TOOL

The Orientation to Rural Practice Tool (Maw, Echkoff, & London, 2002) comprises everything a new practitioner entering a rural community needs to know for effective community practice. This tool is designed as a user-friendly Word document (www.moh.govt.nz/moh.nsf/indexmh/ruralhealth) to enable students to complete the specific information related to their designated community, within the Tool.

RURAL NZ RESOURCES

The textbook *Rural Nursing: Aspects of Practice* (Ross, 2008) provides a broad overview of rural nursing practice in New Zealand. The content includes information on theory development, descriptions of rural practice, and adaptation of practice to fit rural contexts, with inclusion of relevant research. The various chapters have been written by New Zealand rural nurses as a component of their research activities. The content of this textbook is a compulsory educational resource within the BN and is provided free of charge via the Ministry of Health in New Zealand's website http://www.moh.govt.nz/moh.nsf/indexmh/ruralhealth. Additional web-based resources are used for various courses to include online journals and textbooks. These courses provide very timely current information and are readily accessible, especially when students are in rural clinical placement.

Rural Documentary (Film)

Another important resource is a documentary film focusing on rural NZ, and was developed to address the following aims:

First, the film introduces Otago, New Zealand, the local region associated with the educational institution and clinical placement areas. The main urban center, Dunedin, is included. The documentary provides local knowledge while orientating the student to the physical location of Dunedin and Otago and the wider environment, rural Otago. Having been orientated to the location, and the distance from Dunedin to rural Otago settlements, students are introduced to its people, the second aim. Otago has a total population of 205,000 people; the population density is 6.2 people per km. The population is made up of mainly Maori and New Zealand European culture. The Otago region has only 4.8% of New Zealand's population and is, therefore, a more isolated setting. The third aim is to capture the thoughts about rural lifestyle from Otago residents (including children, old-timers, and newcomers). Their comments highlight social and economic issues associated with life in a more remote setting and provide insights about access to health services. This documentary has proven to be an excellent teaching resource that integrates didactic content with nursing practice in a particular rural community.

In summary, on completion of this BN program, students fulfill all the Nursing Council of NZ (NCNZ) competencies for registered nurse. The development of the PBPM, with its underpinning concept "place" from political and social geography perspectives, offers a deeper understanding of rural nursing practice. "Place" provides meaning and experience in reference to rural as a location, locale, and sense of place (Agnew, 1987). The PBPM is responsive to the political and social mandates of New Zealand national government to address the particular nursing needs of rural communities and the nursing workforce. This PBPM curriculum is designed to prepare BN graduates and facilitate their successful transition to rural nursing practice.

REFERENCES

Agnew, J. (1987). *Place and politics*. Boston: Allen and Unwin.

Cresswell, T. (2004). *Place: A short introduction*. Oxford: Blackwell Publishing Ltd.

Fitzwater, A. (2008). The impact of tourism on a rural nursing practice. In J. Ross (Ed.), *Rural nursing: Aspects of practice* (pp. 137–143). Dunedin, New Zealand: Rural Health Opportunities.

Health Workforce Information Programme. (2009). *Health workforce projections modeling 2009 rural nursing workforce*. Wellington, New Zealand: Ministry of Health.

Howie, L. (2008). Rural society and culture. In J. Ross (Ed.), *Rural nursing: Aspects of practice* (pp. 3–18). Dunedin, New Zealand: Rural Health Opportunities.

Jamison, I. (2008). The mobile operating theatre project. In J. Ross (Ed.), *Rural nursing: Aspects of practice* (pp. 81–97). Dunedin, New Zealand: Rural Health Opportunities.

Jones, D. (2007). *The role of agriculture and arm households in the rural economy: Main findings of a report prepared for the OECD Trade and Agriculture Directorate.*

Retrieved December 1, 2010. Available at www.edsconference.com/content/docs/papers/jones.%@OD.pdf

Jones, S., & Ross, J. (2000). Defining the role of a rural health nurse. *Kai Tiaki Nursing New Zealand, July*, 20.

Jones, S., & Ross, J. (2003). *Describing your scope of practice: A resource for rural nurses.* Christchurch, New Zealand: National Centre for Rural Health, Department of Public Health and General Practice, Christchurch School of Medicine, University of Otago.

Maw, H., Echkoff, E., & London, M. (2002). *Orientation to rural practice tool.* Christchurch, New Zealand: National Centre for Rural Health, Department of Public Health and General Practice, Christchurch School of Medicine, University of Otago.

Massey, D. (2005). *For space.* London: Sage.

Ministry of Health. (2001). *Primary health care strategy.* Wellington, New Zealand: Ministry of Health.

Ministry of Health. (2002). *Implementing the primary health care strategy in rural New Zealand*, Wellington, New Zealand: Ministry of Health.

O'Malley, J., & Fearnley, J. (2007). Can generalist nurses be specialists? *Kai Tiaki Nursing New Zealand, 13*(4), 21.

O'Malley, J., Lawry, D., Barber, M., & Fearnley, J. (2009). *Rural nursing workforce strategy: Final report July 2009.* West Coast DHB; Greymouth, New Zealand.

Ross, J. (1996). *Rural practice nurse skills project.* Christchurch, New Zealand: National Centre for Rural Health, Department of Public Health and General Practice, Christchurch School of Medicine, University of Otago.

Ross, J. (1998). Advanced rural nursing practice. *Primary Healthcare, 1*(1), 36–38.

Ross, J. (2008). *Rural nursing: Aspects of practice.* Dunedin, New Zealand: Rural Health Opportunities.

Sedgwick, M. G., & Yonge, O. (2008). Undergraduate nursing students' preparedness to "go rural." *Nurse Education Today, 28*(5), 620–626.

Smith, S., Edwards, H., Courtney, M., & Finlayson, K. (2001). *Factors influencing student nurses in their choice of a rural clinical placement site.* Rural and remote 1: 89. (Online) 2001. Retrieved December 1, 2010 from http://www.rrh.org.au

Statistics New Zealand. (2006). *New Zealand: An Urban/Rural Profile.* Retrieved December 1, 2010 from www.stats.govt.nz/urban-rural-profiles

Vanclay, F., Higgins, M., & Blackshaw, A. (2008). *Making sense of place: Exploring concepts and expressions of place through different senses and lenses.* Canberra: National Museum of Australia Press.

8

Rural Nursing in the Australian Context

Karen Louise Francis and Elisabeth R. Jacob

A ustralia offers diverse nursing career opportunities that include practice in metropolitan as well as in rural and very remote settings ("the bush"). This chapter describes geographical and population features of Australia and examines the nations' rural nursing workforce. A case presentation (Wendy's) highlights an innovative nursing/midwifery baccalaureate degree program, designed to prepare graduates who can effectively transition into rural practice settings and meet the particular health care needs of the people who live there.

An Australian-focused nursing/midwifery case (Wendy) was developed based on discussions with students, graduate nurse coordinators, and faculty involved with nurse education about the transition of students to graduate nurses. Essentially, the case approach facilitates in-depth understanding by presenting a detailed overview of information influencing the process (Stake, 2003). Case studies are used widely in social science disciplines, including nursing as they "... investigate a contemporary phenomenon within its real life context" (Mohd Noor, 2008, p. 1602).

AUSTRALIA: THE LAND AND ITS PEOPLE

Australia is an island continent with the majority of the population (70%) living in the capital cities located on the coastal fringes of the continent. Because of this settlement pattern, health care and other services are concentrated in the high-population areas. In the late 1980s and early 1990s, research identified that people living in less populated areas of Australia (rural and remote) experienced poorer health than

95

people living in the populated metropolitan regions (Wilkinson & Blue, 2002). This disparity in health status was further exacerbated by the higher proportion of indigenous Australians living in rural and remote Australia, who experience similar morbidity and mortality to people in the majority world (developed world). Australia, unlike other nations, traditionally differentiates between rural and remote. This differentiation was largely rationalized on the basis of population density versus land mass (Hugo, 2004).

Australia is a multicultural nation and has an ethnically diverse population with a varying mix of people from different cultures and racial and ethnic groups, including indigenous Australians (Aboriginal and Torres Strait Islanders). Indigenous Australians trace their genealogy to the original inhabitants of Australia prior to British colonization in 1788 (Omeri & Raymond, 2010; Wilson & Grant, 2008). From 1788, the composition of Australia's population has changed, with people of European descent becoming the dominant group. Today, indigenous people comprise 2.5% of the total Australian population, with 32% of this group residing in major cities. Over 40% of the indigenous population live in inner- or outer-regional Australia and more than 20% live in remote or very remote areas (Australian Bureau of Statistics, 2008). Almost a quarter of Australia's total population was born overseas (Year Book of Australia, 2008). Australia today is a multicultural nation that celebrates its rich cultural heritage. To represent the average nurse in Australia, this chapter will discuss the journey of Wendy Jones, a white Australian, baccalaureate graduate nurse/midwife (referred to as graduate nurse in Australia) to registered nurse working in rural Australia.

WENDY'S CASE

Wendy Jones was a 22-year-old female from a rural township in South East Victoria, Australia. The region in which Wendy lived was classified as rural as it is 200 km from the major state capital, Melbourne. She lived in a town with a population of 10,000 people, while the surrounding district had a population of over 50,000 people. Wendy's hometown was designated rural according to the Australian government.

Many definitions have been used in Australia to define rurality including the Accessibility Remoteness Index of Australia [ARIA]; Rural Remote Metropolitan Access Classification Scheme [RRMA]; and the Griffith Service Access Frame (Australian Institute of Health and Welfare, 2008; Humphreys & Rolley, 1991). Each classification system was developed to reflect specific interests. For example, ARIA stressed accessibility in terms of known transport links and available services that could be accessed (Department of Health and Ageing, 2005) while the Griffith Service Access Frame was specifically developed for quantifying the service access of populations in rural and remote areas to educational services. RRMA used distance to larger towns and cities and from other people as a basis for its remoteness index. Each system had value, however. RRMA is a preferred system as it allows for greater variance in the characteristics of the populations studied (Francis, Bowman, & Redgrave, 2002) (see Table 8.1 for RRMA's index of remoteness).

Wendy is the second (middle) child of Tom and Janet. Both Tom and Janet were born and raised in central rural Victoria and on marrying relocated to the south eastern region of Victoria. Tom established a stock and station agency in Timbertown that had a solid reputation throughout the region. Janet held a degree in teacher education. She worked part-time at the local high school since they settled in Timbertown, taking maternity leave when each of the children was born. Wendy had an elder brother, Andrew, aged 25 years and a younger sister, Matilda, aged 19 years. Wendy and her siblings attended local schools in Timbertown, including the high school where their mother Janet worked. Wendy and her siblings enjoyed attending their mother's school; however, on occasion they felt intimidated because everyone knew who they were and that their mum was on staff.

Wendy and her siblings were encouraged to participate in recreational and other social activities that Timbertown supported. Wendy enjoyed playing netball on Saturday mornings and was also a member of the local pony club from the age of 7 years. Like many of her school friends, Wendy joined the local youth group when she started high school at the age of 13 years. The Youth Group was

TABLE 8.1
Australia Definition: Rural Remote Metropolitan Access Zones[a]

ZONE	CLASSIFICATION	CATEGORY
Metropolitan	1	Capital cities
	2	Other *metropolitan* centers (urban center population >100,000)
Rural	3	Large *rural* centers with population 25,000–99,000
	4	Small *rural* centers with population 10,000–24,999
	5	Other *rural* areas with population <10,000
Remote	6	*Remote* centers with population >5,000
	7	Other *remote* areas with population <5,000

[a]Australian Institute of Health and Welfare, 2004, p. 3; Wakerman & Humphreys, 2008.

managed by the local Police and the Local Council. Wendy was involved in volunteer work with an aged care facility organized by the Youth Group and also had the opportunity to assist in a number of fund-raising events supporting the local hospital. These experiences exposed Wendy to the health care system. She admired the work of the health care team, in particular the nurses. Wendy knew many of the nurses who lived locally. Some of her friends' parents, mostly their mothers, were nurses who volunteered to work at pony club, netball, and the local football club games as first-aid officers. Wendy's best friend Kate's mother was the school nurse who delivered health education and promotion information to the high-school students and also provided immunization clinics.

Even as a small child Wendy wanted to be a nurse and dreamed of working in the Australian outback. She went to Alice Springs, located in central Australia, during the final year of her secondary schooling and had the opportunity to visit the Flying Doctors Service (FDA). Wendy met the nursing and medical staff employed by the FDA who related stories of their practice to her. Wendy decided that she wanted to be a health professional and felt that nursing was a career that would be a satisfying job that provided great opportunity for career advancement. To ensure that she understood what becoming a nurse would involve, she searched online for information. Wendy was astounded that there were many different types of preservice nursing courses available and that she could also apply for a direct entry midwifery program (see Exhibit 8.1).

Wendy sought advice from the careers advisor at her school about educational options that would lead to registration as a nurse and or a midwife. The careers advisor helped her to choose the subjects recommended to enter preregistration nursing, such as English, mathematics, and a life science, and suggested that Wendy attend the nursing careers expo hosted by the Royal College of Nursing Australia (RCNA). These careers expos were held in all major cities in Australia once every year. Education providers and health services attended information booths and displays at the expos to provide information on undergraduate and postgraduate nursing education as well as employment opportunities (Royal College of Nursing Australia, 2010a). Wendy and her mother traveled to Melbourne where Wendy talked with a number of universities about their undergraduate preservice programs. She was interested in nursing and midwifery and after talking with a number of rural health services at the expo felt that being both a nurse and a midwife would be beneficial and provide her with a solid foundation for practice in remote settings in the future. She was informed that her options in undertaking nursing would be to complete a double degree in nursing and midwifery,

EXHIBIT 8.1   Australian Preservice Nursing/Midwifery Education Programs

Entry requirements to practice as a registered nurse in Australia require the completion of Bachelor of Nursing degree. This is usually undertaken over 3 years of study and can be taken as a single nursing degree or in a combination program that can include midwifery, paramedic studies, or mental health nursing. The addition of the second degree usually lengthens the program of study to 4 years for the completion of both degrees. The basic degree requires a set number of clinical placement hours and theoretical content as specified by the Australian Nursing and Midwifery Council, which is the body responsible for nursing course accreditation in Australia. Completion of the basic degree and passing the English requirements for international students enables the graduate nurse to register as a nurse.

licensing on completion in both discipline areas or she could do a single degree in nursing and after a period of consolidation (normally 1 year is advocated) following her graduation undertake a postgraduate degree in midwifery. Wendy was keen to practice as both a nurse and midwife in a rural context and felt that undertaking a double degree would enable her career to progress at a faster rate by providing her with multiple skills necessary to work in a rural environment (Francis et al., 2010). Wendy also consulted her friend's parents who were nurses, seeking their advice about nursing as a career and the experiences they had working in rural Australia.

Wendy applied for entry to the Bachelor of Nursing Practice/Bachelor of Midwifery program offered at the local university that had a very good reputation. During the course of her studies she attended a presentation by the RCNA, the peak professional body for nursing in Australia. The RCNA offers student nurse memberships that Wendy felt would be useful in keeping her current on professional issues in Australia. She understood that the RCNA included a number of professional specialist nursing faculties, including a Faculty of Rural Nursing and Midwifery who advocate on behalf of rural nurses and midwives. RCNA members have access to the 3IP program which is an online program that assists members to plan and track continuing professional development needs and activities as evidence supporting currency of practice necessary for licensure (Royal College of Nursing Australia, 2010a) (see Exhibit 8.2).

EXHIBIT 8.2   Australian Nursing and Midwifery Regulatory Board

Nurses in Australia licence with the Nursing and Midwifery Board of Australia (NMBA). In 2009, new legislation was introduced that paved the way for a single regulatory authority to be established, replacing the existing system of State and Territory jurisdictional regulatory authorities. National legislation defining the practice, regulation, and education of health professionals, including nurses and midwives, was introduced replacing state/territory legislation. The NMBA licenses all nurses (registered and enrolled) and midwives in Australia. Licensed nurses and midwives may practice in any jurisdiction and are required to demonstrate that on application for relicensure (annually) their knowledge and practice are current (Nursing and Midwifery Board of Australia, 2010).

Applying for a Graduate Nurse Position

In the final year of her undergraduate degree, Wendy began to investigate what options were available for her to work in as a graduate nurse, post registration. Graduate programs provided support to newly registered nurses and midwifes transitioning from the role of student to registered nurse and/or midwife (Francis & Mills, 2011). Wendy was informed that securing a graduate position required her to register online through the Victorian computer match scheme (Postgraduate Medical Council of Victoria, 2010). This was an online program administered by the Postgraduate Medical Council of Victoria for the Department of Health Victoria, which matched prospective graduates with health services offering graduate nurse positions. This program was similar to that offered in other states in Australia where graduate years were partly funded by the state departments of health. The application process required an online application stating the preferred health services she would like to work in and also require direct applications be sent to each of the four selected health service (Postgraduate Medical Council of Victoria, 2010). To determine which health services best fitted her career plans, Wendy attended a graduate information day at the local university in which health services from both metropolitan, regional, and rural areas presented on what they offered in the graduate year in terms of clinical rotations, support services, and postgraduate opportunities. She was particularly interested in obtaining a graduate year in a health service that provided the prospect to undertake experience in both general ward areas and midwifery. Wendy also attended information days held by each health service where she had the occasion to ask questions of the graduate nurse program coordinators to gain a better understanding of what each graduate program offered. She also spoke with graduate nurses from previous years who had undertaken graduate programs at the health services in which she was interested to find out how supportive the health services were in terms of how many study days where provided, how many rotations to different wards were expected during the 12-month graduate placement, if supernumery orientation was available on each rotation (nurses not allocated workload for a period of time), if preceptors were used to support each graduate nurse, whether educators were available for staff support on each ward, and how smoothly the graduate nurses found the program throughout the graduate year.

Following application for a computer match, Wendy was requested to attend interviews at each of the selected health services. At the interview she was asked questions to determine her understanding of the health service and how she would fit in with the current teams at the organization. Questions were asked to determine her level of critical thinking, understanding of professional practice (Australian Nursing and Midwifery Council, 2008c, 2008d) issues such as the nursing code of ethics (Australian Nursing and Midwifery Council, 2008a, 2008b), equal opportunity, scope of practice, the drugs and poisons act, and other related legislation. The health services then ranked each of the prospective graduates they had interviewed and entered them into the computer match system. Computer match then undertook a process of matching the applicants with their selected health service and then notified both the health service and Wendy of where she had received her graduate year (Postgraduate Medical Council of Victoria, 2010). Each graduate was offered only one position by the computer match system. Government funding to support each graduate position was subsequently provided to the employing health service to ensure that the support needed to assist the transition of the student nurse to graduate registered nurse was available.

GRADUATE NURSE: SCOPE OF PRACTICE

Having undertaken a double degree in both nursing and midwifery, Wendy was looking for a health service that would allow her to use her skills and knowledge in both areas of professional licensure. In considering her career as a nurse and midwife, Wendy planned to apply for a graduate nurse program in her local rural area in Victoria. Wendy had been advised that working in a small rural health service would enable her to work in combined midwifery/general care wards, where she could utilize the full range of skills knowledge acquired during her degree. Initially, she thought that she would like to commence her graduate year in an environment where she could learn from experienced people such as her friend's parents. While she was anxious to make her own way in the world and move out of home, she wanted the security of knowing the local community and having her family on hand for support.

During her studies Wendy was told that rural nurses are generalist/specialists, that their practice is diverse, and that they require a broad knowledge and skill base as they must be able to manage clients from "womb to tomb" (Francis et al., 2002; Hegney, 2010). Wendy's conversations with her friends' parents who were nurses confirmed that they shared this view of their practice. Wendy was surprised to learn that the scope of practice is broader for registered nurses working in rural areas than it is for nurses who choose to work in the city. She accepted that in rural practice contexts the health care team was predominantly composed of nurses and that the proportion of other providers, including medical doctors and allied health professionals decreased with increasing remoteness (Coyle, Al-Motlaq, Mills, Francis, & Birks, 2010; Hegney, 2010). Wendy understood that rural nursing practice differed from the practice of nurses in metropolitan contexts who were able to focus on age and specialty-specific areas. She was aware that rural nurses were described as generalists and expected to manage a broad range of patients with varying conditions and age ranges (Hegney, 2010).

The scope of practice for nurses in Australia was defined as any activity in which the individual nurse was educated, competent, and authorized to perform (Australian Nursing and Midwifery Council, 2007). Wendy learnt that this broad definition of scope of practice enabled rural nurses to practice at a different level than city-based nurses, as in the more remote practice context with smaller numbers of available health care workers; nurses are often the only health service providers (Hegney, 2010). Nurses in these practice contexts took on roles that other specialist health workers would undertake in larger health services, requiring a much broader knowledge and skill base.

MAINTAINING CURRENCY: PRACTICE REQUIREMENTS

Wendy wondered how rural nurses ensured that their knowledge and skills remained current. Talking to the local librarian at a health service, Wendy found that a range of online services were available for rural nurses to assist with health information, professional support, and development. She discovered that the Victorian government funded the Clinicians Health Channel which was an online program that allowed health professionals to access online databases, such as Medline and CINAHL, therapeutic drug guidelines, Cochrane database, and best practice guidelines from the Joanna Briggs Institute (Department of Health Victoria, 2010; The Joanna Briggs Institute, 2010). Other education services available for updating skills and knowledge for staff were health service-based in-service education programs and online services such as "think GP," a website that provided regular education sessions for general medical practitioners. As continuing education was a requirement for renewing of the annual nurses' license for practice in Australia, Wendy decided to continue her membership with the Royal College of Nursing on graduation and planned to subscribe to the 3lP program which is an online service that assists members to plan and document continuing professional development.

Wendy was aware that rural health services recruiting nurses prioritize applicants who have emergency, midwifery, and general nursing experience (Francis et al., 2010). The double degree in midwifery and nursing equipped Wendy with base-level skills covering "womb to tomb" nursing care; however, Wendy was aware that she needed to develop advanced skills in life support and trauma management to have the suite of skills necessary to practice effectively as a rural nurse.

Wendy was looking for a health service that offered postgraduate education in the specialty of emergency care, as this specialty covered content that she felt would supplement her existing knowledge and skill base and allow her to achieve her long-term goal of becoming a nurse practitioner in the specialty field of rural/remote area nursing. Nurse practitioners are masters-prepared advanced practice nurses licensed to practice by the Nurses and Midwives Board of Australia (NMBA, 2010).

Thinking about her career, Wendy investigated work options she could pursue following her graduate year that would support her goal of endorsing as a nurse practitioner in the future. Wendy had been informed at the RCNA Nursing Expo she attended that the state of Queensland offers opportunities for interested nurses to complete a training program prior to appointment to a remote area practice site (Council of Remote Area Nurses Association, 2010; Queensland Government, 2010). The training program oriented new nurses to practice in remote and isolated contexts and was inclusive of clinical skills training. Wendy planned to apply for a position offering this training program after she completed her initial year of practice (graduate year) and a specialist graduate qualification.

Many health services in rural Australia were unable to offer support for specialty education due to their small size and the distance to universities and other education providers. In response to this need, many universities developed postgraduate education that could be completed through distance education modalities. Programs that were inclusive of clinical skill development had methods embedded for students to work in the clinical specialism to develop competency in the skills required for that specialty. Wendy wanted to complete her graduate year in a medium-sized rural hospital that provided emergency care so that she could enhance her skills. She knew that the hospital located in the next township to Timbertown, Summerville had a busy emergency department that would meet her career needs and possibly provide support for her to complete a graduate qualification in emergency nursing.

LIVING AND WORKING IN THE BUSH

Wendy Jones grew up in the bush and had an understanding of rural living, but as a professional working in a rural context she knew from the literature and talking with other health professionals during clinical practice that she would be faced with a range of professional issues (Bourke & Sheridan, 2008). These may have included living and working in isolation (Gibb, 2002), nursing family and friends (Hegney, 2010; McConnell-Henry, Chapman, & Francis, 2010), and working with culturally diverse populations including indigenous peoples (Ellis, Davey, & Bradford, 2010; Omeri & Raymond, 2010; Wilson & Grant, 2008).

Rural health services were often described as being resource-poor environments (Francis & Chapman, 2008; Hegney, 2010) which Wendy understood meant that it was limited in both physical and human resources. In preparation for working in this environment, Wendy looked on government sites and contacted the different health services in which she was interested to find out what support packages were available for nurses moving to rural areas. Some health services provided support for travel to undertake professional development activities and accommodation and relocation allowances for nurses wishing to undertake a graduate year in a rural health service. The Queensland Government offered generous scholarships, relocation allowances, housing support, professional development leave, and bonus payments for nurses who worked in remote areas (Queensland Government, 2010). Organizations such as the RCNA administered scholarships for professional development activities including short nonaward courses, conference, and workshop attendance and undertaking postgraduate specialist education programs (Royal College of Nursing Australia, 2010b).

Having support during the initial year of practice as a registered nurse was an important consideration for Wendy. She planned to investigate at interview for her graduate year if the health service allocated a mentor to new staff as an extra support mechanism. Mentorship in Australia is the pairing of a junior staff member with a senior clinician who is able to advise, coach, council, teach, and guide the mentee as well as connect them with others when appropriate (Mills, Lennon, & Francis, 2006).

In thinking about her transition from a student to a registered nurse, Wendy investigated the various graduate nurse programs available and the different practice models used at the health services she was considering applying to for a graduate nurse position. During her clinical placements she had been exposed to several different models of care, including team nursing, primary care nursing, and community nursing. Team nursing was a frequently used model of care that involved the delivery of total patient care by a team of nurses to a group of patients. The team of nurses was managed by a team leader responsible for the performance of the team on that shift (Coiffe & Ferguson, 2009). Wendy was very familiar with this model of care as it was used extensively in the acute care health services she undertook clinical practice in during her degree. Throughout her undergraduate degree Wendy was told that in most practice environments, nurses work as part of a multidisciplinary team. Multidisciplinary health care teams are groups formed to achieve a common set of objectives (Crookes, Griffiths, & Brown, 2010). Crookes et al. (2010, p. 218) maintain that these objectives are generally related to measureable health outcomes that are ". . . beyond the capacity of individuals or groups from the same disciplines." Wendy's experience as a student nurse prepared her for joining a multidisciplinary team. Good communication skills, understanding and valuing each team member's contribution, and being clear about team member's roles are attributes considered essential for effective functioning of multidisciplinary teams (Crookes et al., 2010).

Nurses in Australia have and continue to practice in diverse settings using models of care that are appropriate, which Wendy felt was an advantage. She knew of nurses who were case managers responsible for the coordination of care for clients in general practice, mental health, and aged care settings and was familiar with nurse-led clinic models (Faithfull & Hunt, 2005; Herber, Schnepp, & Rieger, 2008; McAllister, 2007; Wideman, Pizzello, & Lemke, 2008). Wendy was hopeful that during her graduate year she would have the opportunity to experience a variety of models of care. She was particularly interested in gaining skills necessary to operate nurse-led clinics for ambulatory care patients with chronic illness.

Having investigated all the options and opportunities available for her during her graduate placement, Wendy was excited as she anxiously awaited the results of the computer match system to find out where she would be offered a graduate year contract and begin her career as a registered nurse. She was keen to experience the challenges and opportunities that rural/remote nursing in Australia offer and was confident in the amount of support available to her during her transition to rural nursing practice.

In summary, Wendy's case reflects decision-making activities that nursing graduates engage in when planning their initial graduate year and future careers as licensed practitioners in Australia. This case exemplar could be useful for nursing educators and administrators who design, implement, and evaluate nurse transition to practice models in rural Australia; and, perhaps, in other international rural contexts.

REFERENCES

Australian Bureau of Statistics. (2008). *Experimental estimates of Aboriginal and Torres Strait Islander Australians, June 2006.*

Australian Institute of Health and Welfare. (2004). *Rural, regional and remote health: A guide to remoteness classifications.*

Australian Institute of Health and Welfare. (2008). *Rural, regional and remote health: Indicators of health status and determinants of health.* Retrieved October 20, 2008 from http://www.aihw.gov.au/.

Australian Nursing and Midwifery Council. (2007). A national framework for the development of decision making tools for nursing and midwifery practice. Available from http://www.nursingmidwiferyboard.gov.au/Codes-and-Guidelines.aspx.

Australian Nursing and Midwifery Council. (2008a). *Code of ethics for midwives in Australia.* Retrieved from http://www.nursingmidwiferyboard.gov.au/Codes-and-Guidelines.aspx.

Australian Nursing and Midwifery Council. (2008b). *Code of ethics for nurses in Australia.* Retrieved from http://www.nursingwidwiferyboard.gov.au/Codes-and-Guidelines.aspx.

Australian Nursing and Midwifery Council. (2008c). *Code of professional conduct for midwives.* Retrieved November 17, 2010 from http://www.nursingmidwifery-board.gov.au/Codes-and-Guidelines.aspx.

Australian Nursing and Midwifery Council. (2008d). *Code of professional conduct for nurses in Australia.* Retrieved November 17, 2010 from http://www.nuringmid wiferyboard.gov.au/Codes-and-Guidelines.aspx.

Bourke, L., & Sheridan, C. (2008). Understanding rural health—Key concepts. In S. Liaw, & S. Kilpatrick (Eds.), *A textbook of Australian rural health.* Canberra: Australian Rural Health Education Network.

Coiffe, J., & Ferguson, L. (2009). Team nursing in acute care settings: Nurse's experiences. *Contemporary nurse, 33*(1), 2–12.

Council of Remote Area Nurses Association. (2010). *Remote health practice post graduate nursing programs.* Retrieved November 23, 2010 from http://www.crana.org.au/146-remote-health-practice-postgraduate-nursing-programs.html

Coyle, M., Al-Motlaq, M., Mills, J., Francis, K., & Birks, M. (2010). An integrative review of the role of registered nurses in remote and isolated practice. *Australian Health Review, 34,* 239–245.

Crookes, P., Griffiths, R., & Brown, A. (2010). Becoming part of a multidisciplinary health care team. In J. Daly, S. Speedy, & D. Jackson (Eds.), *Contexts of nursing* (3rd ed.). Sydney: Churchill Livingstone, Elsevier.

Department of Health and Ageing. (2005). *Review of the rural, remote, and metropiltan areas (RRMA) classification discussion paper (without predjudice).*

Department of Health Victoria. (2010). *Clinicians health channel.* Retrieved November 17, 2010 from http://www.health.vic.gov.au/clinicians/

Ellis, I., Davey, C., & Bradford, V. (2010). Cultural awareness: Nurses working with Indigenous Australian people. In J. Daly, S. Speedy, & D. Jackson (Eds.), *Contexts of nursing* (3rd ed.) (pp. 301–313). Sydney: Churchill Livingstone, Elsevier.

Faithfull, S., & Hunt, G. (2005). Exploring nursing values in the development of a nurse-led service. *Nursing Ethics, 12*(5), 440–452.

Francis, K., Birks, M., Al-Motlaq, M., Biggs, J., Miles, M., & Bailey, C. (2010). Responding to a rural health workforce shortfall: Double degree preparation of the nurse midwife. *Australian Journal of Rural Health, 18*(5), 210–211.

Francis, K., Bowman, S., & Redgrave, M. (2002). Knowledge and skills required by rural nurses to meet the challenges of a changing work environment in the 21st century. In P. Heath (Ed.), *National Review of Nursing Education* (pp. 151–215). Canberra: Australian Government.

Francis, K., & Chapman, Y. (2008). Rural and remote community nursing. In D. Kralik, & A. D. Van Loon (Eds.), *Community nursing in Australia.* Carlton: Blackwell Publishing.

Francis, K., & Mills, J. (2011). Sustaining and growing the rural nursing and midwifery workforce: Understanding the issues and isolating directions for the future. *Collegian, 18*(2), 55–60.

Gibb, H. (2002). Educating nurses for rural clinical practice: Working and studying alone. In D. Wilkinson, & I. Blue (Eds.), *The new rural health.* South Melbourne: Oxford University Press.

Herber, O. R., Schnepp, W., & Rieger, M. A. (2008). Developing a nurse-led education program to enhance self-care agency in leg ulcer patients. *Nursing Science Quarterly, 21*(2), 150–155.

Hegney, D. (2010). Dealing with distance: Rural and remote area nursing. In J. Daly, S. Speedy, & D. Jackson (Eds.), *Contexts of nursing: An introduction* (3rd ed.). Sydney: Churchill Livingstone, Elsevier.

Hugo, G. (2004). Australian Census Analytical Program: Australias most recent immigrants 2001. Cat no 2053.0. Australian Bureau of Statisics. Available from http://www.ausstats.abs.gov.au/ausstats/free.nsf/Lookup/2C95BF6FB48F0F2 BCA256ECE007C345E/$File/20530_2001.pdf

Humphreys, J., & Rolley, F. (1991). *Health and health care in rural Australia.* Armidale: University of New England.

McAllister, M. (2007). New models of care in mental health. *Australian Nurses Journal, 48*(8), 37.

McConnell-Henry, T., Chapman, Y., & Francis, K. (2010). Indigenous an remote health: Rural nursing—Looking after people we know. *Australian Nursing Journal, 17*(8), 42.

Mills, J., Lennon, D., & Francis, K. (2006). Mentoring matters: Developing rural nurses knowledge and skills. *Collegian, 13*(3), 9–13.

Mohd Noor, K. B. (2008). Case study: A strategic research methodology. *American Journal of Applied Science, 5*(11), 1602–1604.

NMBA. (2010). *Nursing and midwifery board of Australia.* Retrieved November 17, 2010 from http://www.nursingmidwiferyboard.gov.au/

Nursing and Midwifery Board of Australia. (2010). *Nursing and Midwifery Board of Australia.* Retrieved November 17, 2010 from http://www.nursingmidwifery board.gov.au/.

Omeri, A., & Raymond, L. (2010). Diversity in the context of multicultural Australia: Implications for practice. In J. Daly, S. Speedy, & D. Jackson (Eds.), *Contexts of nursing* (3rd ed.) (pp. 287–300). Sydney: Churchill Livingstone, Elsevier.

Postgraduate Medical Council of Victoria. (2010). Computer matching service Victorian GNP match guide 2010. Available from http://computermatching.pmcv. com.au/public/howto/index.cfm

Queensland Government. (2010). *In many ways it pays to nurse in rural Queensland.* Retrieved November 30, 2010, from http://www.health.qld.gov.au/nursing/ rural_remote.asp

Royal College of Nursing Australia. (2010a). *Nursing and health expo.* Retrieved November 11, 2010, from http://www.nurseinfo.com.au/becoming/ nursinghealthexpos

Royal College of Nursing Australia. (2010b). *RCNA grants.* Retrieved November 17, 2010, from http://www.rcna.org.au/development/development_events

Stake, E. (2003). Case studies. In N. K. Denzin, & Y. S. Lincoln (Eds.), *Strategies of qualitative inquiry* (2nd ed.) (pp. 134–164). London: Sage Publications.

The Joanna Briggs Institute. (2010). *The Joanna Briggs Institute.* From http://www. joannabriggs.edu.au/about/home.php

Wakerman, J., & Humphreys, J. (2008). Rural and remote health—Definitions, policies and priorities. In S. Liaw, & S. Kilpatrick (Eds.), *A textbook of Australian rural health.* Canberra: Australian Rural Health Education Network.

Wideman, M., Pizzello, L., & Lemke, S. (2008). Impact of nursing case management on an underserved population. *Home Health Care Management & Practice, 21*(1), 17–22.

Wilkinson, D., & Blue, I. (2002). *The new rural health* (1st ed.). South Melbourne: Oxford Press.

Wilson, D., & Grant, J. (2008). Culturally competent partnerships with communities. In K. Francis, Y. Chapman, K. Hoare, & J. Mills (Eds.), *Australia and New Zealand community as partner: Theory and practice in nursing* (pp. 113–127). Broadway: Lippincott, Williams and Wilkins.

Year Book of Australia. (2008). *Country of birth.* From wwww.abs.gov.au

9

University HealthSystem Consortium and American Association of Colleges of Nursing Nurse Residency Program

Debra A. McElroy and Kathy McGuinn

This chapter presents background information on nurse transition-to-practice programs and features the University HealthSystem Consortium (UHC) and the American Association of Colleges of Nursing (AACN) UHC/AACN Nurse Residency Program[TM] *model. This model includes learning and work experiences designed to assist new nurse graduates as they transition into their first professional role in rural as well as urban practice settings. The experiences reinforce clinical and leadership skill development for the novice nurse to function as a full partner on the health care team.*

The historic landmark report, *The Future of Nursing: Leading Change, Advancing Health* (IOM, 2011), underscores the urgency for the implementation of nurse residency programs to facilitate the transition of new nurse graduates into a variety of professional roles. Recommendation 3 in this futuristic report reiterates the need to implement nurse residency programs and strongly advocates widespread adoption of nurse residency programs.

> State boards of nursing, accrediting bodies, the federal government, and health care organizations should take actions to support nurses' completion of a transition-to-practice program (nurse residency) after they have completed a pre-licensure or advanced practice degree program or when they are transitioning into new clinical practice areas.

The American Association of Colleges of Nursing (AACN) and the University HealthSystem Consortium (UHC) have recognized this critical need and forged a long-term partnership to support the development and implantation of a 1-year, postbaccalaureate nurse residency program across care settings. Since March 2000, the UHC and AACN have worked to develop strategies to address the nursing shortage, as well as enhance the expertise of the nursing workforce in an effort to reduce practice errors and minimize the burnout caused by stress in underprepared nurses. The UHC/AACN Nurse Residency Program™ has conducted an ongoing multisite research study of program outcomes since 2002, with more than 25,000 first-year nurses enrolled to date. The UHC and AACN continue to be committed to monitoring the efficacy and impact of residency programs.

With 81 UHC/AACN residency sites now active in 29 states, this effort to enhance patient safety is consistent with many other organizational efforts. For example, a study by the National Council of State Boards of Nursing (Smith & Crawford, 2002) found that health care employers perceive that newly licensed RNs are not fully prepared to perform common tasks in the practice setting. The employers view new RNs as especially deficient in recognizing abnormal physical and diagnostic findings, responding to emergencies, supervising care provided by others, and in psychomotor skills. After much study, NCSBN (2010) issued a white paper in support of a 6-month transition program for new graduates with an additional 6 months of support. In addition, the Joint Commission in its *Health Care at the Crossroads* report (2002) cited this specific nurse residency program as an important model for postgraduate nurse training. Further, the American Academy of Nursing (AAN, 2010) announced the addition of the UHC/AACN Nurse Residency Program™ as a newest addition to the Edge Runner program: "Our Edge Runners are nurses who have developed innovative models of care with excellent clinical and financial outcome data." These innovations were developed in response to the unmet health needs of individuals, families, and communities. The *Raise the Voice Board* chairperson, Diana Mason, expressed the importance in these words: "Most models could be scaled up to help our nation transform health care delivery in ways that emphasize health promotion, chronic care management, and care coordination."

The UHC/AACN Nurse Residency Program™ model is based on a standard curriculum, structured as monthly seminar sessions that include a series of learning and work experiences. The residency experience is intended to support nurses entering practice as they transition into their first professional role, and a key concept of the program is to promote the development of nurse leadership at the patient's bedside. The program emphasizes development of the clinical and leadership skills necessary for the advanced beginner nurse to be successful as a full partner on the health care team. The residency program was developed for nurses with direct care roles in the acute care hospital setting, although application of the residency model in other settings is being explored.

It should be noted that the UHC/AACN Nurse Residency Program™ was developed as a postbaccalaureate program and the curriculum assumes that the Essentials of Baccalaureate Nursing Education have been met. These essentials support the program's goal of increasing the number of nurses whose education preparation is a Bachelor of Science in Nursing to enhance the expertise of the nursing workforce, reduce practice errors, and minimize burnout. The reality of the labor workforce often makes it impossible for organizations to restrict hiring to only BSN or higher-degree new graduates. In today's hospitals, bedside nurses are functioning under the same license, often with the same clinical responsibilities, regardless of academic preparation. Recognizing these challenges, this residency model has developed parallel curriculum and strategies for transition support to associate degree nurses, while continuing to promote their advancement to higher levels of nursing education. This approach is supported by Recommendation 4 of the recent Institute of Medicine report referenced earlier, which states, "Academic nurse leaders across all schools of nursing should work together to increase the proportion of nurses with a baccalaureate degree from 50 to 80 percent by 2020."

There are a number of key principles that provide the foundation of the UHC/AACN Nurse Residency Program™ model, which should apply to the development of any nurse residency experience.

PROMOTE TRANSITION FROM ADVANCED BEGINNER TO COMPETENT NURSE

The conceptual framework of this residency model is based on Dr. Patricia Benner's work, *From Novice to Expert*, in which new graduate nurses are identified as advanced beginners, requiring a year to move to competent practice. Dr. Benner outlines the development of the new graduate nurse, and describes the new nurse as not only having gained the necessary theoretical knowledge from academic preparation, but also having the need to develop the clinical, situational, and intuitive skills to function in an effective, independent manner at the patient bedside. The UHC/AACN Nurse Residency Program™ is of 1 year duration and has outcome data demonstrating the gains experienced by nurse residents from a full year of transition support.

FOCUS ON CRITICAL THINKING DEVELOPMENT

The focus of the program curriculum is on the development of the challenging critical thinking issues facing the nurse in the first year of practice rather than instruction on nursing tasks, which organizations are very capably able to address. A study on new graduate competency published in the *Journal of Nursing Administration* in 2008, ranked competencies such as delegation, communication with physicians, conflict resolution, and prioritizing as issues of greatest concern.

The UHC/AACN Nurse Residency Program™ curriculum is evidence based and complements existing hospital and nursing orientation and specialty-care training. One of the primary goals of the curriculum is to improve the residents' critical thinking skills and ability to manage outcomes data to promote patient safety. The focus of the program content is on in-depth development of residents' leadership skills, analysis of evidence through reviews of the literature, application of outcomes data to patient care improvements, and professional development. Both structured and informal sessions incorporate a resident facilitator to oversee resident development and coach residents to clinical success.

CLINICAL/ACADEMIC PARTNERSHIP

A program requirement includes partnership between the hospital or practice setting and an academic partner. The partnership between the hospital and the school of nursing has been of tremendous value to both sides. The hospital benefits from the added expertise of the school's faculty, and assures that the residency experience builds upon, and does not replicate, the new graduate's academic preparation. The school benefits from increased understanding of the difficulties new graduates face in their transition to practice.

USE OF EXPERT NURSES

Expert nurses are an integral part of the program, providing the mentoring and role modeling for professional practice. Inherent in the nurse residency model is an expert nurse who can act as a point of contact for the residents. These expert nurses often function as an advisor and sounding board, helping the residents deal with transition to practice and "reality shock," facilitating attendance at learning opportunities, teaching curriculum content, and serving as a clinical expert to promote the development of critical thinking and leadership skills.

FOSTER PROFESSIONAL PRACTICE AND PROFESSIONAL DEVELOPMENT

Professional development planning is necessary for all nurse residents to guide development and enhance their commitment to the nursing profession. The commitment of the program to evaluate outcomes on an ongoing basis has yielded insights into the value of the residency experience as well as highlighted better-performing organizations who can share their best practices. The program has evaluated retention, with a progressively positive trend of improved retention. In 2009, an impressive average retention rate of 95.6% for the first year of employment for participating organizations was reported. This compares favorably with the average national turnover of first-year nurses of 27.1% as reported in a report issued by PricewaterhouseCooper's Research Institute (2007). Program outcomes data have also consistently shown resident improvement in confidence, competence, ability to organize and prioritize, communication, leadership, and a reduction in stress levels. Finally, the residency outcomes data have shown that there is a statistically significant improvement in months 6–12, a time frame at which most organizations have traditionally ended their preceptor and specialty training support of the new graduate nurse.

OVERVIEW OF THE UHC/AACN NURSE RESIDENCY PROGRAM™ MODEL

The UHC/AACN Nurse Residency is built on an evidence-based curriculum using the *Essentials of Baccalaureate Education for Professional Nursing Practice* (AACN, 2008) as its foundation. Additionally, the Commission on Collegiate Nursing Education (CCNE, 2008) has approved accreditation standards for nurse residency programs based on the UHC/AACN curriculum and model. In April 2010, the CCNE Board of Commissioners granted accreditation to the first two post-baccalaureate nurse residency programs:

▪ University of Colorado Hospital, Denver, Colorado
▪ University of Kansas Hospital, Kansas City, Kansas

The nurse residency, a 1-year program, uses a series of learning and work experiences to support graduate nurses as they transition into their first professional positions. The program is structured using monthly seminar sessions in a "face-to-face" format. The program objectives state that by the end of the residency program, the new graduate nurses will

■ Transition from an entry-level, advanced beginner nurse to a competent professional nurse, as defined in Patricia Benner's "Novice to Expert" theory (1984)
■ Develop effective decision-making skills related to clinical judgment and performance
■ Be able to provide clinical leadership at the point of patient care
■ Strengthen their commitment to nursing as a professional career choice
■ Be able to incorporate research-based evidence into their practices
■ Formulate individual career development plans

All program activities are designed to move the resident forward in their transition to competent, professional nurse. The tools of the program include case scenarios, topical content, and professional reflection. The case scenarios are based on actual complex clinical situations that have occurred in the participating hospitals. Case scenarios focus on Leadership, Patient Outcomes, and Professional Role components. These case scenarios are integrated with specific evidence-based journal reviews and the residents' own personal experiences. Various techniques for improving critical thinking/clinical judgment are used, including comparisons with other cases, personal experiences, differentiation of symptoms and diagnoses, alternative approaches, "what if" discussions, and causal relationships.

The 1-year program culminates with the completion of an evidence-based project by the residents. The projects allow participants to focus on topics about which they are passionate; this experience provides an empowering opportunity where nurses can identify an issue and truly make a difference. These evidence-based practice projects are often presented as posters at the annual UHC meeting. Posters by staff nurses participating in the UHC/AACN Nurse Residency Program™ swept UHC's member poster competition at the 2008 Performance Excellence Forum, taking first, second, and third place.

■ The Methodist Hospital drew the most votes with "Faces of Nurses 2007."
■ The second place went to The Ohio State University Medical Center's "PICC Line Care and Maintenance."
■ The University of Wisconsin Hospital & Clinics' poster, "Nursing Care during Hypothermia," was placed third.

ORGANIZATIONAL IMPACT

Based on academic/practice partnerships, the residency program is a highly effective program, developed by experts from academic health centers and schools of nursing across the country. Partnerships between academic nursing institutions and hospitals provide a strong mechanism for fostering collaboration and innovation around shared education and research interests (AACN, 1999). For example, culture shifts have been noted by participating organizations after implementation of the residency program. Chief nursing officers and residency coordinators report the following outcomes that are mutually beneficial to both the academic and practice partners:

- Decreased preceptor burnout
- Increased understanding and implementation of evidence-based practice
- Increased professionalism
- Development of professional practice opportunities (i.e., Quality fellowships, research)

Effectively transitioning new nurse graduates into acute care settings is essential to ensuring first-year retention and success in the RN role. In addition to improvements in retention rates, organizations see improvement in recruiting for nurses. The human resources department at residency sites report gaining many more applicants than positions. Further, outcomes data demonstrate resident improvement in confidence, competence, ability to organize and prioritize, communication, and leadership as well as a reduction in stress levels.

Since 2002 the program has

- Saved participants more than $6 million a year on first-year nurse turnover expenses (estimated costs of $88,000 price tag on recruiting and retaining a replacement nurse)
- Achieved a retention rate of more than 95% in 2010 compared to a retention rate of 87% in 2004
- Increased stability in staffing levels, thereby reducing stress, improving morale, increasing efficiency, and promoting safety
- Delivered a return on investment of up to 14:1
- Helped many thousands of first-year nurses deliver better patient care by assisting these nurses to:
  - Develop effective decision-making abilities in clinical judgment and performance
  - Gain clinical autonomy at the point of patient care

- Incorporate research-based evidence into their practices to advance safe, high-quality nursing
- Strengthen their commitment to nursing as a career choice

To measure outcomes, the program uses the Casey–Fink Graduate Nurse Experience Survey, a tool that is particularly helpful because it was truly made for new nurses rather than the nursing population as a whole. This tool provides information about clinical skills that might be anxiety-provoking for new nurses. Casey–Fink data are collected at the beginning of the residency program, at 6 months, and at 1 year, so that progress can be measured over time. The strength of these results after 12 months, versus at the 6-month mark, makes a powerful case for the yearlong residency program.

Participating organizations receive an annual analysis of their outcomes measures to gauge their progress. The reports help organizations know how their nurses are feeling in comparison to national data, while also identifying specific areas in which organizations need to provide additional support to the residents. Every year a meeting is held by the UHC, and annual outcomes are reported. The 2010 report contained the following findings:

- Retention of residents is 95.6%, which greatly exceeds that conventionally reported for new graduates. The turnover rate is 4.4%.
- Retention of each graduate nurse/year saves the employing institution an estimated $80,000+ annually per new hire.
- Residents most commonly identify the following skills as the ones they are uncomfortable performing throughout the residency year:
  - Codes/emergency response
  - Starting IVs
  - Ventilator care
  - Chest tube care
  - Death and dying/end-of-life care
  - Tracheostomy care.
- Transition to the professional role is impacted by a combination of the workload and expectations. Peer support is the most satisfying aspect of the program.
- Residents evaluate various aspects of the program on a minimum of 3 on a 4-point scale. Almost 90% would recommend the program to others.
- A total of 80% participated in some evidence-based research activity.

Almost 60% formulated individual development plans.

PROGRAM STRENGTHS AND CRITICAL SUCCESS FACTORS

The lessons learned from implementation of the UHC/AACN Nurse Residency Program™ from organizations across the country include shared experiences at the annual user group meetings, which have provided networking experiences for program participants, and that the ongoing collection of outcomes data have highlighted critical success factors and program strengths that comprise a residency experience that provides value to the nurse and to the institution.

A Strong Return on Investment

The median voluntary turnover rate for first-year nurses is 27.1% and the average total cost associated with that turnover as reported by Jones (2008) is estimated at $88,000 per nurse. The 2009 turnover rate for the UHC/AACN Nurse Residency Program™ was 4.4%, which demonstrates the potential for a positive investment return. In addition, Texas Methodist Hospital reported a significant return on investment for implementation of the UHC/AACN Nurse Residency Program™ (Pine & Tart, 2007).

Resources and Support

Training and ongoing implementation support for program coordinators, academic partners, and staff have been of high value to program participants. This type of support allows different organizations to share their successes and challenges, share strategies for creative delivery of curriculum content, and brainstorm as they seek to integrate new educational models or content. Annual user group meetings provide participants with opportunities to spotlight innovations, share best practices, network with peers, and provide input on program development. The program also provides ongoing program communication, and staff and residents participate in periodic educational web conferences.

Better Patient Outcomes

A higher retention rate also delivers better patient outcomes (Goode & Blegen, 2009). The program helps nurses develop effective decision-making abilities in clinical judgment and performance.

Clinical and Academic Partnership

Organizations have reported that the partnership has revealed increased opportunities for collaboration, and a better understanding of the new graduate experience from both perspectives.

Increased Professional and Institutional Satisfaction

A goal of the nurse residency program is to increase new graduate job satisfaction and reinforce professional commitment to the nursing profession, which will contribute to the lone-range goal of alleviating the nursing shortage. Organizations and program outcomes data report improvement in organizational and professional satisfaction.

The UHC/AACN Nurse Residency Program™ has proven to be an effective model for addressing new graduate nurses' transition needs, promoting high-quality care by providing professional support. The following are the key components of this model that have proven to be *critical success factors* for positive outcomes for nurse residency implementation.

INVOLVEMENT OF EXPERT NURSES IN THE INSTITUTION

These expert nurses are the bridge to competent clinical practice for the new nurse, providing guidance and providing a model for professional growth.

One-Year Program

The standardized curriculum is evidence based and meets national residency accreditation standards. The core content focuses on three critical areas: (1) leadership, which focuses on the management of resources—staff, supplies, and services—as well as the initial clinical survival skills for the new nurse; (2) nurse-sensitive patient outcomes, which build upon the new graduate's academic preparation and enhance knowledge of the clinical and quality considerations of the practice environment; and (3) professional role, which is woven throughout the residency experience and includes key issues such as stress management, end-of-life issues, and ethics. Curriculum is assessed each year, completely reviewed every 3 years, and revised as necessary. Residents are required to complete an evidence-based project that is relevant to their clinical setting (University HealthSystem Consortium, 2010).

Evidence-Based Projects

The residency experience supports new graduate nurse understanding of how to incorporate the principles of evidence-based practice and apply established evidence to daily nursing practice at the bedside. In addition, the project requirement promotes and encourages participation in nursing research. This component of the curriculum has demonstrated tremendous organizational impact, as well as a valuable experience for the nurse resident. Rather than replicating a similar academic exercise, this experience allows the new graduate nurse to respond to conflicting clinical practices that they have observed, to delve into a priority for the unit manager, or provide evidence for a change in policy.

The program has found that the nurse resident competence and enthusiasm for conducting nursing research have impacted on nursing practice in their organizations and helped to support nursing research. Projects such as "The Septic Stethoscope: Exploration of Infectious Disease Prevention Through the Diligent Decontamination of Stethoscopes" examined the pathogens growing on the stethoscopes of patient care providers and also identified a solution to prevent the spread of these pathogens; another looked at "Pre-Filled Syringes: Let's Take Another Look," a project that saved over $37,000 during the initial study and has now been adopted throughout the hospital. An annual call for abstracts for podium and poster presentation at the annual meeting provides opportunity for professional growth.

Ongoing Data Collection

In addition to the retention data discussed earlier in the chapter, the residency program has collected data on a number of survey tools. Specifically measuring new graduate nurse experience, the Casey–Fink measurement tool has consistently shown positive outcomes related to communication, leadership, organizing, and prioritizing. Data are collected at three points within the program year: hire, 6 months, and 12 months.

Qualitative data have been collected since the inception of the program. Residents report on the top three skills and/or procedures that cause discomfort at each point of data collection, providing feedback and program direction. Residents also provide responses to the following topics, choosing either drop-down or free text responses:

- Transition difficulties being experienced
- Most satisfying aspects of work environment

■ Least satisfying aspects of work environment
■ Feedback on how to increase feeling of support and integration

Analysis of nurse resident response has shown an increased sense of camaraderie and a feeling of belonging develops over time that there is a very strong need for manager support and feedback and socialization within the work environment and that ongoing coaching remains a developmental need.

DEVELOPING A NATIONAL MODEL OF TRANSITION TO PRACTICE

The program has provided a national residency model, which allows organizations of all types to promote a similar on-boarding experience for the new graduate nurse.

ADAPTING TO THE RURAL SETTING

A great opportunity in health care has been created by the Patient Protection and Affordable Care Act passed in March 2010 that will provide access to health care for 32 million more Americans. The challenge of health care reform will be to meet this new demand on the nation's health care system, while accommodating the increased need for improving the quality of health care services. The 3 million registered nurses in the United States represent the largest sector of the health professions. Well-educated nurses are critical to the success of attaining the quality measures that have been targeted for improvement. Therefore, health care reform provides an opportunity for the nursing profession to meet the demand for safe, high-quality, patient-centered, and equitable patient services in all settings. Since the nursing profession will play an increasingly important role in primary care, an urgent need exists to expand nurse residency programs to the rural setting.

National organizations have recognized that nursing must prepare for its expanding role, and this includes an education model that requires a residency experience. To position themselves to meet this requirement, rural hospitals must explore collaboratives and partnerships with regional health care providers and other creative approaches to garner the resources necessary for providing such an experience. Increasingly, new graduate nurses are receiving their first practice experience in settings other than the acute care hospital. In addition, health care reform has called for organizations to become "Accountable Care Organizations," assuring that patients have consistent and well-communicated health care across the continuum of health settings. Many alternative settings such as long-term and ambulatory care are exploring the benefit of supporting new graduate nurse transition as they prepare for meeting health care demands of the future and potential nursing workforce shortages on the horizon.

In summary, regardless of the practice setting, be it urban or rural, all recent nursing graduates as well as nurses who are seeking new roles or specialty practice can benefit from a nurse residency program. The core content of the UHC/AACN Nurse Residency Program™ that includes critical areas of leadership, patient outcomes, and professional role is applicable to all practice settings. In particular, case studies and content on rural contexts would be useful for rural nurse transition programs. Information and findings describing rural-focused transition-to-practice programs should be disseminated. Such information is needed to inform us about successful transition models, lessons learned, and creative ways to prepare novice nurses to practice effectively and safely in a variety of rural settings.

REFERENCES

American Academy of Nurses. (2010). *Raise the voice campaign gains three new edge runners.* Retrieved from http://www.aannet.org/files/public/AAN%20 Announces%20New%20Edge%20Runners_8_24.pdf

American Association of Colleges of Nursing. (1999). *The essential clinical resources for nursing's academic mission.* Washington, DC: AACN.

American Association of Colleges of Nursing. (2008). *The essentials of baccalaureate education for professional nursing practice.* Washington, DC: Author.

Benner, P. (1984). *From novice to expert: Excellence and power in clinical nursing practice.* Menlo Park, CA: Addison Wesley.

Commission on Collegiate Nursing Education. (2008). *Standards for accreditation of post-baccalaureate nurse residency programs.* Retrieved from http://www.aacn. nche.edu/Accreditation/pdf/resstandards08.pdf

Committee on the Robert Wood Johnson Foundation Initiative on the Future of Nursing at the Institute of Medicine. (2011). *The future of nursing: Leading change, advancing health.* Washington, DC: National Academies Press.

Goode, C., & Blegen, M. (March 2009). *The link between nurse staffing and patient outcomes.* Presented at UHC Performance Excellence Forum, Orlando, FL.

Jones, C. (2008). Revisiting nurse turnover costs: Adjusting for inflation. *Journal of Nursing Administration, 38*(1), 11–18.

Pine, R., & Tart, K. (2007). Return on investment: Benefits and challenges of a baccalaureate nurse residency program. *Nursing Economics, 25*(1), 13–39.

PricewaterhouseCoopers Health Research Institute. (2007). *What works: Healing the healthcare staffing shortage.* New York, NY: PricewaterhouseCoopers, 6.

Smith, J., & Crawford, L. (2002). *Report of the Findings of the 2001 Employers Survey.* Volume 3. Chicago: National Council of State Boards of Nursing.

The Joint Commission. (2002). *Health care at the crossroads: Strategies for addressing the evolving nursing crisis.* Retrieved from http://www.jointcommission.org/assets/1/18/health_care_at_the_crossroads.pdf

University HealthSystem Consortium. (2010). *The UHC/AACN Nurse Residency Program.* Oak Brook, IL: Author.

10

National Council of State Boards of Nursing's Transition-to-Practice Regulatory Model

Josephine H. Silvestre and Nancy Spector

The background and components of the National Council of State Boards of Nursing (NCSBN) Transition-to-Practice (TTP) model are highlighted in this chapter. This model lends itself to rural and urban health care settings for transitioning newly licensed nurses, at all educational levels, specifically practical nurses and associate degree, diploma, baccalaureate, and other entry-level graduates.

Anecdotally, a recent graduate employed in a setting without a transition-to-practice (TTP) program was heard saying: "I am frightened for my patients and for my own license as I soon will be turned loose with only a resource person and expected to take a full load after only 5 days of orientation in my new assigned unit" (North Carolina, 2009, p. 35). The need for TTP programs is discussed in other chapters of this volume. A long-term project undertaken by the National Council of State Boards of Nursing's (NCSBN's) Board of Directors' long-term project to develop a regulatory model for TTP is examined in more detail in the next section of this chapter (Spector & Echternacht, 2010).

In 2007, NCSBN's Board appointed a Transition-to-Practice Committee, which included members from state Boards of Nursing and a representative from the American Organization of Nurse Executives (AONE). The committee members reviewed published and unpublished data on TTP programs and developed an evidence-based transition model to assist the Boards in their missions of public protection. Feedback was sought from state Boards of Nursing on a regular basis. Additionally, there was collaboration with more than 35 stakeholders.

123

Committee members presented the model to the organization and listened to their concerns and suggestions.

Significant changes based on the feedback were made. One of the main alterations was recategorizing modules to be congruent with the Institute of Medicine (IOM) (Greiner & Knebel, 2003) and Quality and Safety Education for Nurses (QSEN) (Cronenwett et al., 2007) competencies. Stakeholders and the Boards of Nursing recommended conducting a multisite study using the model to analyze the effect on patient outcomes. The transition committee also heard stakeholders' concerns regarding the need for preceptor education.

Funding for the implementation of transition programs was raised repeatedly by collaborators, and this is particularly an issue for small, rural facilities. Consultants for the project developed a business plan for facilities that want to implement a TTP program, which can be found at https://www.ncsbn.org/1603.htm. Furthermore, NCSBN is actively pursuing financial support for this initiative.

During the planning meetings with stakeholders, the role of regulation was clarified. Based on outcomes of the multisite study, NCSBN membership will have the opportunity to vote on the model during the NCSBN's 2014 annual meeting. However, even if the model is adopted by NCSBN, each state's Board of Nursing must decide whether or not to implement the NCSBN's model. This TTP regulatory model affects only newly licensed nurses, but not their employers. In other words, the state's Board of Nursing does not have legal authority over facilities that employ nurses, but has authority over the nurses. Therefore, if the NCBSN model is adopted as designed, newly licensed nurses will need to show documentation to their Board of Nursing of successfully completing a TTP program, in order to renew their licenses after their first year in practice.

THE MODEL

The NCSBN's TTP regulatory model was designed to be robust. That is, the model is appropriate for all health care settings that hire newly licensed nurses, including practical nurses and associate degree, diploma, baccalaureate and other entry-level graduates. There are several effective transition models focusing on rural settings (Bratt, 2009; Molinari, Monserud, & Hudzinski, 2008) but the NCSBN's model was designed to accommodate novice nurses in both the rural and urban context.

The NCSBN's model is flexible enough so that many of the current nurse TTP programs meet its requirements. Likewise, the model can be modified to fit the needs of a particular geographical region or setting. For example, a large urban medical center could partner with a local nursing program to develop their transition program. Smaller hospitals could facilitate new graduates by accessing a national website. NCSBN is developing didactic learning modules and a social networking functionality where new graduates could be connected to preceptors online. In both cases, the institutions would meet the standards.

In NCSBN's TTP model, the new graduate must first successfully pass the National Council Licensure Examination (NCLEX®), obtain employment, and then enter the transition program. An institutional orientation is required before entering the transition program, which would include being instructed on the policies, procedures, and role expectations of the workplace. The orientation is *separate* from the TTP program, a formal program designed to support new graduates as they progress into practice.

The NCSBN's model is dependent on a well-developed preceptor–nurse relationship, where preceptors are prepared for the role. Preceptors work with new graduates for the first 6 months of the yearlong transition program. The level of oversight will decrease as the newly licensed nurse becomes more experienced and develops self-confidence, thus fostering independence.

Successful programs reviewed by NCSBN incorporated preceptorship experiences (https://www.ncsbn.org/1603.htm). Preceptors (mentor, coaches) need preparation to function in this role with the novice nurse. Often, preceptors feel unprepared and unsupported for this role. For example, in one study of 86 preceptors, researchers found that nurses reported feeling unprepared to precept new graduates and needed support and recognition (Yonge, Hagler, Cox, & Drefs, 2008). The Vermont Nurse Intern Program (VNIP, 2010) is one model of preceptor education. Other preceptor models are described in the literature (Molinari & Monserud, 2008; Nicol & Young, 2007; Phillips, 2006). There is evidence that team preceptorships are also successful (Beecroft, Hernandez, & Reid, 2008) and would be acceptable in the NCSBN's model. In regions where preceptors are not readily available, a national web site is planned to connect preceptors with novice nurses as is done in Scotland's Flying Start program (Roxburgh et al., 2010). Such strategies could provide new nurses with opportunities for feedback, reflection, and support even when preceptors are not geographically accessible. "Preceptor burnout" is a reality that must be addressed by an institution. The most effective strategy is to offer a preceptor development program. One can hope, however, that novice nurses will see the importance of learning from seasoned, dedicated preceptors, and, in turn, serve as future preceptors for new nurses.

During the last 6 months of NCSBN's TTP program, the institution would empower the nurse and allow a novice to evaluate policies and procedures to determine if these could be implemented more effectively. During this period, the new nurses will be encouraged to reflect on lessons learned from specific situations and experience a performance appraisal where strengths and future learning needs will be identified. The institution could also include the new nurses in the review of sentinel events or near misses to develop problem-solving skills. The new graduate will be assigned to committees and participate in grand rounds to understand interdisciplinary dynamics. Finally, at the end of the program, the institution will host a celebration to recognize the new nurse's successful completion of the transition program and to recognize preceptors.

Experiential Learning of Five Modules

The transition modules are based on the Institute of Medicine's (Greiner & Knebel, 2003) competencies and the Quality and Safety for Nursing Education initiative (Cronenwett et al., 2007):

- Patient-Centered Care
- Communication and Teamwork
- Evidence-Based Practice
- Quality Improvement
- Informatics

The concepts are not taught as deficit education but rather with the assumption that students need to experientially learn the content since nursing is a practice profession (Johnston & Kanitsaki, 2006). The concepts should be incorporated into clinical experiences, along with role modeling by the preceptor, to assist the novice nurse to learn how to think like a more experienced "expert" nurse.

Patient-centered care

Patient-centered care emphasizes specialty content and prioritizing/organizing care. Specialty content in a transition program is linked to self-report of lower practice errors (NCSBN, 2007). Other research supports integrating specialty practice into transition programs (Beecroft, Kunzman, & Krozek, 2001; Benner, Sutphen, Leonard, & Day, 2010; Beyea, Slattery, & von Reyn, 2010; Halfer, 2007; Joint Commission, 2002; Keller, Meekins, & Summers, 2006; Pine & Tart, 2007; Roxburgh et al., 2010; VNIP, 2010), including those with an emphasis on rural nursing (Bratt, 2009; Molinari et al., 2008). A related element is prioritizing and organizing one's work. Prioritizing and organizing is a part of clinical practice that is often a weakness for novice nurses (Berkow, Virkstis, Stewart, & Conway, 2008; Halfer, 2007; NCSBN, 2004, 2006a; Williams, Goode, Krsek, Bednash, & Lynn, 2007), most likely because of lack of experience. Specifically, the UHC/AACN residency program measured nurses' abilities to organize and prioritize before and after the residency experience, and found significant increases by the end of the program. Prioritizing and organizing was integrated throughout most of the transition programs that focused on specialty content. Boards of Nursing also identified boundary issues as important (e.g., diffuse professional/personal boundary issues, and appropriate use of social media) as an important area to stress in all TTP programs.

Communication and teamwork

Communication and teamwork are essential in any TTP model. The IOM report on Health Professions Education (Greiner & Knebel, 2003) stressed teaching health care students to collaborate across professions. McKay and Crippen (2008) found that in hospitals where collaboration occurs, there is a 41% lower mortality rate compared to mortality rates of 58% when this behavior was not present. Similarly, enhanced communication in hospitals has been linked to nurse satisfaction, lower costs, and greater responsiveness of health care providers (McKay & Crippen, 2008).

Most of the reports of transition programs reviewed recommended a purposeful integration of communication, including interprofessional relationships, into transition programs (Beecroft et al., 2001; Beyea et al., 2010; Halfer, 2007; Keller et al., 2006; Pine & Tart, 2007; Roxburgh et al., 2010; Williams et al., 2007), including those programs specifically designed for rural settings (Bratt, 2009; Molinari et al., 2008). The communication and teamwork module for the TTP should also include information on role socialization, delegating, and supervising in the clinical setting, and this is part of NCSBN's model.

Evidence-based practice

Another essential experiential component of a TTP module focuses on evidence-based practice (Cronenwett et al., 2007; Greiner & Knebel, 2003; NCSBN, 2006a, 2006b). In reviewing the literature, evidence-based practice was integral to most of the existing TTP programs. For example, the Texas Launch into Nursing Program assigns new nurses to participate in an evidence-based project and then present the results to the hospital unit on which they work (Keller et al., 2006). The NCSBN's model includes these concepts in light of overwhelming support for incorporating evidence-based practice into transition programs (Beecroft et al., 2001; Bratt, 2009; Pine & Tart, 2007; Roxborgh et al., 2010; Williams et al., 2007).

Quality improvement

Quality improvement has been incorporated into NCSBN's TTP program as one of the modules. With health care institutions focusing on safety and improving their systems, novice nurses need experiential learning related to quality improvement processes, such as Six Sigma. Berkow et al. (2008) surveyed educators and practice leaders about the emphasis of 36 competencies taught in nursing programs, compared to how prepared new nurses were related to those competencies. They found that quality improvement, priority setting, and delegation were not emphasized enough in nursing education and concluded they are best learned in a practice setting with experiential learning, such as a TTP program. Additionally, Barton, Armstrong, Preheim, Gelmon, and Andrus (2009) conducted a national Delphi to determine the progression of quality and safety competencies and identified the following knowledge and skills for introduction in the advanced phase of a nursing curriculum, which also would include TTP programs (p. 329):

- Give examples of tension between professional autonomy and system functioning
- Explain the importance of variation and measurement in assessing quality care
- Describe approaches for changing processes of care
- Participate in a root cause analysis of a sentinel event
- Practice aligning the aims, measures, and changes involved in improving care
- Evaluate the effect of change

Informatics

Originally, informatics was integrated within the Communication, Teamwork, and Evidence-Based Practice modules. However, based on feedback from reviewers, a distinct module was assigned for this content in light of the future of telecommunication and technology within the health care system. In this module, the newly licensed nurses learn how to identify the electronic information at the point of care and learn how to access information that is not readily available, but needed. The Technology Informatics Guiding Educational Reform initiative (TIGER, 2010) and confidentiality of information are emphasized in the NCSBN TTP module.

Cross-Cutting Threads in the NCSBN Program

Safety, clinical reasoning, and reflection are threaded throughout all modules. These values are taught, expected, and measured.

Safety
Safety and risk management are essential components of any TTP program and therefore is a cross-cutting theme in all the NCSBN modules. Johnstone and Kanitsaki (2006, 2008) in Australia have reported on the importance of experientially teaching risk management to new nurses. Cronenwett et al. (2007), using the expertise of national health care leaders across disciplines, have described safety in detail, as a competency, and this could be used in transition programs. This consensus opinion document, QSEN, can be considered excellent evidence for this transition model. The Massachusetts Board of Nursing (Board of Registration in Nursing, 2007) findings on nursing home errors called attention to addressing safety issues in transition programs, based on their review of discipline of new practical nurse graduates. Likewise, an NCSBN study (NCSBN, 2007) found that, according to self-reports, practice errors made by new graduates were prevalent. Many of the successful transition programs focus on safety (Beecroft et al., 2001; Beyea et al., 2010; Bratt, 2009; Halfer, 2007; Pine & Tart, 2007; Roxburgh et al., 2010; Williams et al., 2007).

Clinical reasoning
Clinical reasoning, sometimes referred to as critical thinking or clinical judgment, is another essential aspect of a TTP model and will be integrated in all the NCSBN modules. As the Carnegie study on nursing education (Benner et al., 2010) points out, this is where nurses learn to "think like a nurse." The Dartmouth program (Beyea et al., 2010) is exemplary as it uses simulation to assist novice nurses in making decisions during common clinical events or events that are uncommon, but life threatening. Transition programs that specifically report integration of clinical reasoning/critical thinking include Beecroft et al. (2001), Bratt (2009), Halfer (2007), Keller et al. (2006), Mississippi (2010), Pine and Tart (2007), VNIP (2010), and Williams et al. (2007), and this includes the programs with a rural focus. However, interviews with project managers of transition programs indicated that all programs examined attempt to integrate clinical reasoning.

Feedback and reflection

Feedback and reflection are other important cross-cutting themes in NCSBN modules and should be formally structured during the 6-month transition program, as well as during the 6 months that follow. If new nurses do not receive feedback on their practice, along with an opportunity to reflect, their practice will not improve. As in Bjørk and Kirkevold's (1999) study, without those opportunities, new graduates are at risk of making the same mistakes time and time again. It is very important for preceptors to be taught how to provide constructive feedback and how to foster reflective practice. (Beyea et al., 2010; Bratt, 2009; Halfer, 2007; Keller et al., 2006; Pine & Tart, 2007; Roxburgh et al., 2010; Williams et al., 2007). Journaling and personal inventories have been described as successful strategies to foster personal reflection.

IMPLEMENTING THE NCSBN'S TTP MODEL

Following obtaining approval from appropriate Institution Research Boards (IRB), the NCSBN will conduct a longitudinal, multisite, randomized study to evaluate its TTP model. The primary objective of this study is to determine whether newly licensed nurses' participation in NCSBN's TTP model improves patient safety, leads to higher-quality outcomes, and improves nurse retention. The secondary objectives are (a) to determine whether NCSBN's preceptor module adequately prepares nurses for the preceptor role, (b) to identify the challenges and potential solutions of planning and implementing the transition model within the organization and across the state/jurisdiction, and (c) to determine the cost–benefit analysis to implement the TTP model at a health care organization by evaluating the return on investment based on new nurse turnover rates. The study will compare an experimental group that participates in the TTP program with a control group that does not on the following variables:

- Patient safety (through analysis of infection rates, decubiti, post-op thrombosis, falls with and without injury, failure to rescue, adverse events/incident reports)
- Competence of the new nurse
- Experiential knowledge of the new nurse
- Stress perceived by the new nurse
- Patient satisfaction
- New nurse job satisfaction

- Retention (actual turnover rates and reports by new nurses of intent to leave/stay)
- Self-reports by new nurses of errors, near misses, and failure to rescue patients

Study Overview

The study will consist of two phases. Phase I is designed to examine the internal validity of the model and will include registered nurses from hospitals. Phase II is designed to evaluate the external validity and will include licensed practical/vocational nurses from hospitals as well as registered nurses from other health care settings, including long-term care, schools, correctional facilities, etc. States submitted applications to participate in the study, and three states/jurisdictions were selected: Illinois, Ohio, and North Carolina. The selection was based on each state being able to provide at least 250 new graduates for Phase I of the study, and the selection committee also looked at the diversity of sites within the state so that urban medical centers, suburban community hospitals, and rural settings will all be represented. Further, the committee sought a willingness for each site to designate coordinators to assist with data collection.

A state coordinator will be hired by NCSBN to act as the liaison for communication between NCBSN and the study sites and will ensure that new nurses, preceptors, and site coordinators are adequately trained on the study procedures. Additionally, the state coordinator will assist in identifying the study sites for Phase II. The site coordinator will assist with the identification of new nurses and preceptors for the study and will be the primary contact person for the new nurses, preceptors, and state coordinator. The coordinator will also assist in the collection of institutional data from her/his hospital and ensure that it is entered into the online database.

Study sites in each state will be randomly assigned (using a stratified assignment methodology) to the experimental group or the control group. Those randomized as a study site will use NCSBN's TTP model as their only method of TTP for the duration of the study. The TTP program in this study will be used as an adjunct to the organization's current orientation program (institutional policies, procedures, protocols, etc.) and is not meant to replace it. The new nurses and preceptors in the experimental group will actively participate in the online training modules and will also be asked to complete periodic surveys related to her/his transition to practice. The sites in the control group will implement the usual process of on-boarding new graduates and will not complete the online training modules but will be asked to complete the surveys. Complete details for IRB approval, design, sample selection, preceptor training, data collection, instruments, and procedures for the study can be obtained from the NCSBN.

In summary, the multi-institutional study will be useful to determine the degree to which the NCSBN's standardize model impacts patient safety, quality of care, and nurse retention. Data are also needed to determine if the NCSBN's preceptor module prepares the expert nurses to appropriately serve as a preceptor to a more novice colleague. Findings from the study could identify challenges along with potential solutions of planning and implementing the transition model at the organizational level and across states. Research-based evidence is critical for making economic decisions regarding the design, implementation, and sustainment of TTP programs by health care organizations in urban as well as rural settings.

REFERENCES

Barton, A. J., Armstrong, G., Preheim, G., Gelmon, S. B., & Andrus, L. C. (2009). A national Delphi to determine developmental progression of quality and safety competencies in nursing education. *Nursing Outlook, 57*, 313–322.

Beecroft, P., Hernandez, A. M., & Reid, D. (2008). Team preceptorships: A new approach for precepting new nurses. *Journal for Nurses in Staff Development, 24*(4), 143–148.

Beecroft, P. C., Kunzman, L., & Krozek, C. (2001). RN internship: Outcomes of a one-year pilot program. *JONA, 31*(12), 575–582.

Benner, P., Sutphen, M., Leonard, V., & Day, L. (2010). *Educating nurses: A call for radical transformation*. San Francisco: Jossey-Bass.

Berkow, S., Virkstis, K., Stewart, J., & Conway, L. (2008). Assessing new graduate nurse performance. *JONA, 38*(11), 468–474.

Beyea, S. C., Slattery, M. J., & von Reyn, L. J. (2010). Outcomes of a simulation-based residency program. *Clinical Simulation in Nursing, 6*(5), 169–175.

Bjørk, I. T., & Kirkevold, M. (1999). Issues in nurses' practical skill development in the clinical setting. *Journal of Nursing Care Quality, 14*(1), 72–84.

Board of Registration in Nursing, Division of Health Professions Licensure, Massachusetts Department of Public Health. (2007). *A study to identify evidence-based strategies for the prevention of nursing errors*. Massachusetts: Author.

Bratt, M. M. (2009). Retaining the next generation of nurses: The Wisconsin Residency Program provides a continuum of support. *The Journal of Continuing Education in Nursing, 40*(9), 416–425.

Cronenwett, L., Sherwood, G., Barnsteiner, J., Disch, J., Johnson, J., Mitchell, P. et al. (2007). Quality and safety education for nurses. *Nursing Outlook, 55*, pp. 122, 131.

Greiner, A. C., & Knebel, E. (Eds.). (2003). *Health professions education: A bridge to quality*. Washington, DC: The National Academies Press.

Halfer, D. (2007). A magnetic strategy for new graduates. *Nursing Economics, 25*(1), 5–11.

Johnstone, M. J., & Kanitsaki, O. (2006). Processes influencing the development of graduate nurse capabilities in clinical risk management: An Australian study. *Quality Management in Health Care, 15*(4), 268–278.

Johnstone, M. J., & Kanitsaki, O. (2008). Patient safety and the integration of graduate nurses into effective organizational clinical risk management systems and processes: An Australian study. *Quality Management in Health Care, 17*(2), 162–173.

Joint Commission White Paper. (2002). *Health care at the crossroads: Strategies for addressing the evolving nursing crisis.* Retrieved November 15, 2009 from http://www.jointcommission.org/NR/rdonlyres/5C138711-ED76-4D6F-909F-B06E0309F36D/0/health_care_at_the_crossroads.pdf

Keller, J. L., Meekins, K., & Summers, B. L. (2006). Pearls and pitfalls of a new graduate academic residency program. *JONA, 36*(12), 589–598.

McKay, C. A., & Crippen, L. (2008). Collaboration through clinical integration. *Nursing Administration, 32*(2), 109–116.

Mississippi. (2010). Accessed from http://www.monw.org/

Molinari, D. L., & Monserud, M. (2008). Rural nurse job satisfaction. *Journal of Rural and Remote Health, 8*(1), 1055. Retrieved from http://www.rrh.org.au/articles/defaultnew.asp?IssueNo = 8x

Molinari, D. L., Monserud, M., & Hudzinski, D. (2008). A new type of rural residency. *The Journal of Continuing Education in Nursing, 39*(1), 42–46.

NCSBN. (2004). *Report of findings from the 2003 practice and professional issues survey: Spring 2003.* Chicago: Author.

NCSBN. (2006a). *Evidence-based nursing education for regulation (EBNER).* Chicago: Author. Retrieved October 17, 2008 from https://www.ncsbn.org/Final_06_EB NER_Report.pdf

NCSBN. (2006b). *A national survey on elements of nursing education.* Chicago: Author.

NCSBN. (2007). *The impact of transition experience on practice of newly licensed registered nurse.* Data presented at February, 2007, Transition Forum, Chicago, IL.

Nicol, P., & Young, M. (2007). Sail training: An innovative approach to graduate nurse preceptor development. *Journal for Nurses in Staff Development, 23*(6), 298–302.

North Carolina. (2009). *Phase I study of North Carolina evidence-based transition to practice initiative project.* Accessed from http://ffne.org/file_library/Phase%20I%20 Findings%20Summary.pdf

Phillips, J. M. (2006). Preparing preceptors through online education. *Journal for Nurses in Staff Development, 22*(3), 150–156.

Pine, R., & Tart, K. (2007). Return on investment: Benefits and challenges of a baccalaureate nurse residency program. *Nursing Economics, 25*(1), 13–18.

Roxburgh, M., Lauder, W., Topping, K., Holland, K., Johnson, M., & Watson, R. (2010). Early findings from an evaluation of a post-registration staff development programme: The Flying Start NHS Initiative in Scotland, UK. *Nurse Education in Practice, 10*(2), 76–81.

Spector, N., & Echternacht, M. (2010). A regulatory model for transitioning newly licensed nurses to practice. *Journal of Nursing Regulation, 1*(2), 18–25.

TIGER. (2010). *The TIGER initiative.* Accessed from http://www.tigersummit.com/ Home_Page.php

Vermont Nurse Internship Program (VNIP). (2010). Accessed from http://www.vnip.org/

Williams, C. A., Goode, C. J., Krsek, C., Bednash, G. D., & Lynn, M. R. (2007). Post-baccalaureate nurse residency 1-year outcomes. *The Journal of Nursing Administration, 37*(7/8), 357–365.

Yonge, O., Hagler, P., Cox, C., & Drefs, S. (2008). Listening to preceptors. *Journal for Nurses in Staff Development, 24*(1), 21–26.

11

Northwest Rural Nurse Residency

Deana L. Molinari and Tamara Hollinger-Forrest

The Northwest Rural Nurse Residency is a combination distance education and clinical supervision yearlong program that transitions novice nurses to competent team members. The collaborative model was developed by rural directors of nursing and a school of nursing to provide transition-to-practice competence standards, quality content, and local control. Education for residents, preceptors, and chief nursing officers is provided. Local support roles and processes are described and program administration tips are provided.

The Northwest Rural Nurse Residency (NWRNR) is a collaborative transition-to-practice (TTP) project serving small hospitals and agencies across the United States. The Idaho State University School of Nursing (ISU-SON) and rural health care facilities work collaboratively to assist new nurses to change roles from student to competent professional. The employer and school depend on each other to meet program goals. The resident relies on the facility for employment, competency measurement, guidance, and supervision, and trusts the school of nursing for standards and educational content.

Many individuals and at least two business organizations collaborate for the new graduates' benefit. The rural employer adapts the NWRNR's components to meet the new employee's needs. The agency markets, maintains, and administers the program. Local supervisors manage preceptor and resident processes. The ISU-SON delivers the flexible TTP program.

The ISU-SON provides the evidence-based continuing education curriculum and provides processes based on national residency standards. The ISU clinical coordinator facilitates rather than regulates the program. The coordinator assists managers with administration issues, acts as a safe liaison for residents, tracks participant progress, and assists preceptors with program issues. The NWRNR provides national standards and measurement tools.

Residents complete 64 hours of didactic instruction as well as 104 hours of clinical supervision. New nurses choose from a buffet of elective courses in addition to the 28 hours of core curriculum. The preceptors aid new employees in choosing electives and reflecting on both career and residency goals. Each resident's curriculum is customized according to self-assessment and job descriptions data.

The freedom to choose electives is like a double-edged sword. In the past, academic institutions presented "one-size fits all" information transfer sessions. The NWRNR offers a program that is locally customized. The ability to customize a program costs an agency leadership. Administrators build a supportive culture in order for the program to work.

Administrators design support systems and then need to encourage and evaluate participants. Programs with less flexibility require less leadership (Molinari & Monserud, 2009). Preceptors require policies, a selection process, documentation systems, and recognition. An evaluation over time indicates that administrative and preceptor leadership are key to residents' success. Residents cannot learn alone as they become lost in caregiving tasks. New nurses depend on leaders to provide an educational scaffold. Employees need to know why the residency is important to the employer, the patient, and themselves. They need the resources to succeed and finally need to know that the nurse manager is holding them accountable throughout the learning process. Simple progress inquiries during informal contacts are a social method of encouragement.

The program's flexibility also extends to large hospital networks and state organizations. Larger facilities usually have more educational supports than small agencies. Several multifacility organizations adopted the program in order to support critical access hospitals, clinics, and long-term care providers who are often left out of organized TTP education.

HISTORY

The purpose of the NWRNR is to increase new rural nurses' retention, critical thinking, socialization, and patient care quality. The residency originated in 2004 when the chief nursing officers in Idaho and Washington collaborated to solve the high turnover rate of new graduates. The program was built on several principles. Nurses learn the rural nurse specialty best:

- In their own facilities
- From rural experts
- When socialized into the community as well as the facility
- If taught to think rather than act
- When local leaders administer the program
- When the rural nursing specialty practice is recognized
- When preceptors are fostered
- When nurses set goals and measure outcomes

The residency changed as data were gathered. Appreciative inquiry provided the evidence on which to base the changes (Chapter 19). The simple asynchronous distance education program alterations include more than content differences. The curriculum now highlights rural crisis assessment and management. The program lengthened to 1 year. Residents now attend in synchronous cohorts. Both preceptors and residents are mentored. Networking and competency measurement were emphasized. Curriculum now includes standards developed by the Institute of Medicine (IOM), the National Council of State Boards of Nursing (NCSBN), and the American Association of Colleges of Nursing (AACN).

THEORETICAL FOUNDATIONS

Since there was no new graduate transition theory in 2004, several combined theories formed a conceptual foundation. Patricia Benner's work *From Novice to Expert* (Benner, 1984), transformative learning theory (Mezirow, 2000), and rural nurse competency measures developed in Nova Scotia and Alaska created the foundation. The theories basically posit that individuals choose to grow from novice to expert through a series of transforming experiences and that growth needs to be routinely measured. Appreciative inquiry and participatory action research methods were employed to develop and monitor the progress of the NWRNR. Rapidly occurring innovations were based on evidence gathered from data in the ongoing research study and the literature. Data are gathered from the first day of participant enrollment.

COMPETENCY MEASUREMENT

Two types of competency are measured during the year: clinical skills and nursing role. During the first week of the residency, preceptors administer a clinical skills checklist developed by northwest chief nursing officers. The residents rate their confidence in completing specific clinical tasks. Benner states that novice nurses are anxious to differentiate between black and white concepts, and, therefore, appreciate checklists. In order to become competent, novices require a lot of practice in patient assessment and management. The residency teaches crisis assessment and management in six nursing subspecialties: obstetrics, pediatrics, medical surgical, geriatrics, mental health, and trauma.

Residents self-assess practice knowledge by employing a nursing suite at the bedside. The software on a mobile device prevents reliance on memory, provides the latest best practices, medication information, laboratory tests, patient education tips, procedures, definitions, and evidence. In effect, new nurses carry a nursing library in their uniform pockets.

Using an electronic nursing suite teaches novices to ask questions and gives reliable answers. The software reduces errors and lateral violence according to the participants: errors due to easy access to the answers, lateral violence because the novice asks questions of the software rather than peers.

Role competencies take more time to measure than skill competencies. The NWRNR uses two tools over the year. Chapter 15 presents the Alaskan competency measurement approach. Another competency matrix adapted from the work of the Registered Nurses Professional Development Centre in Halifax, Nova Scotia is provided in the appendix along with an adaptation of the Quality and Safety for Educational Nursing group's knowledge, skills, and attitudes competences.

Preceptors use the clinical skills checklist ratings to develop a lesson plan for the clinical supervision period. The 10 most frequent and high-risk clinical skills with the lowest confidence perceptions are chosen to improve. At the end of the clinical supervision, preceptors employ the same clinical skills checklist to measure nurse capabilities. Preceptors write a narrative report describing the new graduate's task and role progress.

CRITICAL THINKING

Critical thinking is the foundation of safe practice, and so elements of the critical thinking process are taught and measured. Due to the profession's disparate definitions and expectations of critical thinking, both preceptors and residents are taught the same critical thinking process model. Using one model increases communication and standardizes measurement. The Perceptive, Affective and Cognitive Critical

Thinking model (PAC) enables preceptors and residents to communicate clearly (Molinari & Dupler, 2005).

The PAC model measures thinking processes and not thinking outcomes. The measurement tool is a matrix enabling self-assessment as well as remediation. NWRNR promotes clinical reasoning as well, which is taught as part of the core curriculum. Preceptors using the PAC model praise the ease of facilitation of discussion, and the residents report increased understanding of how to think critically so as to increase clinical reasoning outcomes. Critical thinking increases with practice, thus core classes are based on patient care scenarios. Preceptors assess novice nurse thinking using the talk-aloud thinking method and can increase information gathering and processing.

SUPPORTIVE ROLES AND RESIDENCY ELEMENTS

Many people are needed to nourish new nurses. The administrator, preceptor, and peers all play a role in developing a nurse's competence and confidence. The Idaho State University's School of Nursing employs a program coordinator, a clinical coordinator, an educational information technologist, and an administrative assistant. Teachers are hired according to their specialties. The hospital or agency needs a motivated supervisor, talented preceptors, and supportive peers.

Chief Nursing Officer

The chief nursing officer (CNO) may be the busiest person in a small rural facility as patient care and administration duties fill the day. The residency challenges a CNO's values, priorities, and time management. The main role is changing culture. Supervisors use change theories to move an organization from a "survival of the fittest" mentality to nourishment, accountability, and reward. The recent reports by the Robert Wood Johnson Foundation and the Institute of Medicine (2011) may help to pressure change but will not develop a nourishing culture without the supervisor's influence (Parsons & Cornett, 2011). Instituting new programs takes dedication, time, and repeated efforts.

Preceptors

Each resident requires a competent preceptor to transition from academic learning to professional development.

The preceptor is the key to this change. The complex clinical educator position requires specific personal characteristics and professional skills available in a small minority of nurses. Novice and advanced beginner nurses report valuing clinical teachers who are empathic, warm, respectful, humorous, flexible, fair, dependable, consistent, and enthusiastic (Molinari, Monserud, & Hudzinki, 2008). Preceptors are required to demonstrate knowing the latest knowledge and current practice; as well as, the ability to model communication skills, recognize assumptions and logically reason through clinical challenges. NWRNR residents describe successful preceptors as actively involved in the resident's daily routine. The new nurse feels less anxiety when the preceptor is routinely available (Molinari et al., 2008). In addition, the preceptor's positive attitude, effective listening skills, and corrective feedback improve the resident's job satisfaction (Wormsbecker, 2008). The complex role requires preparation.

New experts in NWRNR earn a rural nurse preceptor certificate after the completion of all program requirements: 16 hours of education based on national standards and the literature, 104 hours of mentoring, and a scenario-based problem-solving test. The program provides flexibility for hospitals that prefer to train their own preceptors using different curricula. Nurses who provide proof of education and pass the test are eligible for mentoring, student assignments, and preceptor resources.

Selection

Choosing the right people to coach new employees is the administrator's challenge and the beginning of organizational change. Applicants who love teaching and possess clinical expertise are preferred. In fact, some studies show that recent residency graduates make supportive preceptors. The selection process demonstrates the agency's values.

Some preceptors report that new employees are simply assigned, as if they were patients, rather than being interviewed for a new job description. The application and interview process can celebrate the complexity of clinical coaches. An application process indicates the nurse's interest. If a rural nurse finds him- or herself assigned to an unwanted role, resentment can prevent adequate performance. Precepting is more than just another task for an experienced nurse. An effective preceptor is the difference between an eager new employee and an unsafe nurse with a high potential for turnover. Organizations risk turnover of expert nurses if they do not support them.

Residents describe successful preceptors as actively involved in the resident's daily routine. The new nurse feels less anxiety when the preceptor is routinely available (Molinari et al., 2008). In addition, the preceptor's positive attitude, effective listening skills, and corrective feedback improve the resident's job satisfaction (Molinari & Monserud, 2008).

Support

Preceptors are the key to an educational cultural change. New preceptors are novices as well as clinical experts requiring ongoing assistance. Building a nourishing organizational culture consists of many elements. Some elements can be quickly implemented while others require ongoing attention.

Preceptors require a clear description of their role, precise documentation, procedures for unsafe practice, lists of resources, and expectations. Some call this the preceptor's bill of rights.

Residencies depend on the expert teaching and mentoring of clinical instructors. Preceptors role model nursing practice as well as teach practice principles. When preceptors are insufficiently motivated, educated, or fostered, residents are forgotten in the pressures of patient care.

Since the role is complex, a mentor is provided for the novice preceptor. The preceptor's mentor works with the novice preceptors for one year. Their purpose is to walk with the novice clinical educator through the residency experience. The mentor serves as a reminder, counselor, and problem-solver. The NWRNR clinical coordinator circulates monthly preceptor journal articles and discussions of safety, quality, and clinical education issues.

Education is an important support. Some agencies do not educate preceptors and simply expect successful practice. Many facilities provide an initial education program. Still other programs measure preceptor competencies.

The NWRNR educates, measures competency, and mentors preceptors. A 16-hour education program and a knowledge achievement test are followed by mentoring during the preceptor's first teaching experience. Class sessions include applying rural nurse theory to practice, team work, reality shock, emotional competence, prioritization, Benner's stages of novice to expert, critical thinking processes and clinical reasoning, competency measurement processes, communication techniques, conflict management, learning preferences and processes, teaching strategies, personal growth, and analyzing issues/concerns related to precepting experiences.

Competence measurement is another support that enables self-assessment. The NWRNR provides a postknowledge survey that assesses knowledge, skill, and attitude development. Annual preceptor conferences can increase preceptor knowledge and improve skills. The

NWRNR uses a simulation workshop with competence measurement to increase knowledge.

Encouragement of personal growth through goal setting, recognition of personal novice status, and journal keeping are also helpful. Preceptors need to self-assess personal growth as they monitor new employees' growth. Setting personal goals enables novice preceptors to recognize the experiences' value rather than focusing on the challenges of the position. Journal keeping assists preceptors to monitor both personal and employee progress.

Administrators who include the preceptor role in a clinical ladder and performance evaluations also ensure preceptor progression beyond the initial certificate process. Recognition for the work can honor clinical teachers. Rural agencies can recognize preceptors through a variety of methods.

- Mentioning accomplishments in newsletters, newspapers, bulletin boards, or websites.
- Differential payment while teaching.
- Limiting workload during teaching periods
- Organizational parties
- Name tag preceptor pins.

Some agencies provide a pin or logo on the name tag telling others of the preceptor's status.

Requiring accountability is another strategy for nourishing an educational culture. Measuring preceptor competence and residents' satisfaction will encourage continued preceptor growth. There are many ways to grow as a clinical teacher.

NWRNR preceptors are given electronic library database access for evidence-based practice. Preceptors receive monthly articles from peer-reviewed journals that can be discussed on a discussion forum for personal growth and development.

NWRNR supports preceptors by providing administrative processes, competence measurement strategies, and curriculum resources. The preceptor website provides instruction about how to develop new task competencies, role competency measurement tools, and other documentation aids needed to conduct a homegrown residency. An 8-month quality and safety workbook enables preceptors to teach and measure competence.

Preceptors enjoy the yearly simulation workshop. The workshop is presented via audio/video web-based instructional technology to both preceptors and residents over 2 days. Workshop attendees participate in crisis assessment and management simulations. For instance, a virtual rural community hospital requires participants to manage five patients' crises and communicate with an interprofessional team. The combination of novices and experts increases participation. Preceptors coach residents while residents want to appear knowledgeable during the difficult situations.

PROGRAM DEVELOPMENT TIPS

Program coordinators at NWRNR and rural facilities learned best practices during the residency development and delivery process. A few of these are presented below.

- Appreciative inquiry program development strategies similar to those described in Crusoe's chapter 19 empower organizations to quickly build strength. Nursing staff members with few resources can develop a residency or preceptor program by self-assessing, dreaming, and collaborating. Groups find more energy to improve organizational strengths than when groups try to correct weaknesses. Since change is difficult, an optimistic attitude eases the emotional burdens of shifting priorities or processes. Setting realistic change goals keeps nurses moving forward. Periodically reviewing progress enables a new round of self-appreciation and goal setting. Change seems easier when staff feel supported and appreciated. The process provides evidence on which to base change.
- Data gathering assists with cultural change. Collecting data about the program as well as the participants provides evidence for change. Program data can be collected and analyzed. The data can answer important questions. How many errors do new employees report compared to long-term employees? Do residents make fewer errors? How many preceptors does the organization support? How do the skill levels and continuing education courses compare? How many hours are spent supporting new employees? What are the costs of turnover? Agencies can also measure resident and preceptor practice competency. The NWRNR provides administrators with preceptor progress reports to minimize problems occurring from preceptor/resident disconnects, shift changes, or inadequate performance.
- Residents are given the opportunity to evaluate the preceptor early in the residency. Sometimes designated preceptors are not effective or for some reason the preceptor and resident is not a good match.

Preceptor changes need to be made quickly to avoid inconsistency in the resident's experience.

■ Providing monthly articles to preceptors focuses energies and attention to the needs of the new nurse with an emphasis on communication and critical thinking. Article topics include self-evaluation, becoming a successful preceptor, patient safety, healthy environment, team work, and stages of development. These articles provide insight into challenges of both the preceptor and new nurse resident and techniques to overcome those challenges.

■ An early discovery was the fact that managers, preceptors, and residents held different perspectives about the goals and outcomes of a residency program. Therefore, an orientation of all participants in each agency is conducted before the first educational activity. NWRNR staff learn the unique qualities of each hospital and make recommendations as to how to best structure the residency program. Each hospital has unique challenges. For example, some rural hospitals have a difficult time coordinating a new resident nurse with one preceptor. Other hospitals schedule the new nurse to work a night shift and the preceptor works a day shift. Or perhaps working the night shift prevents participation in live educational classes. Some hospitals expect new nurses to complete courses during off-duty hours. The one-on-one orientation informs everyone of best practices so that planning and development support optimal outcomes.

■ Web-based resources archive educational programs, program resources, and handouts as well as provide discussion forums. The web houses a centralized library of surveys, case scenarios, tests, and measurement tools. The site also links to the online library database.

■ Program staff created one manual to assist both preceptors and residents. The manual contains a basic overview of the program, expectations of the preceptor and resident, class topics, competency measurement aids, and the 1-year time line. The main focus of the first 4 months of the residency is completion of core classes and the clinical experience. Preceptors develop a learning plan based on the resident's and organization's needs. The remaining 8 months of the program emphasize the Quality and Safety for Education in Nursing (QSEN) competencies. Preceptor and resident use a workbook for monthly sessions. During the session, goals are set, resources outlined, and competencies measured from the last month using a rubric. The QSEN competencies include:

■ Patient-Centered Care
■ Teamwork and Collaboration

- Evidence-Based Practice
- Quality Improvement
- Safety
- Case Management
- Informatics
- Career Management

Asking residents to seek out general information about a topic is as important as learning agency or hospital information and practices. Preceptors are encouraged to help residents base their practice on several levels of evidence and to apply knowledge gained from the literature. This is done in practical ways. For example, during the month when evidence-based practice is stressed, a specific patient care issue can serve to focus learning. Residents can review hospital protocols, patients/families/caregivers can be interviewed, or participation in relevant committees can increase knowledge of various levels of evidence. Residents can make reports to decision makers if practice issues are identified. When preceptors and residents use the workbook, agency systems change.

- Since new employees prefer to learn by discussion and stories rather than by searching the web, the Resident Workbook provides discussion topics for preceptor/resident interaction, peer-reviewed articles, websites, and discussion topics. Preceptors can offer the important information residents prefer and make a difference in nurse achievement. Each workbook section contains a definition of the monthly topic, resources, discussion questions, and an assessment rubric.

In summary, collaboration is the key to rural nurse competence. When providers work with educators to improve health care, both money and reputations are saved. The NWRNR initiative evolved from collaborative processes and evidence. The program is intricately connected to its partners. Every new nurse is an opportunity for improving the profession. Data about each nurse strengthen organizations and improve TTP programming. Data analysis in the NWRNR seeks out methods to expand best practices.

Strength recognition unites NWRNR with resilient rural agencies. Small hospitals and clinics might experience difficulties in providing sustainable residencies without collaboration while the NWRNR would fail to exist without rural providers' clinical strengths. Cooperation based on organizational strengths allows educational leaders and health care providers to create one supportive TTP structure.

TTP collaborations include intraorganizational strategies as well as interorganizational strategies. Much support is needed for transitioning nurses to competent team members. Administrators work with bedside care experts to educationally nourish all nurses. The result is job satisfaction, which creates retention. Likewise, when new graduates partner with clinical preceptors, the synergy increases safe patient care. Collaboration is the key to transition to practice, patient safety, and leading the future of health care.

REFERENCES

Benner, P. (1984). *From novice to expert: Excellence and power in clinical nursing practice.* Menlo Park: Addison-Wesley.

Committee on the Robert Wood Johnson Foundation Initiative on the Future of Nursing at the Institute of Medicine. (2011). *The future of nursing: Leading change, advancing health.* Washington, DC: National Academies Press.

Hauck, A., Quinn, M. T., & Fitzpatrick, J. J. (2011). Structural empowerment and anticipated turnover among critical care nurses. *Journal of Nursing Management, 19*(2), 269–276. 21375631.

Mezirow, J. (2000). *Learning as transformation: Critical perspectives on a theory in progress.* San Francisco: Jossey Bass.

Molinari, D. L., & Dupler, A. (2005). Online critical thinking in problem-solving groups. In G. Berg (Ed.), *Encyclopedia of international computer-based learning.* Hershey Penn: Idea Group, Inc. (*Invited*).

Molinari, D. L., & Monserud, M. (2008). Rural nurse job satisfaction. *Journal of Rural and Remote Health, 8*(1), 1055. Retrieved from http://www.rrh.org.au/articles/defaultnew.asp?IssueNo=8x

Molinari, D. L., & Monserud, M. (2009). Rural nurse cultural self-efficacy and job satisfaction. *Journal of Transcultural Nursing, 20*(2), 211–218.

Molinari, D. L., Monserud, M., & Hudzinski, D. (2008). The rural nurse internship: A new type of nurse residency. *Journal of Continuing Education in Nursing, 39*(1), 42–46.

Parsons, M. L., & Cornett, P. A. (2011). Sustaining the pivotal organizational outcome: Magnet recognition. *Journal of Nursing Management, 19*(2), 277–286. 21375632.

Wormsbecker, K. J. (2008). Job satisfaction in rural and remote nursing: Comparison of registered nurses in nurse practitioner vs. non-nurse practitioner roles. *Thesis.* http://library2.usask.ca/theses/available/etd-05282008-143740/

12

Vermont Nurses in Partnership Model

Susan A. Boyer

Vermont has significant rural regions with small health care facilities. A collaborative process resulted in the development of the Vermont Nurses in Partnership (VNIP), a transition-to-practice model, that includes a formal preceptor program. VNIP targets recent nursing graduates who successfully completed the NCLEX and are beginning employment. The emphasis of the VNIP is developing a supportive and sustainable hospital culture. This chapter explores the origins and activities of the VNIP that evolved into a nationally recognized transition-to-practice approach for nurses.

Based on Vermont nursing workforce research (Kaeding, 1998), a collaborative group of Nurse Leaders in the state established an internship framework that supports safe, effective transition for new graduates who successfully complete the NCLEX and start employment in complex, high-acuity health care settings. Developers of the VNIP designed a model that could be adapted in a variety of settings and agencies. The unique components of the VNIP include statewide standardization of competency assessment; collaboration between academia, regulation, and practice settings from across the continuum of care; development of clinical coaching plans; and intensive preceptor development and support. The VNIP program conducted its initial pilot project in 2000. Since then, the program has evolved and expanded within the state, and has been adopted by several other regional and statewide initiatives.

PHILOSOPHICAL UNDERPINNINGS

The VNIP was developed in response to research and strategic planning that was conducted by the Vermont Organization of Nurse Leaders in 1999. This multidisciplinary, collaborative, leadership group took a proactive approach to the nursing shortage, which was already impacting on Vermont health care settings. A small grant from the Southern VT Area Health Education Center funded a part-time Director's position, which led the work into the initial internship pilot project.

The mission statement for the VNIP internship set the purpose: "to create a formal and sustainable nurse internship program that provides the clinical experience necessary to support the novice's entry into practice, their growth along the continuum of expertise, and their professional practice within the complex and demanding field of healthcare." The project goals included (a) providing support for the transition from new graduate to a self-confident, adaptable, and independent professional; (b) collaboration between the Board of Nursing, Academic Centers and Practice sites from across the continuum of care; (c) statewide implementation; and (d) working toward sustainability of a nationally recognized Nurse Internship Program.

Development of the Model

The consensus was the preferred decision-making approach; thus, a small directive group was never identified. Instead, all interested nurse leaders were invited to participate to whatever degree was feasible for them. Individual workgroups formed to target the development needs related to

- Model and/or competency expectations
- Teaching plans
- Outcomes and sustainability
- Preceptor program

Each group developed relevant documents, framework, and/or a plan specific to their content focus and then the information was shared statewide. Cyber communications allowed feedback from all participants. The project director collated the editing, comments, and suggestions, and then re-sent them to the entire group, providing further opportunity for comment prior to finalizing the document, presentation, or process.

At the initial VNIP meeting, it was determined that three levels of internship were needed: (1) student (extern program) for expanded undergraduate clinical experience; (2) graduate-level (transition-to-practice) internship—to provide an organized, supportive transition to practice that included educational support, competency development, and skills evaluation; and (3) specialty care internships—to provide additional education and support for work in a specialty care area such as OR, ICU, home care, long-term care, etc. The decision to address the graduate-level internship for the initial pilot project was based on the logistics of employment versus student, and who might support the costs of the venture. Another driving force was the urgent need to shift the workplace to one that emphasizes nurture and support for the new graduate.

Before program development could begin, the important decision of "internship" versus "residency" model required resolution by the planners. The Vermont program needed to be inclusive of associate degree-prepared nurses and would be targeting the very initial transition—novice to advanced beginner on Benner's continuum of development. The driving forces for this initiative included acute care- and community-based agencies, which shared a priority of cost containment. With strictly limited resources, the planners decided on an internship framework that would provide support for a nurse during the crucial transition period—wherein initial evidence is collected that validates the individual as safe and effective. It was further decided that the internship would be based in a preceptor delivery model. As a result, two programs were required—an internship program for the new graduates and a preceptor program for the development and support of clinical staff preceptors (Foundation for Nursing Excellence, 2009).

The duration of the internship was another crucial question that needed to be addressed. Regrettably, in 1999, the literature search did not provide much guidance, revealing that internships ranged anywhere from 2 weeks to several months. There was no evidence of consistency in the pattern or length of the program; nor was there evidence to support decisions for duration. With that in mind, the planners accessed the best evidence available at the time—the expertise and experience of the many managers and educators that were involved in the project. This group of experts agreed that 10–12 weeks was probably a realistic and workable time frame for most new nurses. Current nursing literature validates findings of the preliminary efforts of VNIP planners, reinforcing the need for (at a minimum) 10–12 weeks for the nurse internship for transition to practice (del Bueno, 2005; Duchscher, 2008, 2009).

DEFINING COMPETENCIES

The difficult work of developing competency expectations received an immense "jump start" from Dr. Lenburg's Competence Outcomes Performance Assessment (COPA) model (Lenburg, 1999a, 2009, 2010). The COPA model brought two significant transitions to the Vermont internship: (1) It provided an outline of the eight core competencies, which clearly defined the role of the nurse in the clinical setting. (2) It created a shift in mindset to target performance outcomes statements, which clearly define the performance expectations in clinical practice (Armstrong, 2009; Robert Wood Johnson, 2010; Lenburg, 1999b). This emphasis replaced the previous one that targeted the minutiae of nursing—the tasks and procedures that are a component of providing care.

The COPA model is a research- and theory-based approach for defining the expectations for the new nurse in the clinical setting. Significantly, this model caused a reevaluation of all orientation tools with the priority of incorporating Critical Thinking, Ethical Comportment, Human Caring relationships, Leadership, and Management as they occur in daily patient care in each clinical practice area. While previous orientation and/or internship tools resembled a "grocery list" of clinical tasks and procedures, the COPA model prioritized critical thinking aspects of what a nurse does in the clinical setting. The competency framework has evolved to a perspective that targets statements that incorporate clinical reasoning, nursing judgment, skilled know-how, and are now delving into aspects of ethical comportment (Benner, 2009).

An ongoing challenge is writing "competencies" that clearly define clinical expectations in a clear, objective, measurable, and pertinent manner. The COPA model helped in this realm by replacing learning objectives with performance outcomes statements. Traditional learning objectives provide the instructor with guidance related to what to teach, whereas performance outcomes statements target actual practice in the care setting. By using the COPA model as a theory- and evidence-based framework, we were able to write clearly defined expectations that target this clinical performance.

Another unique challenge within the VNIP project was the intent to create an internship that could be utilized in multiple settings, not just a single agency or health care system. The work was inclusive of the full continuum of care; thus, there were nurse leaders from public health, long-term, and home care settings assessing if the selected criteria fit within their practice arenas as well. This supported a development process that was inclusive; thus, the resulting tools "fit" when they were taken for specific customization for use in these areas. The final competence verification form outlines the core role of the generalist registered nurse in the direct care setting. Each specialty unit/service then developed an additional listing of clinical performance expectations that are unique to that specialty, and these forms are used concurrently.

IMPLEMENTATION STRATEGIES

The VNIP program prioritized experiential, reflective learning for the new care provider. To accomplish this, the clinical preceptors needed extensive instruction related to Critical Thinking. They require not just an understanding of what Critical Thinking is, but also "what does it look like" in actual practice, and especially "how do they foster its development in the novice care provider?" Program goals targeted clinical performance at the top of "Bloom's taxonomy," and so many of the competency statements used action verbs within the realms of analyze, synthesize, prioritize, and evaluate. VNIP planners recognized as vital that learners move toward integrating related skills and naturalization of the more common tasks, rather than simply following directions. The emphasis within the affective domain was to move beyond responding or reacting to, on toward adopting behavior and internalizing values systems. Two items that impacted on this development were (1) writing clearly defined expectations at the highest possible action verb level and (2) preparing preceptors as effective clinical instructors that can foster reflective learning within the clinical setting. With this second challenge in mind, VNIP updated preceptor development and support to meet the challenges faced in 21st-century health care.

The VNIP Preceptor program (Boyer, 2008, 2010; VNIP, 2008) is a formal, postlicensure educational program designed to increase the capability of experienced nurses as relates to teaching, evaluation, interpersonal, and communication skills. The skills learned in these intensive workshops are used by specialty care area personnel for continued development of experienced staff in OR, ICU, psychiatric, home care, public health, and other special care areas. The concepts and process also increase the effectiveness of the preceptor's work with nurse students. The research-and theory-based course curriculum addresses the role and responsibilities of the preceptor and intern, Transition

Shock© theory (Duchscher, 2008, 2009), stages of Benner's model of novice to expert (Benner, 1984), developing clinical judgment (Benner, Sutphen, & Day, 2009), principles of teaching and learning, learning styles, team building, personality style, effective communication, conflict management, generational (Weston, 2006) and cultural issues, competence of new RNs in clinical practice (Lenburg, 2009, 2010), evidence collection, delegation, accountability, promoting critical thinking in the novice, and issues or concerns related to the difficult "preceptee."

The Protector role of the preceptor was introduced in 2001 and the revised roles and responsibilities were shared nationally in 2003. This transition shifted emphasis to the Protector and Evaluator roles, while retaining the Educator role as a core responsibility. First and foremost, the nurse accepts the role of patient protector when they become licensed as a nurse. It is the philosophy of VNIP that preceptors then accept the responsibility for protecting the learner, the agency, and colleagues when they take on the role of "preceptor." Protection of our profession occurs as well, as preceptors assure safe care for consumers and maintain public confidence in nurses.

The second most crucial job of the preceptor is that of collecting evidence. *Essentially, a preceptor's job is to gather evidence that the new staff member provides care in a safe and effective manner, according to the protocol.* However, not every person can produce such evidence on arrival— thus, a preceptor is also expected to develop performance capability, or function as an "Educator," wherever capability is missing. Instead of considering this goal as an afterthought, administrators of nurse internship programs must take into consideration that teaching to address the learning needs of an individual is a time-consuming priority. Whenever assigning another task to someone, it is important to remember that completing it will require time and resources. Thus, the time required to precept a novice nurse mandates reduced patient assignments. Time must be reallocated by the expert for observing, supporting, showing the ropes, assessing knowledge level, evaluating, and documenting competence. Emphasis consistently remains on the provision of safe and effective care based on all applicable protocols.

A pilot project of the VNIP was implemented in the summer of 2000. Four agencies participated and each reported on successes and challenges associated with the workload and outcomes. Based on these data, the model was modified and recommendations were put forth to successfully implement the program. In the summer of 2001, a second series of pilot programs were implemented. Each agency that used the framework approached it with different resources. Specifically, some agencies had centralized educators, others were limited to a few unit-based educators, yet others had no one in the educator role. Planners of the VNIP found that despite the difference in support systems, the program was evaluated as "successful." The variety of resources created variances in the approach, thus giving results similar to running multiple pilots at the same time. The findings identified essential resources and techniques for successful and cost-effective implementation of the VNIP program within an agency.

CLINICAL COACHING PLANS

Another notable feature of VNIP is inclusion of Clinical Coaching Plans—having specific written plans for the teaching/learning that occurs in the clinical setting between the preceptor and new graduate. VNIP is developing a textbook of "Clinical Coaching Plans" for preceptors similar to textbooks containing standardized nursing care plans. The plans include specific performance expectations that should be demonstrated by the novice nurse to the preceptor to validate capability or competence. The plans need to include teaching and learning activities as well as strategies to promote and assess critical thinking and clinical judgment.

RECOMMENDATIONS

Based on the pilot projects and implementation of the VNIP for almost a decade, the following recommendations are offered:

■ The need for three distinct programs that address the needs of new graduate, new-to-specialty, and reentry nurses: both registered nurse (RN) and licensed practical nurse (LPN) graduates.
■ Offer internships with a minimum of 10-week duration (not including the basic agency orientation).
■ Include at least 40 hours of didactic instruction that is provided by the participating agencies and institutions. Recommended topics (among others) include Quality Improvement, Protocols, Medication Administration, Cultural Competence, Managed Care, and Pain Management.
■ Nurses who are in the intern role should not be considered as part of the day-to-day staffing mix.
■ The VNIP core competency form is used to delineate and document an intern's performance. This form details performance outcomes expectations that are based on the COPA model and apply to all nurses providing direct care.
■ Interns should be paired with a primary preceptor.

- Preceptors should receive intensive preparation for their role via instruction that addresses all the core topics identified by VNIP.
- The primary preceptor is responsible for educational planning, selecting the patient assignment that serves intern learning needs, weekly conferences, and communications with colleagues, manager, and other preceptors.
- Preceptors are facilitators while they coach, teach, and evaluate the intern through their daily clinical experiences on the unit.
- Patients assigned to interns should be part of their preceptor's assignment and preceptors progressively allocate patient care activities to the intern.
- On a weekly basis, the intern, preceptor, and/or clinical educator should meet to establish and evaluate goals and foster the development of critical thinking abilities.
- Delivery of the internship requires release time that supports educational preparation, didactic instruction, goal setting, weekly conference, and support group meetings. Approximately 200 hours of educator time are required for each internship cohort and/or session.
- Whereas four is the preferred limit, each cohort will consist of not more than five interns starting at the same time on a single direct care unit.
- Initial internship experiences should be offered during the day shift, 8 hour days, Monday through Friday. During this timeframe there are more available staff, and more opportunities for experiences offered with a multidisciplinary team.
- Generally, 12 hour shifts are less effective as they are associated with fatigue and reduction in continuity of repetition/practice.
- Interns are hired for a minimum of 32 hours per week through completion of competency requirements. Part-time internship was unsuccessful due to reduction in days of repetition/practice.
- Interns should take NCLEX prior to starting the internship.
- Specialty care internships may require up to 12 months for completion of specialty service competencies (American Association of Colleges of Nursing, (n.d.)).

OUTCOMES

Data collected over time for the VNIP reveal the following outcomes:

- Recruitment: Of all interns, 48% were recruited from out-of-state schools and/or residences for the initial pilot.
- Retention: The tertiary care center tracked retention data prior to, and following internship implementation

■ The 1999 Preinternship rate was 75% retained until December 31 of hiring year
■ With the internship, the rate rose to 93% of new graduates who completed the VNIP program.
■ Position vacancy rate: One Vermont agency has maintained a 0% vacancy rate for nursing positions for the last 3 years. They became involved with the original VNIP pilot due to their vacancy rate being consistently 20% and higher on the medical-surgical unit. They now experience no recruitment or advertising costs, reduced turnover rates, nursing students vying for positions after program completion, and decreased orientation costs due to fewer new hires.
■ Turnover: While "the inability to handle the intense working environment, advanced medical technology, and high patient acuity results in turnover rates of 35–60% in the first year of employment" (Halfer & Graf, 2006, p. 150), from 2003 through 2007, the VNIP turnover rate remains <10% for new graduates completing the internship.

The VNIP program is in its 12th year of implementation and a number of benefits have been identified, specifically, the broad-reaching influence the VNIP framework has had on programs emerging in other regions of the United States. Planners of the VNIP program encourage taking a statewide and/or a regional approach and using components of existing programs rather than "reinventing the wheel." The VNIP framework has demonstrated that a single tool can be used effectively for competency assessment in multiple settings. This framework supports moving away from orientation to the "minutia of nursing practice," meaning the tasks and procedures, and instead focusing on core nursing concepts and clinical judgment development across a variety of situations. VNIP has standardized the approach and model used for new graduates in diverse settings—inclusive of inpatient, acute care, home health, long-term care, and public health settings within and beyond the state of Vermont across the continuum of care.

FUTURE PLANS

As for the future, VNIP is currently involved in several regional and state initiatives that utilize components and/or the entire VNIP framework for initial transition-to-practice programs. Program planners strive continuously to write clearly articulated, concise, and precise performance outcomes expectations that are clinically relevant. These efforts have evolved from writing a "grocery list" of tasks to the development of performance statements that outline safe, effective care and the application of nursing judgment in the clinical practice setting. In turn, shifting from behavioral learning objectives to written performance outcomes expectations is projected to impact on the development and preparation of the preceptors as well.

VNIP has standardized the new graduate competency assessment tool and process in practice settings statewide. Many agencies utilize the same competency tool and evaluative process for all new hires, from new graduate to traveler. Currently, there are several schools of nursing that are adapting these same performance expectations to fit their clinical documentation tools. Imagine a system of nurse development and competency assessment that follows the same process and expectations from school, to initial practice, and on through each new specialty.

VNIP is recognized as a national "best practice" model for preceptor development and support. The Venn diagram in Figure 12.1 of the preceptor's roles of Protector, Evaluator, Educator, and Facilitator has been widely distributed and influences preceptor instruction across the nation. VNIP expanded its data collection and has invited multiple regional initiatives to submit "transition-to-practice" evaluation data through the validated survey tools linked on the VNIP web site. This option could lead to benchmarking at regional, national, and "agency-type" levels. Planners will continue to evaluate the VNIP framework across clinical settings to be inclusive of education, research, regulation, and practice. Longitudinal data collection continues to determine outcomes for individuals who participate in the program as well as for institutions that are part of the VNIP program. Using concepts from

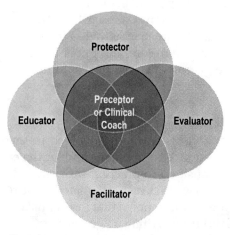

FIGURE 12.1 Preceptor roles

Dr. Lenburg's COPA model, the VNIP will continue to evaluate the competency assessment tool and its validity and reliability with the recent nurse graduates and traveler nurses.

In summary, for institutions—whether rural or urban—considering a nurse transition-to-practice program, it is prudent to begin with the end in mind, that is, defining the desired outcomes. Collaboration with partners desiring the same outcome is important. Then, thoughtful deliberation is critical to determine the resources that are needed to achieve those outcomes. Albert Einstein expressed this approach in the following way: "Any intelligent fool can make things bigger, more complex, and more violent. It takes a touch of genius, and a lot of courage, to move in the opposite direction" (Teach & Murff, 2008).

REFERENCES

American Association of Colleges of Nursing. (n.d.). *Nurse residency program executive summary.* Retrieved October 20, 2010 from University Health System Consortium—UHC 2001 Spring Road Suite 700 Oak Brook, Illinois 60523-1890, Available from http://www.aacn.nche.edu/education/pdf/NurseResidency-ProgramExecSumm.pdf

Armstrong, G. S. (2009). Using quality and safety education for nurses to enhance competency. *Journal of Nursing Education, 48,* 686–693.

Benner, P. (1984). *From novice to expert: Excellence and practice power in clinical nursing.* Menlo Park, CA: Addison Wesley.

Benner, P., Sutphen, M., Leonard, V., & Day, L. (2009). *Educating nurses: A call for radical transformation.* Carnegie Foundation for the Advancement of Teach. San Francisco: Jossey-Bass.

Boyer, S. (2008). Competence and innovation in preceptor development — Updating our programs. *Journal for Nurses in Staff Development, 24*(2), E1–E6.

Boyer, S. (2010, June 15). *Vermont nurses in partnership.* Retrieved July 14, 2010 from http://www.vnip.org/

del Bueno, D. (2005). A crisis in critical thinking. *Nursing Education Perspectives, 26*(15), 278–282.

Duchscher, J. (2008). A process of becoming: The stages of new nursing graduate professional role transition. *The Journal of Continuing Education in Nursing, 39*(10), 441–450.

Duchscher, J. B. (2009). Transition shock: The initial stage of role adaptation for newly graduated Registered Nurses. *Journal of Advanced Nursing. 65*(5), 1103–1113.

Foundation for Nursing Excellence. (2009). *Evidence-based transition to nursing practice initiative in North Carolina; Summary of phase 1 findings.* Raleigh, NC: NC Center for Nursing Excellence, Available from http://www.ffne.org/

Halfer, K., & Graf, E. (2006). Graduate nurse perceptions of the work experience. *Nursing Economics, 24*(3), 50–155. Available from http://www.medscape.com/viewarticle/541778.

Kaeding, T. (1998). The Report on Nursing, December, 1998. Report Commissioned by the Vermont Association of Hospitals and Health Systems. Available from http://www.vahhs.com/lucie/Vonl/VONL%20Presentation.htm

Lenburg, C. (Sept. 30, 1999a). The framework, concepts and methods of the competency outcomes and performance assessment (COPA) model. *Online Journal of Issues in Nursing*, 4(2), Manuscript 2. Available from www.nursingworld.org/MainMenuCategories/ANAMarketplace/ANAPeriodicals/OJIN/TableofContents/Volume41999/No2Sep1999/COPAModel.aspx

Lenburg, C. (Sept. 30, 1999b). Redesigning expectations for initial and continuing competence for contemporary nursing practice. *Online Journal of Issues in Nursing*, 4(2), Manuscript 1. Available from www.nursingworld.org/MainMenuCategories/ANAMarketplace/ANAPeriodicals/OJIN/TableofContents/Volume41999/No2Sep1999/RedesigningExpectationsforInitialandContinuingCompetence.aspx

Lenburg, C. (2009). The COPA model: A comprehensive framework designed to promote. *Nursing Education Perspectives, 30,* 312–317.

Lenburg, C. (2010). Competency outcomes and performance assessment for contemporary nursing education. In L. Caputi (Ed.), *Teaching nursing: The art and science*, Volume 2, (2nd ed.). (pp. 175–215), Glen Ellyn, IL: College of DuPage Press.

Redesigning expectations for initial and continuing competence for contemporary nursing practice. (n.d.).

Robert Wood Johnson Foundation. (2010). *QSEN—Quality and Safety Education for Nurses.* Retrieved September 30, 2010 from http://www.qsen.org/

Teach, R., & Murff, E. (2008). Are the business simulations we play too complex? *Developments in Business Simulation and Experiential Learning, 35,* 205–211.

VNIP. (2008). *Core curriculum for clinical coaching.* Burllington, VT: Queen City Printers.

Weston, M. (2006, May 31). *Integrating generational perspectives in nursing, 11*(2), Manuscript 1. Retrieved October 20, 2010, from *OJIN: The Online Journal of Issues in Nursing*: http://www.nursingworld.org/mods/mod982/generatio nabs.htm

13

North Carolina: Regionally Increasing Baccalaureate Nurses and Evidence-Based Transition-to-Practice Program

Mary P. "Polly" Johnson, Vincent P. Hall, and Joyce W. Roth

North Carolina (NC) implemented two innovative programs in an effort to address the projected shortage of registered nurses across the state. The state's (NC) nursing leaders were concerned about the nursing workforce, especially registered nurses (RNs), in rural communities. The Regionally Increasing Baccalaureate Nursing (RIBN) was designed to increase BSN-prepared nurses; the other program addressed retaining new graduates. The development of a statewide evidence-based transition-to-practice program for novice nurses began with the creation of preceptor education.

As in other parts of the nation, a significant segment of the experienced nursing workforce is nearing retirement age in North Carolina (NC). Furthermore, the majority of RNs currently entering the workforce were educated in community colleges. The state has 25 Associate Degree in Nursing (ADN) programs located in nonmetropolitan areas of NC.

Soon, the state must confront issues associated with a smaller and relatively inexperienced nursing workforce that is expected to care for patients with increasingly complex needs. These challenges are of particular concern in rural and medically underserved regions of the state. More precisely, of the state's 100 counties, 60 are non-metropolitan areas having about one-third of the state's residents (Sheps Center, 2010). Within these nonurban counties are 50 hospitals, about 170 long-term care facilities (NC Division of Health Services Regulation, 2010), and an array of public health and other types of community-based services. In an effort to proactively address short- and long-term nursing workforce needs, the NC Institute of Medicine (NCIOM) Taskforce published the *Nursing Workforce Report* (NCIOM, 2004a). This hallmark document listed 16 recommendations focusing on development and sustainment of nursing faculty; recruitment and retention of nurses in the workforce; nursing education programs; and transition from graduate to RN to professional practice. In response to the NCIOM recommendations, the Foundation for Nursing Excellence (FFNE) assumed leadership in developing two nursing initiatives, the RIBN model and an *Evidence-Based Nurse Transition-to-Practice Program*. These initiatives addressed two NCIOM (2004b) recommendations:

- Increase the production of BSN-educated nurses to achieve a ratio of 60% BSN:40% ADN/diploma nurses.
- Study options to improve school-to-work transition experiences.

Currently, there also is a critical shortage of faculty in the state; in turn, this restricts expanding student admissions into nursing education programs. For example, in October 2009, there were reported to be 127 full-time and 74 part-time unfilled faculty positions (NC Board of Nursing [NCBON], 2010a). Among others, one factor contributing to faculty shortages is that the existing pool of nurses in the workforce are not academically prepared to assume faculty positions. At minimum, a Master's Degree in Nursing (MSN) is the academic requirement for nursing faculty to meet accreditation standards.

Demographically, of all nurses holding the MSN degree in NC, 80% completed the BSN degree as their educational entry level into the workforce. Yet, in 2009, of all new RN graduates in NC, more than two-thirds (66%) were only prepared at the ADN level (NCBON, 2010b). Of these, the majority resided in rural and/or medically under-served areas of the state, and, on graduating, returned there to work as RNs (Cecil G. Sheps Center, 2008). Completion of a 2-year ADN program is a relatively "quick fix" to increase the number of RNs in NC's workforce. However, only 15% of nurses prepared at the ADN level are likely to pursue additional education, specifically BSN and MSN degrees, the essential academic requirements for the nursing faculty role (Bevill, Cleary, Lacey, & Nooney, 2007). Coupled with insufficient nursing faculty, NC's nursing education pattern results in few(er) nurses with the BSN and higher degrees who are available for advanced roles in clinical practice, research, management, and public health. These educational patterns place NC nursing on a serious and declining workforce trajectory.

REGIONALLY INCREASING BACCALAUREATE NURSES MODEL

Over the years, administrators of nursing education programs have dili-gently worked to improve student articulation from ADN to BSN pro-grams with varying degrees of success in establishing and sustaining such partnerships. Given the important role community colleges have in educating the NC nursing workforce and placement of graduates in rural settings, the RIBN partnership was implemented. The novel approach allows students in the ADN program a dual enrollment with the BSN program. The RIBN partnerships provide mutual access for both academic entities to valuable resources, including faculty expertise, laboratories, libraries, and diverse student populations. The ultimate goal of the RIBN is to effectively respond to the NC nursing workforce deficits as stated in the NCIOM recommendations. This goal is also consistent with the recommendation put forth in the recent Institute of Medicine (IOM) report, *The Future of Nursing: Leading Change, Advancing Health* (2011).

A pilot RIBN project was implemented (2008) in Western NC (WNC). The Robert Wood Johnson Foundation (RWJF) and Northwest Health Foundation (NWHF) awarded a 2-year Partners Investing in Nursing's Future (PIN) grant to The Jonas Center for Nursing Excellence in New York City. The Jonas Center implemented the multiregional RIBN project that included WNC and metropolitan New York. Subsequently, FFNE, Western Carolina University (WCU), and Asheville-BuncombeTechnicalCommunity College (AB Tech) partnered to develop the WNC-RIBN project. Project planners reviewed and adapted the Oregon Consortium for Nursing Education (OCNE) model to the NC context (Tanner, Gubrud-Howe, & Shores, 2008). In Oregon, the OCNE model was implemented at the state level and included all public university and community colleges having nursing education programs. While the statewide approach may seem to be ideal, it may not be realistic for states with both significant rural regions and large numbers of universities and community colleges such as the case for NC. Hence, NC implemented the RIBN model on a small scale hoping that these programs could serve as the "seed" that would lead to other BSN programs collaborating with community colleges across the state (Sizemore, Robbins, Hoke, & Billings, 2007). As a result, the NC RIBN model was implemented at the regional level. The NC model provides the framework for community colleges to partner with private and public universities to offer an accessible BSN program to students in rural areas of the state.

Essentially, the NC RIBN model is a seamless educational track to obtain the BSN but it is a rigorous and intense 4-year program.

Admission requirements for the RIBN program are more stringent than for the ADN offered at a community college or the BSN offered at a university. Admission requirements and the RIBN curriculum are available online at the following websites: http://ffne.org/file_library/ WNC%20RIBN%20Admission%20Criteria%20Fall%202011%20v2.pdf and http://www.ffne.org/file_library/WNCRIBNPlanCurriculumNar rative.pdf.

In the first 3 years of the RIBN program of study, a student completes courses at a local community college along with web-based university courses. This arrangement helps to keep the cost lower for the student. At the end of the third year of study, the student is awarded the ADN degree and is eligible to sit for the RN National Council Licensure Examination (NCLEX-RN). To matriculate into the upper-division courses at the university in the fourth year of the RIBN program, the student must have successfully passed the NCLEX. Students may work as RNs after the third year and during the fourth year of the program if they wish to.

Courses in the final year of study focus on professional nursing practice, leadership, gerontology, community/public health, and evidenced-based practice. The RIBN curriculum is concept based and utilizes teaching techniques such as unfolding case studies to support learning. Emphasis is placed on clinical reasoning and integration of didactic content with clinical experiences (Benner, Sutphen, Leonard, & Day, 2010).

A critical retention point for students in the RIBN program occurs after completion of the third year and successful completion of the NCLEX. On entering the workforce, it is not unusual for an RN to opt out of completing course requirements for the university-based BSN courses. Leaders of the RIBN model currently are exploring strategies to help retain students in the program during this critical period. Input is being sought from local advisory boards composed of regional health care leaders who advise and support the RIBN project and its students. A Student Success Advocate (SSA) has also been hired to market the RIBN program; advise students before, during, and after admission and assist students in obtaining financial aid and accessing academic services that can support an individual's academic success.

Overall, North Carolina organizations made great strides in implementing the program at select sites. To date, WNC partners of the RIBN have successfully

▪ Established [dual] entrance admission requirements for the community college and university.

- Received approval from both educational institutions for the 4-year WNC RIBN curriculum.
- Reviewed 20 applications for the first cohort of 16 students to be admitted (Fall Semester 2010).
- Obtained approval from NC Nurse Scholars Commission for the RIBN as an official academic BSN track. This approval qualifies students for the merit-based loan program making them eligible for up to 4 years of funding.
- Implemented ongoing evaluation to identify success indicators for program development.
- Developed and disseminated guidelines to adapt the RIBN model in other states http://www.ffne.org/index.php?action=page&page_id=6.

With the successes of the RIBN in WNC, the FFNE established five additional regional partnerships, including public and private community colleges and universities. Offering the first 3 years of the program at community colleges creates an economically feasible academic opportunity for students in rural and medically underserved areas. In turn, this is projected to increase the number of nurses with a BSN degree who are more likely to pursue advanced education and, hopefully, increase the number of nursing faculty and nurses in advanced practice roles.

NC EVIDENCE-BASED NURSE TRANSITION-TO-PRACTICE MODEL

In 2005, the FFNE collaborated with the state's Area Health Education Centers (NCAHEC) and the Center for Nursing to design and implement an evidence-based transition-to-practice model for nurses. The Agency for Healthcare Research and Quality (AHRQ) provided the financial support for a conference having as its goal the identification of essential core competencies for newly licensed nurses as they prepare to transition to practice (NCFFNE, 2006). Representatives from these three groups along with other invited nursing leaders from practice, education, and research became the Steering Committee for the Transition-to-Practice project. Subsequently, the literature was examined for evidence that could be used to develop the NC project. An Advisory Panel comprised NC health care employers, staff development, educators, regulators, professional associations, philanthropic foundations, newly licensed RNs, and the public offered unique perspectives from across the state. Generous funding for the project was provided by the Blue Cross Blue Shield of NC Foundation, the Duke Endowment, and Kate B. Reynolds Charitable Trust.

PHASE I

The first phase of the project entailed obtaining longitudinal data on competence and confidence of newly licensed RNs after 2, 4, and 6 months of practice. The Newly Licensed RN survey, developed with data from the AHRQ-funded conference (2005), provided information related to competence development, practice errors, risk of practice breakdown, as well as confidence development of the new nurse. Following Institutional review board (IRB) approval, the sample consisted of newly licensed nurses and their preceptor in three rounds of data collection. The findings revealed a statistically significant finding that the better the quality of the new nurse/preceptor relationship, the higher the perceived competency levels by the new RN. The data indicated a low competence score in clinical reasoning and judgment by the new nurse in all three rounds of data collection after an average length (~8-week) orientation program. Of the three types of orientation, none was superior relative to development of the new nurse, and more than 19% of nurses in the study in all three rounds of the study reported that they "often" or "always" felt overwhelmed (FFNE, 2008a).

PHASE II

In the second phase, the Steering Committee undertook a more extensive review of the literature, focusing on the roles, responsibilities, and preparation of preceptors (coaches, mentors) to enhance the development of newly licensed nurses, increased satisfaction with their work, and hopefully, also improve retention rates (Alamada, Carafoli, Flattery, French, & McNamara, 2004; Ardoin & Pryor, 2006; Butler & Felts, 2006; Delaney, 2003; Godinez, Schweiger, Gruver, & Ryan, 1999; Orsini, 2005; Ronsten, Andersson, & Gustafsson, 2005; Schumacher, 2007; Smith & Chalker, 2005). The literature further supported the importance of preceptor preparation in successful transition to work programs (Floyd, Kretschmann, & Young, 2005; Hyrkas & Shoemaker, 2007; McNiesh, 2007; Moseley & Davies, 2008; Sorensen & Yankech, 2008; Yonge, Hagler, Cox, & Drefs, 2008).

With that evidence, surveys were sent to NC health care nurse administrators in acute care, long-term care, public health, and home health to obtain information about preceptor preparation practices as well as their use of simulation to assess new nurse competence. Respondents were asked to specify their institutional requirements for an RN to serve as a preceptor, that is, academic and experiential preparation requirements, expectations of the preceptor, and strategies the preceptor used to assess competence and confidence development of the new nurse (i.e., preceptee). Findings from the survey revealed that only a few agencies in NC were using simulation in any way to assess new nurses' competence. More importantly, the survey revealed that there was no consistent preceptor preparation in the state (FFNE, 2008b).

In 2009, the FFNE convened two invitational working conferences, one focusing on the use of simulation to assess new nurse competence and the other addressing preceptor preparation and development. Participants identified essential content and concepts that should be included in a preceptor preparation program along with strategies for use of simulation to assess progression of preceptees. Focus groups with new nurses supported the importance of the new nurse/preceptor relationship and underscored the current lack of consistency in preceptor preparation.

Based on feedback provided by participants at the invitational conferences, the Steering Committee developed preceptor education tools. The preceptor package consists of three web-based modules and three low-fidelity simulation experiences. The learning modules were developed by staff educators who prepare preceptors in both rural and urban health care facilities. The learning modules address (a) dimensions of the preceptor role, (b) communication in the preceptor role, and (c) the transition process of new nurses. Quality and Safety Education for Nurses competencies provide the framework for the modules and include information on "best and promising" practice models (Cronenwett, Barnsteiner, Johnson, & Taylor, 2007). The self-paced learning modules are interactive, integrate reflective exercises, and include web links for supplementary resources such as the TeamSTEPPs: http://www.ahrq.gov/qual/teamstepps.

The posttests are also a useful tool to document strengths and opportunities to enhance an individual's preceptor development. The Steering Committee pilot tested the preceptor preparation package and sought feedback to tailor the program to the needs of NC health care facilities.

PHASE III

In the third phase of implementing the transition-to-practice program, nine hospitals were selected to participate, representing both rural and urban regions, ranging in size from 58 to 712 inpatient beds. In early 2010, 180 preceptors in these facilities completed the web-based modules and were awarded two continuing education (CE) contact hours for each module. Of the total, 75 preceptors completed 6 hours of "facilitated" simulation experiences to learn how to assess competencies of a novice nurse's (preceptee) techniques and skills. The simulated experiences focused on patient hand-off, response(s) to an adverse event(s), interprofessional communication, prioritization of care, and generational differences.

Preliminary evaluation of the learning modules and the simulation experiences indicate that both have been highly effective development tools for preceptors. Evaluation data were collected from participants, facilitators, and the project director to identify the effectiveness and gaps in modules and simulation experiences. New and experienced alike, preceptors reiterated the value of the modules' content, instructional methods, and simulation experiences. Additional data will be collected from hospitals in the pilot study after 2 months of working with newly licensed nurses from preceptors, nurse managers, and preceptees to further evaluate the effectiveness of the learning package. Similar to Phase I, data will be collected over the first 6 months of a new nurse's employment to assess effects of the program on his or her competence and confidence development, risk for error, and retention in the workplace. The analysis of the data for the project is projected to be completed in 2011.

Based on extensive feedback from preceptors, administrators, and preceptees, the web-based learning modules and simulation exercises will be revised. Additional modules will be developed to address identified learning needs. The FFNE plans to offer the materials in 2011 for a nominal fee to individual nurses as well as health care systems in NC, nationally and internationally. The standardized evidence-based preceptor development program and nurse transition program is cost effective and designed to be accessible to health professionals in rural areas.

In summary, North Carolina's journey to plan for and build an adequately sized and appropriately prepared nursing workforce in rural and urban areas of the state has just begun. Two initiatives, the RIBN and transition to practice, have garnered statewide interest. This educational model has been replicated in five regional community colleges and university partnerships. There are plans to admit the first student cohort in 2012. Nurse administrators, preceptors, and novice nurses speak highly of the accessible standardized and user-friendly learning tools. Nursing leaders in NC believe these initiatives can positively impact on the projected nursing workforce needs in rural and urban communities in NC, as well as nationally and internationally. Information on these projects continues to be updated and is available at www.ffne.org.

REFERENCES

Almada, P., Carafoli, K., Flattery, J. B., French, D. A., & McNamara, M. (2004). Improving the retention rate of newly graduated nurses. *Journal for Nurses in Staff Development, 20*(6), 268–273.

Ardoin, K. B., & Pryor, S. K. (2006). The new grad: A success story. *Journal for Nurses in Staff Development, 22*(3), 129–133.

Benner, P., Sutphen, M., Leonard, V., & Day, L. (2010). *Educating nurses: A call for radical reform.* San Francisco, CA: Jossey-Bass.

Bevill, J., Cleary, B., Lacey, L., & Nooney, G. (2007). Educational mobility of RNs in North Carolina: Who will teach tomorrow's nurses?: A report on the first study to longitudinally examine educational mobility among nurses. *American Journal of Nursing, 107*(5), 60–70.

Butler, M. R., & Felts, J. (2006). Tool kit for the staff mentor: Strategies for improving retention. *Journal of Continuing Education in Nursing, 37*(5), 210–213.

Cecil G. Sheps Center for Health Services Research, University of North Carolina at Chapel Hill. (2008). A Study of Associate Degree Nursing Program Success—Evidence from the 2002 Cohort, 38–42.

Cecil G. Sheps Center for Health Services Research, University of North Carolina. (2010). Informal report of highest degrees earned by RNs practicing in North Carolina in 2008.

Cronenwett, L., Barnsteiner, J., Johnson, J., & Taylor, D. (2007). Quality and safety education for nurses. *Nursing Outlook, 55*(3), 122–131.

Delaney, C. (2003). Walking a fine line: Graduate nurses' transition experiences during orientation. *Journal of Nursing Education, 42*(10), 437–443.

Floyd, B. O., Kretschmann, S., & Young, H. (2005). Facilitating role transition for new graduate RNs in a semi-rural healthcare setting. *Journal for Nurses in Staff Development, 21*(6), 284–290.

Foundation for Nursing Excellence. (2006). *AHRQ grant final progress report: Building an evidence-based transition to practice project.* Retrieved from http://ffne.org/file_library/AHRQ%20Grant%20Final%20Progress%20Report.pdf

Foundation for Nursing Excellence. (2008a). *Progress report phase I study of North Carolina evidence-based transition to practice initiative project.* doi: http://ffne.org/file_library/Phase%20I%20Findings%20Summary.pdf

Foundation for Nursing Excellence. (2008b). *Survey of clinical agencies.* Unpublished data.

Godinez, G., Schweiger, J., Gruver, J., & Ryan, P. (1999). Role transition from graduate to staff nurse: A qualitative analysis. *Journal for Nurses in Staff Development, 15*(3), 97–110.

Hyrkas, K. S., & Shoemaker, M. (2007). Changes in the preceptor role: Revisiting preceptors' perceptions of benefits, rewards, support and commitment to the role. *Journal of Advanced Nursing, 60*(5), 513–524.

McNiesh, S. (2007). Demonstrating holistic clinical judgment: Preceptors perceptions of new graduate nurses. *Holistic Nursing Practice, 21*(2), 72–78.

Moseley, L. G., & Davies, M. (2008). What do mentors find difficult? *Journal of Clinical Nursing, 17*(12), 1627–1634.

North Carolina Board of Nursing. (2010a). *North Carolina trends in nursing education: 2004–2009.* Retrieved from http://www.ncbon.com/content.aspx?id=1090

North Carolina Board of Nursing. (2010b). *Currently licensed RNs*. Retrieved from http://www.ncbon.com/LicensureStats/LicStat-RNWSTAT.asp

North Carolina Division of Health Service Regulation. (2010). *State medical facilities plan*. doi: http://www.ncsmfp.org/20101.html

North Carolina Institute of Medicine. (2004a). Task Force on the North Carolina Nursing Workforce Report.

North Carolina Institute of Medicine. (2004b). Task Force on the North Carolina Nursing Workforce Report, 104–107.

Orsini, C. H. (2005). A nurse transition program for orthopaedics: Creating a new culture for nurturing new graduates. *Orthopaedic Nursing, 24*(4), 240–248.

Ronsten, B., Andersson, E., & Gustafsson, B. (2005). Confirming mentorship. *Journal of Nursing Management, 13*(4), 312–321.

Schumacher, D. L. (2007). Caring behaviors of preceptors as perceived by new nursing graduate orientees. *Journal for Nurses in Staff Development, 23*(4), 186–192.

Sheps Center (2010). Center for Health Services Research, University of North Carolina at Chapel Hill. *North Carolina Health Professions 2009 Data Book*, 126–128. http://www.shepscenter.unc.edu/hp/publications/2009_HPDS_DataBook.pdf

Sizemore, M. H., Robbins, L. K., Hoke, M. M., & Billings, D. M. (2007). Outcomes of ADN-BSN partnerships to increase baccalaureate prepared nurses. *International Journal of Nursing Education Scholarship, 4*(1), 1–18.

Smith, A., & Chalker, N. J. (2005). Preceptor continuity in a nurse internship program: The nurse intern's perception. *Journal for Nurses in Staff Development, 21*(2), 47–54.

Sorensen, H., & Yankech, L. R. (2008). Precepting in the fast lane: Improving critical thinking in new graduate nurses. *Journal of Continuing Education in Nursing, 39*(5), 208–216.

Tanner, C., Gubrud-Howe, P., & Shores, L. (2008). The Oregon consortium for nursing Education: A response to the nursing shortage. *Policy, Politics, and Nursing Practice, 9*(3), 203–209.

Yonge, O., Hagler, P., Cox, C., & Drefs, S. (2008). Listening to preceptors part B. *Journal for Nurses in Staff Development, 24*(1), 21–26.

14

Washington State: Rural Outreach Nursing Education Program

Helen Hing Kuebel and Karen L. Joiner

A persistent challenge in rural regions of the state of Washington (WA) is recruiting nurses. Another challenge is retaining Registered Nurses (RNs) after they relocate from an urban community. In response to a statewide hospital executive request for nursing education delivered in rural communities, Lower Columbia College located in Longview, WA, responded with the Rural Outreach Nursing Education (RONE) program. This chapter explores components of the transition-to-practice program along with strategies to retain nurses in rural communities.

The first step in the development of the RONE entailed surveying Washington's critical access hospitals (CAHs) and reviewing state data collected to determine the state's need for RNs in rural areas. The assessment was undertaken by the University of Washington and Washington's Center for Nursing. Cost comparisons were documented comparing the cost of hiring "travel nurses" versus costs of financially supporting a nursing education program that could be available in a rural community. Both the Western Washington Area Health Education Center (AHEC) and the Eastern Washington AHEC were instrumental in surveying CAHs to determine their nursing needs as well as interest in developing a solution to make education more accessible for local individuals wishing to pursue nursing education. The survey also included an inquiry to identify local nurses holding a master's degree who could potentially serve as clinical instructors.

PLANNING AND IMPLEMENTATION OF RONE

Partnerships are important in developing outreach programs. Community colleges often have the flexibility as well as the technology to deliver distance education and to pursue such partnerships. In the development of RONE, after the education partner was identified, a statewide committee was formed to leverage resources and to secure grants to plan and implement the program. Since nursing is a popular occupation, institutions of higher education, in particular community college councils, were interested in addressing the educational needs in their catchments. The planners of the RONE initiative organized a statewide "steering committee" with members representing Lower Columbia College, the Washington Center for Nursing, the Rural Hospital Association, several CAHs, AHECs, migrant and community health centers, the state board for community and technical colleges, and the state labor relations council. An educational pipeline was delineated, identifying students in high school who could progress to the Licensed Practical Nurse (LPN), to the Associate Degree in Nursing, and then the RN-Baccalaureate in Science in Nursing (BSN). The model allowed students to stop after the first year at the LPN level. The RONE model was designed to be flexible; if a community decides not to repeat the project, it could be discontinued.

The education partner has the responsibility to secure regulatory and accreditation board approvals prior to implementation. The local college should develop a timetable that includes curriculum development and implementation along with needed resources (funding, personnel, time) for each phase. The education partner must consider boundary issues since most institutions of higher learning in a state are assigned specific geographical areas for the recruitment of students and the offering of programs. Accessing rural communities via technology may involve crossing another institution's service area. Turf can become a political issue and therefore attention to academic boundaries is important. Likewise, college administrators should be fully informed about the project's progress, be aware of the fiscal requirement, and be supportive for the project to succeed.

The rural outreach option must adhere to academic standards consistent with those of the main campus, including robust learning outcomes, evaluation measures, and a budget to support the program. Also, for accreditation purposes, the curriculum must be consistent with that of the main campus and adapted with web-based learning opportunities. Faculty must meet academic and clinical accreditation standards. With respect to technology to offer distance education, a web-based learning management system with campus support as well as off-site technical support is essential for the learning activities that include online assignments for theory courses, clinical discussions, along with high-fidelity simulation experiences. It is important for campus-based faculty to visit the rural outreach students at least twice a year. Policies must be developed regarding minimal computer technology and software by students and faculty involved in the project. Preferably, the project must have a website that reflects accurate information about the program admission criteria, application deadlines, expectations of students enrolled in the program (e.g., schedules, time, and technology requirements) and costs associated with the program.

Simulation experiences can enhance learning; however, RONE does not replace simulation for clinical assignments. Rather, patient simulation activities are viewed as homework that supports clinical experiences. It is helpful to use a simulation curriculum that is fully developed such as the one developed by Medical Education Technologies (METI). Additional online learning enhancements used for the RONE project are the learning packages available for purchase through Assessment Technologies, Inc. (ATI). Both METI and ATI are examples of learning support programs and technology that are available to nursing programs. The authors of this chapter have no relationship to endorse either of these companies; rather, the examples are illustrative of materials that RONE used successfully. Additional elements in planning and implementing the programs include the following:

- Develop a timetable and list of activities for each of the Steering Committee members.
- Obtain letters of commitment from the hospital and other local partners; include details about the financial support for clinical faculty over 2 years for the Associate Degree in Nursing program.
- Recruit a local rural mentor for students, that is, a hospital-based person who is available to answer questions and assist students. This individual does not replace college academic advisement.
- Support recruitment and academic advisement for students in rural areas. For RONE, a minimum of two students and a maximum of 4–5 students are optimal for a successful rural program.
- Undertake complete Community Asset Mapping, that is, identify the strengths and resources in a community, including individuals with expertise in particular areas, local events, and activities that could be used for clinical experiences (i.e., health fairs, child care centers, and senior activities), local industrial, and ethnic support councils. This information will assist in deciding on the size of the cohort.
- Assess rural partner's resources for offering on-site courses such as computers for testing, classroom space, patient/client census, and other local clinical learning opportunities. Often, all the clinical objectives cannot be achieved in the local community (e.g., psychiatric,

obstetrical, and critical care). "Clustered" clinical learning activities in a larger institution in another city was one strategy used to meet students' educational requirements.

■ Formal legal contracts need to be in place between the education partner with hospitals and other clinical sites; include specific details such as space, technology, financial commitments for clinical instructor(s), and other project requirements (i.e., travel, technology support, liability, etc.).

■ Establish an evaluation matrix that includes timeframes and benchmarks for the program, to include feedback from faculty, students, and partnering institutions. This information also assists rural partnering institutions to determine if they wish to start or continue the nursing education program. If the rural program option is a different program from the campus-based option, are the intended outcomes for the two consistent? Are admission criteria similar? Is the NCLEX pass rate compiled separately for the two? These criteria must also be addressed in program reports to regulatory and accreditation agencies (e.g., State Board of Nursing, National League for Nursing Accrediting Commission [NLNAC], American Association of Colleges of Nursing [AACN]).

■ Discuss with RNs at the CAH the defined program goals, clinical assignments, and student objectives. It is essential that the staff understand the role of a clinical instructor versus that of a staff nurse for the project.

Recruit and orientate qualified clinical faculty in the local area. Along with clinical supervision, the faculty will be expected to proctor on-site as well as online exams.

Clinical Instructor Responsibilities

All new instructors for the RONE project are required to attend a 2-day program orientation held at the campus in Longview, Washington. Prior to being employed by the college, an applicant's references are checked and an unencumbered Washington RN license is verified. Other documentation is also reviewed, such as immunizations and cardiopulmonary resuscitation card.

1. Discussion with the Nursing Program Director to review student rights and responsibilities:
   ■ Lower Columbia Community College (LCC) Program overview
   ■ Student "due process" and liability issues, patient safety, confidentiality, etc.
   ■ LCC Student Handbook

- Nursing Student Handbook, clinical expectations of student and faculty
- Instructor identification
- Documentation of student performance
- Nursing program student forms/documents
- Review of rural partners' contracts relative to clinical faculty roles, responsibilities (i.e., nurse educator role vs. staff nurse role)
- Review LCC faculty contract, salary, and faculty handbook
- Articulate expectations of proctoring online and in-class exams (i.e., ATI supplemental tests, course-related exams)
- Use simulation scenarios (METI) when available as clinical homework to enhance student learning
- Partner RONE clinical faculty with the on-campus eLearning classroom instructors and the eLearning nursing coordinator

2. Review of didactic and clinical objectives for each semester by campus-based course coordinators:
   - Establish communication procedures and schedules for clinical and online didactic courses
   - Review course syllabi and textbooks. Provide textbooks and other relevant course materials to clinical faculty
   - Explain student's assignments relative to didactic and theoretical content
   - Review course and clinical grading policies; expectations for student achievement at different levels
   - Articulate policies for patient assignments for students
   - Discuss policies regarding student's clinical placements. The RONE clinical instructor must work with the local hospital to ensure that a student, if not employed by the hospital, meets all agency requirements (i.e., immunizations, etc.). If questions arise, the clinical instructor should contact the LCC Nursing eLearning Coordinator

3. Explain precise number of supervised hours and objectives for each clinical course
   - Meet with students on the first clinical day to review academic and institutional policies and faculty/student communication protocols. Inform students about your philosophy of nursing as related to LCC program philosophy. Supplies and materials will be sent to the instructor and student as needed for new nursing skills
   - Discuss strategies for student "demonstration/return demonstration" of essential nursing skills
   - Schedule regular meetings with campus-based course coordinator to discuss individual student's learning needs and progress in online courses. Discussions can be via telephone and/or e-mail

■ Plan for a preconference and structured postconference with students for each clinical day or week (depending on assignments/schedules)

■ Assign patients to a student, based on his or her learning needs. Clinical faculty are expected to know assigned patient's diagnoses, medications, and treatments, and relate these aspects of nursing care to a student's clinical decision making and development of critical thinking

■ Read all assigned course materials. Be able to relate this information to students' clinical assignments

■ Maintain daily documentation on each student's clinical performance and his or her ability to relate theory to the assignment

■ Individualize instruction and supervision to help a student learn how to apply nursing knowledge in dynamic patient care situations (with *equal emphasis* on cognitive, affective, and psychomotor learning domains)

  ■ Building student's critical thinking skills/clinical decision-making skills

  ■ Developing student's professional attitudes

  ■ Developing student's technical skills

■ Understand that patient, student, and instructor safety are paramount in all clinical experiences

■ Grade care plans and written assignments; return to student in timely manner

■ Schedule weekly meetings with students or as needed. Meet with each student and complete midrotation conferences. Complete formal written midterm evaluations based on clinical evaluation tool (included in the syllabus) and meet with student to discuss progress/grade

■ Schedule conference with each student at the completion of clinical hours to discuss formal written evaluation

■ Proctor ATI tests and theory tests (required password to access web-based exams)

■ Submit final grades to campus-based course coordinator. Clinical courses are graded as Pass/Fail

■ Distribute student perception of (adjunct) faculty evaluation forms as directed by Office of Instruction. These forms are completed by students, and returned to the Department Chairperson, the Nursing Program Director, and Dean, who review the anonymous forms and then return them to the individual faculty member

■ Evaluate effectiveness of clinical agency as a student learning site. This written document is to be filed with the agency contract in the

LCC Nursing Program Office. The forms are sent to the instructor at the end of the semester

LESSONS LEARNED

Online delivery of courses can be an effective strategy but there are inherent challenges. Most importantly, always have an alternative plan should the technology not function properly. For example, in rural areas there may not be high-speed internet connections; telephonic dial-up connections may require long-distance charges, or an older computer and software may not be able to access or download large electronic files. Consequently, a student may only be able to access the internet at the hospital or perhaps the local library (at times when it is open to the public). For that reason, assignment due dates should take into consideration potential technology challenges. Regarding exam proctors, have preapproved individuals who are familiar with the technology and the students in case the clinical instructor cannot be available.

The RONE administrators recommend offering a detailed program orientation for each nursing student at the beginning of every quarter and for each course. Maintain a log of problems that arise and how these were resolved. Note gaps and repetitive content. What went well? What needs improvement? Qualitative anecdotal comments can enhance quantitative program evaluation measures. Invite students in the rural outreach program to the main campus for important events to expose them to other faculty, students, and the college. Finally, remember to celebrate the students' success in their home community and on the main campus.

EVALUATION

The evaluation of the RONE project required the time for students to complete the program and complete the licensure examination. As mentioned earlier, similar evaluation elements are used for the outreach program as those used for the campus-based program. Additionally, the outreach programs evaluated the following criteria:

- *Faculty*: Completed quarterly by students
- *Clinical sites*: Completed by clinical facility
- *Students*: ATI assessment data by cohort, and compared with campus-based classes; simulation surveys and "point of leaving" surveys
- *Resources*: Student advising, technology, and other off-site resources

In summary, the RONE project was developed to meet the nursing needs of rural communities across Washington. Nursing education was made more accessible for a limited number of students who lived and worked in a rural community, and strategies were developed to retain nurses in these settings. Details about RONE can be obtained from the authors and from the following website: www.lowercolumbia.edu/nursing

15

Alaska Frontier: Statewide Competency Development Initiative

Cynthia J. Roleff, Julie McNulty, and Jill Montague

Successful nurse transition-to-practice programs depend on appropriately prepared and supported preceptors. Rural health care providers experience challenges associated with environmental and geographical factors. In this chapter, the authors describe the remote Alaskan health context along with substantiating the need for a nurse preceptor preparation program. Highlighted herein is the description of a statewide collaborative group process to develop and implement both a face-to-face and distance education preceptor program. The approach is to measure expected behaviors. The group developed competencies for the rural nurse "generalist" and nine other nursing specialties. The outcomes of the group process and standardized competences are described.

Alaska spans a large geographical area that is twice as large as the state of Texas (Figure 15.1) and has a population density of fewer than 700,000 residents (US Census Bureau, 2009). The health care delivery system in Alaska is comprised of medical centers located in urban areas (e.g., Anchorage, Juneau, and Fairbanks) and a network of smaller "hub" facilities located in outlying rural communities. In turn, these hubs are referral facilities for ill patients who live and work in the more remote villages (Figure 15.2 shows one of these systems). It is not unusual for a village or even a hub community to be inaccessible by road (ground transportation), and only accessible by boat or air transportation. As for the rural "hub" facilities, these tend to be small and unable to offer most specialty services such as pediatrics, obstetrics,

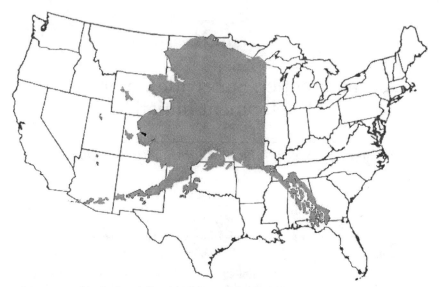

FIGURE 15.1   Alaska in relation to other mainland states

oncology, orthopedics, neurology, etc. Consequently, when a village resident becomes seriously ill, he or she must be evacuated to the nearest "hub" hospital either by a small plane, boat, four-wheeled all-terrain vehicle, or snowmobile. Once at the hub facility, the patient may then need to be referred and transported to a distant urban-based medical center to obtain a more complex level of care.

Coordinating and implementing evacuation processes for a sick patient can be a complex logistical nightmare. It is not unusual to experience extensive transportation delays associated with inclement weather. Consequently, nurses who work in rural and remote Alaska health care facilities must know how to stabilize and treat patients while awaiting transportation as well as provide support during the transport. It is unrealistic to expect a recent graduate to be proficient with these complex nursing skills or to have the confidence to function in such an austere environment. Consider the following comments by J. M. about her experience as a Registered Nurse (RN) in rural Alaska.

[Upon] Graduation from nursing school in 1989 I was apprehensive about my first job, fearing that I did not know enough to practice safely. During my last semester at the University of Alaska, Anchorage [UAA] a presenter from the Alaska Native Medical Center [ANMC] spoke to the class about a 5-month internship program for new graduates.

The Alaska native health care system
Typical referral patterns

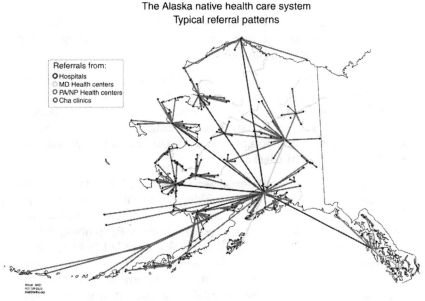

Referrals from:
○ Hospitals
○ MD Health centers
○ PA/NP Health centers
○ Cha clinics

FIGURE 15.2 Alaska native health care system

I applied and was hired by a hospital in rural Alaska. I spent the first 5 months at ANMC taking part in the comprehensive nursing internship. We spent one or two days a week in classroom sessions. The majority of the time we were on the units with preceptors. We spent a month working in various hospital units, including OB, pediatrics, surgery, medical floors and the emergency room. I was privileged to work with some of the best nurses in the hospital. The [pay back] commitment was fulfilled by working for 19 months at the sponsoring rural facility. Another new graduate and I went to work in a remote Native community in rural Alaska. After completing the ANMC internship, I felt more prepared for the adventure that awaited me. I had completed ACLS, PALS, and NRP training, and had experience in all of the acute care areas.

Working in bush [remote] Alaska was a unique experience in that my co-workers and patients were my neighbors and friends. I worked with individuals from all over the United States as well as those who were born and raised in the community. More than half of the nurses were travelers [on temporary assignment from other states]. My preceptor had lived and worked in the local community for several years. She was the person I went to with my questions and was the most experienced nurse on the unit. Although she was an excellent preceptor, there was no formal structure to guide the process [my learning and skill progression].

I worked on the adult unit of the 50-bed hospital which was built on stilts. All the building's water and sewer pipes are above ground due to year-round permafrost in the ground which prohibits digging and maintaining essential public utilities.

Medivacs [transports of a patient to another, usually larger facility] are not unusual. Hospital staff often volunteered to accompany a patient to Anchorage either as a planned or an emergency transport. While the flights were very stressful, visiting Anchorage was enjoyable . . . shopping, going to a movie, and taking advantage of activities not available in rural Alaska.

One of my more memorable experiences happened on a day I was not scheduled to work. I had been working for about three months and lived in housing that was adjacent to the hospital. It was winter and very, very cold; about minus-100 degrees Fahrenheit, taking into consideration the wind-chill factor. I was called in to work by the friend who had completed the internship with me. Upon reporting to the hospital, I was asked to accompany a patient via air Medivac to the Anchorage hospital. The patient was an elderly woman with pneumonia. She was vented, sedated and paralyzed. Having had little critical care experience, needless to say, I was overwhelmed. I was greatly relieved to hear a physician would be accompanying me on the flight.

The patient was loaded into an orange basket used for transport, then into the ambulance. We drove to the small local airport to catch the evening flight to Anchorage. In this small hospital there was no Medivac team, no respiratory therapist, and only one staff member who really understood how to work with the ventilator. Among the hospital staff that day the anxiety level was high; the goal was—get the patient to Anchorage as quickly and as safely as possible.

Upon arriving at the local airport a forklift raised the patient, the physician and me up to the plane's cargo door. Nine passenger seats were folded flat and the stretcher was placed on top. The physician and I sat next to the stretcher, unbuckled. I remember thinking: "I thought a plane couldn't take off when someone was not buckled-up." Other passengers then entered the plane and took seats next to us. Fortunately there were no delays in the plane's departure that day. (Oftentimes in the winter, a plane may need to remain on the runway waiting for weather to clear which could be several days. Sometimes, flights coming in to rural Alaska must return to Anchorage due to unsafe landing conditions.)

That trip to Anchorage was the longest 1 hour and 10 minute flight I have ever been on. We had to 'bag' [manually ventilate] the patient during the entire flight. I spent the whole time bracing my body so I could remain sitting and not dislodge the breathing tube. On arrival in Anchorage we travelled by ambulance to ANMC. I was very relieved when we arrived in the ICU, and the patient was handed over to the nurse and respiratory therapist. My biceps hurt from bagging the patient for more than 2 hours.

Reflecting back on this adventure on my first job made me realize how little I knew. Years later, I ended up working with the respiratory therapist who was on duty that day. She was amazed that I did not have a stethoscope for that transport. I told her, it wouldn't have done much good as it was impossible to hear anything in the plane or in the back of an ambulance, necessitating palpable blood pressure measurement. My goal was met when the patient safely arrived in Anchorage even though I had not received any formal orientation or preceptorship [experience] in flight nursing. (J. M., Personal Communication, November 20, 2010).

The experiences of J. M. in rural Alaska are not unique, reinforcing that recent graduates need support to help transition from the student role into a competent RN in the workplace. There is a national effort to facilitate this transition. Recently, a landmark report by the Institute of Medicine (IOM) and the Robert Wood Johnson Foundation (RWJF) recommended implementing nurse residency programs (IOM, 2010). Currently, the National Council of State Boards of Nursing (NCSBN, 2010) is implementing the *Transition to Practice Model* designed to promote public safety by supporting newly licensed nurses during their critical entry period and progression into practice while promoting competency development. Regarding nursing competencies, numerous initiatives followed the Institute of Medicine Report (IOM, 1999), *To Err Is Human: Building a Safer Health System*. Nationally, emphasis is being placed both on initial and on continuing competency in practice.

Nurse leaders in Alaska have worked on the above issues for decades. More recently, a statewide group was formed to collaboratively work on these common concerns. The initial two areas the group decided to focus on were preceptor development and competency assessment. This chapter describes the Alaska experience in achieving improved preceptor education and implementing standardized nursing competency assessment.

ALASKA'S NURSE PRECEPTOR INITIATIVE

A successful internship or residency program for nurses requires appropriately prepared and supported preceptors. Regardless of the setting, be it rural or urban, preceptor programs tend to be plagued by lack of training, coupled with staffing patterns and workloads that are competing priorities for the nurse preceptor. The lack of time is most often identified by nurse preceptors as a deterrent to properly precepting new staff (Carlson, Pilhammer, & Wann-Hansson, 2010; DeWolfe, Laschinger, & Perkin, 2010). Even when a preceptor finds the experience intrinsically rewarding, role ambiguity, work overload, and time constraints are major stressors. These deterrents can be ameliorated by formalizing the preceptor role, delineating responsibilities, and by providing support and recognition for preceptors (Omansky, 2010).

Challenges that typically beset preceptor programs are magnified in Alaska due to the often harsh environment, vast geographical distances, and difficulty recruiting and retaining staff in remote areas. Alaska facilities, over the years, have implemented a variety of nurse preceptor programs with varying levels of success. A major challenge for Alaska hospitals is the high proportion of traveling nurses who work for short periods of time in a facility, and sometimes comprise 50% or more of the total nursing staff. Travelers are not the best preceptor choice as they are often unaware of the cultural and geographic issues affecting patient care and because they are not permanent staff members. Thus, the pool of experienced nurses able to serve as preceptors is very limited. The same few permanent staff nurses are expected to fulfill multiple roles and "keep things running" in the facility. It is not unusual for a preceptor to work with a new graduate while being the charge nurse, carrying a full patient load, participating on committee work, and supervising travelers all in the same shift!

In an effort to address these nursing concerns, the Alaska State Hospital and Nursing Home Association (ASHNHA) sponsored a statewide education conference in 2004 focusing on the development of nurse preceptors. Attendees arrived from across the state and were, for the most part, nurse educators. Susan Boyer was the keynote speaker and disseminated information about the Vermont Nursing Internship Program (VNIP, http://vnip.org/) and its competency assessment model. There was consensus for implementing the VNIP preceptor training curriculum and competency model as it seemed appropriate for Alaska's context. In order to do so, the Alaska Coalition of Educators–Health Care (ACE-HC) was established with representation from private, for-profit, nonprofit, tribal, and military health care facilities. The Coalition collaborated with the Director of the University of Alaska, Anchorage (UAA) School of Nursing (SON), the Executive Director of the Alaska Board of Nursing, and many chief nurse executives from across the state.

With funding support from ASHNHA, the ACE-HC scheduled teleconferences to develop the Alaska version of the VNIP program. The original VNIP curriculum was based on Alspach's (2000) seminal work. Some of those materials were already in use by ANMC for its nurse preceptor training program, and they took the lead in offering the program statewide, even traveling to rural sites to offer the workshop to nurses in those facilities. Soon, the hospital at Elmendorf Air Force Base collaborated with ANMC to expand the program and offer it to a multi-disciplinary audience. Meanwhile, Bartlett Hospital in Juneau and Fairbanks Memorial modified their preceptor education programs to reflect the same model.

Other smaller facilities attempted to start preceptor programs of their own, but were not able to bring them to fruition. Insufficient funds to support program development and lack of administrative support were cited as reasons for failure. Rural facilities without a nurse educator had an even harder challenge since that key leadership role was not formally in place. In response to the difficulties faced by small facilities, some sent nurses to Anchorage for preceptor training. That proved unsustainable for the majority due to travel costs and staffing issues. Overall, those who did attend the workshops provided positive feedback about the offerings but expressed concerns that the model probably would be difficult, if not impossible, to implement in small communities due to the organizational structure, financial constraints, and staffing shortages. The Coalition recognized this dilemma and began brainstorming about possible solutions (see final section).

DEVELOPMENT OF ALASKA NURSE COMPETENCIES

The Coalition also recognized that to support the preceptor and preceptee, a solid competency assessment process was critical. The ACE-HC and ASHNHA partnered with the Rasmuson, Northwest Health, and Robert Wood Johnson Foundations in 2007 and established the Alaska Partners In Nursing (PIN) project (Robert Wood Johnson Foundation, 2010). This initiative supported consultative services, teleconference meetings, and stipends for individuals to attend the much-needed face-to-face meetings in Anchorage to work on developing a statewide competency program. PIN funding sustained the momentum through allowing consistent contact for both communication and accountability of member participants. Consequently, notable progress was made in developing nursing competency outcomes.

Dr. Carrie Lenburg met with ACE-HC to discuss her Competency Outcomes and Performance Assessment (COPA) model (Lenburg, 1999). ACE-HC adopted the COPA model, which focused on assessment processes to develop competent nurses and ensure patient safety (Lenburg, Klein, Abdur-Rahman, Spencer, & Boyer, 2009). The model proposes creating a relevant, standardized, streamlined, and focused competency assessment process, which was exactly what the Coalition was looking for. The PIN project supported a nurse educator to work with rural institutions to compile a preliminary competency list. Information was collected from all participating facilities to compile a list of competencies deemed appropriate for a beginning rural nurse generalist. ACE-HC members revised items on this list to reflect practice-based outcomes in accordance with the COPA model. The following question assured unwavering focus: "What do I need to see the new nurse do that will make me confident that he/she can practice without my supervision?" The COPA model contains eight core practice competencies that include assessment and intervention, communication, critical thinking, teaching, leadership, management, human caring and relationships, and knowledge integration.

Individual competencies within each of the eight broad categories also contain critical elements that must be met for the preceptee to pass that particular item. For example, one critical thinking competency was "Upon completion of training, the nurse will use resources effectively." Critical elements to be evaluated included "Responds to significant changes in patient status per protocols and orders" and "Notifies charge nurse or manager of significant changes or needs on unit." When the preceptee demonstrates these elements, the preceptor can sign off that competency.

The competency documents were designed to be flexible enough to be used by facilities across the state. The critical elements vary depending on the services provided by a facility or specialty unit. For example, one facility or unit may require a medication test and another may not. Or, if there is a medication exam, the information on the exam will vary by the specialty area of practice. An agreed-upon list of references was included for each competency, including commonly used nursing textbooks, internet resources, professional organizations' standards of practice, along with state and institutional policies and procedures.

By the end of 2007, ACE-HC finalized competencies for the rural nurse "generalist" and nine nursing specialties (intensive care, emergency department, medical–surgical, newborn, obstetrics, operating room, post anesthesia care unit, pediatrics, nurse leadership). The generalist competencies were used successfully for nurse preceptor programs as well as for orienting recently hired nurses to a facility. The nurse leadership module was designed for those who may function in the role of charge nurse, house supervisor, manager, etc. The other specialty competency modules were developed as modules to allow for flexibility at various institutions, depending on the multiple areas a rural nurse would be expected to cover. For example, a nurse in a rural setting may be required to function primarily on a unit that takes medical and surgical patients of all ages, act as house supervisor, plus cover the emergency room. This nurse would complete the generalist competency plus the modules for nurse leadership and medical–surgical, pediatrics, and emergency room nursing. All the competency forms are available at www.ashnha.org.

OUTCOMES

ACE-HC pilot tested the generalist competencies in three Alaska health care facilities. The feedback received from staff nurse preceptors was overwhelmingly positive. They appreciated having one document with focused, clearly stated competencies and expectations as opposed to having to complete a large pile of checklists. The initial intent for competency development was for rural use, but the findings revealed that these documents were highly relevant for nurses in urban-based facilities as well. Partly, this finding is attributable to the high number of rural residents who receive care in urban health care facilities, but it also indicates that core competencies for a nurse remain fairly consistent across settings.

The Coalition modified the competency documents, based on preceptor feedback on a number of items. First, preceptors found the instruction page useful but its placement on the front page overwhelming and confusing. Now, only short instructive reminders are at the beginning of the forms, while the full instructions are at the end. Second, preceptors stated that they felt they may miss sharing important information with this pared-down, highly focused assessment. In response, a column was added to the documents containing anecdotal (noncompetency related) information that preceptors and preceptees may refer to and use as a teaching guide. Third, the term "RN" was changed to "nurse" since the competencies are applicable to licensed practical nurses (LPNs) too. In the few instances where a critical element or competency is not appropriate for an LPN, it is noted. Fourth, feedback from outpatient clinics indicated that the competency package did not meet their needs since outpatient nursing tasks are significantly different and the nature of the job requires leadership attributes for all nurses. In response, ACE-HC developed an outpatient nurse generalist competency. In addition to all these changes, the Coalition identified and developed a nurse educator competency.

As with most changes and new initiatives, there was initial resistance; however, resistance dissipated as the processes evolved. At this time, approximately half of Alaska's acute care facilities have adopted a portion or all of the nurse competency process. One small rural hospital even had each one of their nurses complete the competencies regardless of their length of employment at that site. A nurse, who worked there for decades, walked to the educator's office, held up the package, and exclaimed "it's about time!" (S. F., personal communication, December 12, 2008). The process is also now being used for nurses who travel to another participating facility for training. The documents are simply carried and used from one site to another by the nurse.

At this time ACE-HC has available and in use the nurse generalist, ambulatory care, and 10 specialty competencies forms that are available online, and is disseminating the information through publications and presentations in local, regional, and national venues. The Coalition is planning work on competencies related to discharge planning, mental/behavioral health, and on implementation guides for nurse educators and nurse administrators. They are also working to strengthen sustainment of the competency and preceptor programs.

Recently, ACE-HC partnered with the Anchorage Area Health Education Center (AHEC) and the University of Alaska Southeast to create a multidisciplinary distance education preceptor course. They plan for the course to be web based, using synchronous and asynchronous components, and organized into learning modules roughly modeled after the program in place at Bartlett Hospital in Juneau. This approach will allow access to training to many who otherwise would not be able to obtain it due to financial or staffing constraints. The goal of the course is to provide preceptors in rural settings the additional training, support, and networking they need to ensure excellence in their precepting practice. Live courses will continue to be offered as well.

In summary, in spite of the challenges of being a vast and remote frontier state, Alaska made great strides in statewide standardization of competencies and other preceptor supports. The conditions of J.M.'s experience, at the beginning of this chapter, are not the same today. Many of the same challenges exist, but in addition to internship programs, Alaska now has preceptors supported with the education and practical competency tools needed to further strengthen the nursing workforce.

REFERENCES

Alspach, G. (2000). *Preceptor handbook for professional healthcare staff.* Aliso Viejo, CA: American Association of Critical Care Nurses.

Carlson, E., Pilhammar, E., & Wann-Hansson, C. (2010). Time to precept: Supportive and limiting conditions for precepting nurses. *Journal of Advanced Nursing, 66*(2), 432–441.

DeWolfe, J., Laschinger, S., & Perkin, C. (2010). Preceptors' perspective on recruitment, support, and retention of preceptors. *The Journal of Nursing Education*, *49*(4), 198–206.

Institute of Medicine (IOM). (1999). *To err is human: Building a safer health system*. Retrieved November 21, 2010 from http://www.iom.edu/Reports/1999/To-Err-is-Human-Building-A-Safer-Health-System.aspx

Institute of Medicine. (2010). *The future of nursing, leading change, advancing health: Committee on the Robert Wood Johnson Foundation initiative on the future of nursing*. Washington, DC: The National Academies Press.

Lenburg, C. (1999). The framework, concepts and methods of the competency outcomes and performance assessment (COPA) model. *Online Journal of Issues in Nursing*. Retrieved November 19, 2010 from http://www.nursingworld.org/ojin/topic10/tpc10_2.htm

Lenburg, C., Klein, C., Abdur-Rahman, V., Spencer, T., & Boyer, S. (2009). The COPA model: A comprehensive framework designed to promote quality care and competence for patient safety. *Nursing Education Perspectives*, *30*(5), 312–317.

National Council of State Boards of Nursing. (2010). *Transition to practice modules*. Retrieved November 21, 2010 from https://www.ncsbn.org/2010_TransitiontoPractice_Modules_Oct1810.pdf

Omansky, G. (2010). Staff nurses' experiences as preceptors and mentors: An integrative review. *Journal of Nursing Management*, *18*(6), 697–703.

Robert Wood Johnson Foundation Partners Investing in Nursing's Future program. (2010). *Pin takes aim at nursing workforce development*. Retrieved November 22, 2010 from http://www.rwjf.org/pr/product.jsp?id=43229

US Census Bureau. (2009). Retrieved November 21, 2010 from http://www.census.gov/popest/datasets.html

16

New Mexico: Nurse Residence Collaborative Model

Anna von Dielingen

Implementation of a centralized, statewide residency program positively impacted on the nursing culture in New Mexico (NM), a state that has significant rural and frontier regions within its boundaries. The NM Center of Nursing Excellence developed partnerships with both academicians and health care providers to generate ideas for the improvement of practice outcomes, including the needs and preferences for transitioning novice nurses into the workforce. The selection process used for a rural residency program and outcomes of the implementation are discussed.

New Mexico (NM) covers an area of more than 120,000 square miles having about 2 million residents. Of the state's 33 counties, 28 are classified as rural. Almost the entire state (90%) is designated as a Health Professions Shortage Area (HPSA) compared with the United States as a whole (25%). Of NM residents, about one-third (670,403) live in areas designated as rural or remote, and at least 614,960 citizens are underserved when it comes to primary care health care providers (www. hrsa.gov). Regarding nursing, NM has a profound shortage based on its nurse-to-patient ratio. Of the 50 states and the District of Columbia, NM ranks 49th, having 614 nurses per 100,000 people (www.state healthfacts.org) with high turnover rates in rural settings. Disparate demographics and lack of nurses were two incentives for nursing leaders to implement a rural nurse residency program in NM.

GETTING STARTED

Collaborative initiatives were underdeveloped in NM due to nursing recruitment and retention challenges. Two major initiatives were the Robert Wood Johnson Foundation Colleagues in Caring (1998) and the establishment of the NM Center for Nursing Excellence (NMCNE) (2002). The NMCNE was instrumental in statewide coalition building among nurse leaders and other health-related organizations to "get things done" around the state's challenging nursing situation. In 2009, NMCNE coordinated a conference targeting nursing faculty with the President of the National Council of State Boards of Nursing (NCSBON) as its keynote speaker. The NCSBON President focused on nurse residency programs in general and NCSBON's residency model in particular. The event generated meaningful discussion and consensus among attendees to implement a nurse residency program that fits the health care system in rural NM. In turn, NMNCE established the Practice and Work Environment (P-WE) committee comprising nurses from acute and long-term care facilities, nurse educators, researchers, administrators, along with representation from local agencies and state organizations. The P-WE completed a comprehensive literature review on the topic of "newly licensed nurses and their transition into nursing practice." Next, the committee undertook an extensive reviewe of ~30 nurse residency programs that were offered nationally and internationally.

Of these programs, four models seemed to hold potential for NM. These were compared and contrasted using a matrix that included the following criteria:

- Curriculum plan/organization
- Based on evidence and standards
- Facility requirements for program implementation
- Characteristics of students who could be admitted to the program
- Required resources; cost ratio of facility:nurse
- Length of the program
- Time requirements (didactic/clinical)
- Clinical topics/content
- Preceptor requirements/training
- Support personnel/materials
- Ratio of residents/interns to preceptors
- (Suggested) preceptor compensation
- Outcomes/retention statistics
- Evaluation/comments from hospitals using the program
- Appropriateness of commercially available product for statewide use in NM

Additionally, experts from the four residency programs spoke to members of the P-WE committee in NM. While all four models had excellent features, the Northwest Rural Nurse Residency Program (NWRNR) seemed to be best suited for the NM context. As a result, the NWRNR coordinator presented details of this model in Albuquerque to attendees from across the state (primarily chief nursing officers from acute rural facilities). The P-WE committee approved the implementation of the NWRNR model in NM. The reasons for this choice included, among others, that this model integrated rural nursing theory, research, and evidence-based guidelines. It also included quality and safety, and NCSBON standards, and promoted critical thinking. The program delivery modalities fit NM context, with the use of electronic communication and internet connectivity to make the program accessible to residents and preceptors who lived and worked in rural and remote regions of NM. A convincing feature of NWRNR was its flexibility, designed to accommodate the needs of a particular institution or organization. For instance, NM needed a course on cultural aspects of health among the Navajo, Zuni, Apache, and Pueblo Native American tribes; modules are currently under development for these populations.

MARKETING AND ADAPTING THE NWRNR TO NM

The NMCNE and P-WE committee assumed leadership to market the program to health care leaders in the state and adapted the NWRNR model to fit the NM context. NM targeted marketing strategies to the Board of Nursing, Organization of Nurse Executives, Nursing Council, state and local governmental officials, NM Primary Care Association, NM Association for Home Care and Hospice, NM Health Care Association, nursing faculty, educators, hospitals, and administrators of the Navajo Nation and Indian Health Services. Ultimately, the goal of the leadership was to disseminate information about the program and elicit "buy-in" from organizations that support the professional development of newly licensed registered nurses (RNs).

Regarding program administration, NMCNE arranged with the NWRNR coordinator to serve as the residency program's regional administrator. A part-time on-site program director was hired to manage local concerns; this position was funded by the NMCNE. Responsibilities of the NM coordinator center on marketing and delivering the program, communicating with participant facilities, residents, and preceptors. The NM coordinator collects, analyzes, and disseminates data. The NM program director interfaces with the off-site NWRNR coordinator to tailor the program for the various enrollees, residents, and preceptors. Ultimately, the NM coordinator is projected to assume more responsibilities while the NWRNR will have a lesser role as the nurse residency program evolves and expands.

IMPLEMENTING THE PROGRAM IN NM

There is an application process for interested individuals. Newly licensed registered nurses and nurses who are returning into the nursing workforce in acute and long-term care facilities are admitted into the residency program. The program admits three cohorts during the year and enrollment of facilities and residents has increased gradually in the first year. The first cohort (admitted February 2010) consisted of two enrolled facilities (Hospital A, Hospital B). Hospital A initially planned to have two resident nurses and one preceptor. The intensity of course expectations resulted in residents dropping out of the program coupled with the chief nursing officer experiencing a family emergency, which eroded administrative support for this new program.

Hospital B enrolled two preceptors and two residents who are successfully completing course assignments. On completing the operating room experience, one resident noted: "There were areas of the program that did not fit my role in the OR . . . but the experience was well worth the time." Early on, a surgeon acknowledged the resident nurse's talent and requested her participation with his surgical procedures.

For the second cohort (started June 2010), two hospitals, in addition to hospital B, enrolled in the residency program (total of three facilities). Hospital B continues to have two residents and two preceptors while the other two have been less successful. The less successful hospitals are both located in an urban area situated within a rural county; one has 200 beds and the other has 168 beds. The challenges in the facility with 168 beds were on retaining preceptors who withdrew for a variety of personal reasons and recruiting students. The larger facility had adequate resources with seven preceptors to offer on-site specialized educational programs for newly licensed nurses. Of the seven preceptors, five were also completing ICU, OB-L&D, or Floating RN courses. The nursing administration overtly supports residency programs; however, this facility's nurses practice specialty skills rather than the rural nurse generalist specialty. For this reason, the NM residency program may not be suited for a large, urban hospital setting.

The third NM cohort (started October 2010) supported six facilities. Of these, Hospital B (described above) continues to successfully enroll and support nurse residents and preceptors. Two small, rural Indian Health Services facilities with two residents and two preceptors each enrolled. Another hospital, located on the Navajo Nation, enrolled four residents and four preceptors. Two other rural acute care hospitals (one being Hospital A) are enrolled, each with two residents and two preceptors. All six facilities are progressing favorably without attrition of preceptors or residents.

At the time of this writing, the fourth NM residency cohort (started January 2011) enrolled three facilities, all re-enrolling: Hospital B as mentioned above, a Navajo Nation hospital and an Indian Health Services (IHS) facility. A Director of Nursing from the participating IHS facility stated that without the support of the NWRNR they would not continue to hire recently graduated nurses.

Nursing in the Navajo Nation (NN) parallels that of other rural NM care providers. A critical issue for the NN, however, is that due to retirement within 5 years the turnover rate of experienced nurses is projected to be at least 50% (this is anecdotal information provided by NN chief nursing officers). Given this prediction, nurse leaders from three NN facilities attended meetings focusing on the NWRNR model and have enthusiastically embraced plans to implement the residency in their communities. As it exists, the NWRNR is considered to be a Participatory Action Research design since it entails data collection and funding from Health Resources and Services Administration (HRSA). A proposal describing the residency program must, therefore, be reviewed and approved by the NN Institutional Review Board (IRB). During the approval process, on-site educational activities are provided to residents and preceptors but surveys from NN participants are excluded from data analysis by NWRNR.

Annually, NWRNR offers a national simulation workshop to residents and preceptors enrolled in the residency program. NM participated in this workshop for the first time in 2010. For the workshop, synchronous and asynchronous online web discussions were scheduled along with exercises on computerized mannequins. In light of the excellent learning, NM programs of nursing are offering this workshop across the state to accommodate the needs of residents and preceptors in the nurse residency and other newly licensed nurses across rural NM.

OUTCOMES OF THE NM RESIDENCY PROGRAM

Short- and long-term outcomes of the NM residency program are necessary to assess impacts relative to the costs of starting and sustaining a program. To collect appropriate statistics and measure outcomes of the residency program, the NM leadership collaborated with the coordinator of the NWRNR program. The criteria to be evaluated with each cohort and in total (over time) included demographic data of residents and preceptors, recruitment and retention statistics, level of satisfaction, along with evaluation of an individual's clinical competence and professional development. These data also provide relevant NM information about newly licensed registered nurses employment patterns, turnover rates, as well as facilities that participate in the residency program. In July 2010, a survey was sent to all chief nursing officers of acute care facilities ($N = 42$) in NM to collect data on hiring and turnover of newly licensed registered nurses for 2007–2009. Twelve ($n = 12$) nursing officers responded to the survey, reporting an average retention rate of about 91% at year one and 85% at year two. While the retention seems to be relatively good, one must keep in mind the high cost in time and other resources of recruiting, hiring, and orienting a new (hire) RN to the facility or specialty unit. These findings supported the need for additional data on recruitment and retention of nurses in other kinds of facilities in NM, and the need for comparisons among rural and urban institutions.

FUTURE DIRECTIONS

Overall, there is consensus that developing an NM residency program (adapted from the NWRNR model) is a well-received idea. Residency participant satisfaction is high, that is to say, enrolled facilities, preceptors, and nurse residents are pleased with the process and outcome. While enthusiasm is evident, challenges in sustaining and expanding a program such as this must be addressed.

As with most, if not all, initiatives, procuring funding can be problematic. Financial support for the NM nurse residency program is provided by several entities. The Con Alma Health Foundation has a mission to improve health care delivery and provided funding to market the residency program to NM health care facilities. The NM Board of Nursing funded a 1-year grant to support the NM coordinator position with administrative assistance; this provides resources to seek additional local, state, and federal funding support. Collaborative efforts are underway with the NWRNR coordinator to obtain a federal grant to expand that nurse residency program in NM. The goal is to fully transition from the NWRNR model to the self-sustaining New Mexico Rural Nurse Residency (NM RNR). During this grant period, the NM RNR plans to expand the rural nurse residency model to other clinical entities, such as public health and nurse practitioners who practice in rural and remote regions.

Opportunities exist for leaders and participants in the NM nurse residency program to collaborate with numerous NM health care groups. For example, at the University of New Mexico Hospital simulation symposium (December 2010), the NM rural nurse residency coordinator made a presentation on the use of simulation that has relevance for online nurse residents similar to the NWRNR simulation workshop. Such offerings are also an effective strategy to disseminate information about the NM nurse residency program and serve as a recruitment strategy. Other areas include collaborating with programs of nursing education across the state to promote the residency program as well as share resources to implement this program in more remote regions.

The P-WE committee of the NMCNE continues to be active and is planning a statewide nurse preceptor conference based on findings from a needs assessment of current preceptors from across NM. The P-WE committee's goal is to highlight and support preceptors' contributions in developing an NM nursing workforce and thereby improve health care access for underserved and vulnerable populations. There are numerous research topics that continue to emerge, associated with the residency program; thus, opportunities exist for researchers and program participants to work together to develop a body of knowledge related to marketing, course delivery, organization of the content, and preceptor development.

Three lessons learned in the short time the program has been in existence include

- Nursing administrators and managers must be involved and supportive of a nurse residency program for the initiative to be seen as significant, valuable, and "take root." Role modeling behavior can motivate and promote a culture of change and support among nurses—from novice to expert.
- A thorough research of existing residency programs to identify models that your institution's context and culture is a required preliminary process. There are many to choose from. "Good fit" is essential for implementing and sustaining a successful program.
- When implementing a residency program, celebrate the program participants and their success. Such efforts can go a long way to get "buy in" from staff within the facility. For example, in one facility on the Navajo Nation, a pharmacist stated that this department would do anything necessary to support the residency program. Within this facility, marketing materials were posted in hallways to promote the nurse residency program to staff as well as patients and visitors. In another facility, administrators allowed dedicated time for preceptors to mentor newly hired and licensed colleagues. Preceptors felt appreciated; in turn, this supportive attitude was reflected by coworkers.

In summary, implantation of a residency program with a centralized, statewide model has positively impacted on the nursing culture in NM. It has brought statewide nursing leadership together to focus on a critical nursing issue—meeting the nursing needs of NM, particularly in rural and frontier professionally underserved regions. Collaboration has led to new partnerships, generated ideas, and facilitated creative insights regarding newly licensed RNs' transition into the nursing workforce. NM is pleased with its success.

BIBLIOGRAPHY

Jones, C. B., & Gates, M. (2007). The cost and benefits of nurse turnover: A business case for nurse retention. *The Online Journal of Issues in Nursing, 12*(3). Retrieved September 4, 2011 from http://cms.nursingworld.org/MainMenuCategories/ANAMarketplace/ANAPeriodicals/OJIN/TableofContents/Volume122007/No3Sept07/NurseRetention.aspx

Roth, J. F. (2008). The North Carolina evidence-based transition-to-practice initiative. *Policy, Politics, & Nursing Practice, 3,* 215–219.

Stroth, C. (2010). Job embeddedness as a nurse retention strategy for rural hospitals. *Journal of Nursing Administration, 1,* 32–35.

Ulrich, B., Krozek, C., Early, S., Ashlock, C. H., Africa, L. M., & Carman, M. (2010). Improving retention, confidence, and competence of new graduate nurses: Results from a 10-year longitudinal database. *Nursing Economics, 6,* 363–375.

17

The Oregon N2K Initiative: From Incumbent Worker to Nurse

Gary W. Wappes

*T*his chapter describes a statewide initiative in Oregon to address the growing nursing shortage, particularly in rural regions of the state. At the beginning of the millennium, the state's nursing leaders developed the Nursing 2000 (N2K) strategy to address institutional nursing shortages through partnerships among nursing educational programs and health care institutions. Described herein are the details of student selection, curriculum design, select student cohorts characteristics, and program outcomes.

During the early years of the new millennium (2001–2002), the state of Oregon's health care providers experienced a crisis in the nursing profession that was common across the United States. Nurses and their supporting professionals (Licensed Practical Nurses, Certified Medical Assistants [CMA], and Certified Nursing Assistants [CNA]) provided over 60% of all health care services delivered in hospitals. And yet, there were critically dangerous shortages of nurses in the American health care system nationwide. The state's problem was already acute and growing worse.

> There is currently a multi-dimensional shortage of registered nurses in Oregon ... [that] is adversely affecting patient care, the safety and morale of the nursing workforce, and is driving up the cost of care. ... Unless measures are taken immediately, we can anticipate a severe shortage by 2010, and probably sooner.
>
> —*Northwest Health Foundation, 2001, pp. 8, 20*

We reviewed data on current openings for Licensed Practical Nurses, Medical Assistants, Nurses' Aides, and Registered Nurses. The Oregon Employment Department released a study in 2002 indicating current vacancy rates in key positions. Those current vacancy rates included Licensed Practical Nurses: 250–500, Medical Assistants: 60–90, Nurses' Aides and related: 900–1,300, and Registered Nurses (RNs): 1,400–1,800.

Further validating the need was a report indicating that 60% of Oregon Association of Hospitals and Health Systems members reported 474 current nursing vacancies at the time of their 2002 survey (Oregon Workforce Investment Board, 2002). In Oregon, limited capacity in the higher-education system to produce more nurses presented yet another barrier to overcoming the crisis. The state's community colleges, producing more than 75% of graduating RNs, consistently reported limitations in their enrollment capacity. In fact, nursing education program administrators reported that up to five qualified individuals applied for each available student slot in their programs. In spite of the demand, schools of nursing were unable to significantly expand their programs due to budgetary restrictions, difficulty in recruiting and retaining qualified faculty, and, in some cases, limited sites for student clinical experiences (Northwest Health Foundation, 2001). An Oregon Workforce Investment Board study in 2002 illustrated the problem in this way:

> One of the most important reasons for today's worker shortages is training capacity … This challenge may be particularly acute in health care because required clinical experience often complements classroom training, and licensing and certification rules may limit training flexibility. For some occupations, and especially in rural areas, there are also critical shortages of trained faculty— either now or predicted in the near future, due to scheduled retirements.

While major health systems in metropolitan areas are better able to effectively compete for newly graduated nurses, systems in rural areas struggle to recruit and retain health professionals, especially nurses. Particularly disadvantaged are critical access hospitals (CAHs) located in more remote rural communities, facilities providing care to institutionalized residents and patients such as state psychiatric facilities hospitals, and federally qualified community health centers that require additional skills such as fluency in a second language. Employers aggressively seeking to increase the racial and ethnic diversity of their nursing workforce also experience difficulty finding such candidates among new nurses graduating from traditional nursing programs.

Employers are eager and willing to support current employees who are qualified for entry into nursing education programs. However, daunting barriers remain. Many of these employees are in low-paying, entry-level jobs. The financial hardship of extended time away while attending school is often an overwhelming barrier. Furthermore, particularly in rural communities, potential students are geographically isolated from site-based educational programs and are unable to attend without relocating. And finally, the limited number of available slots in nursing schools makes entry very competitive (or unpredictable in schools utilizing lottery entry systems). The group reasoned that a nursing prerequisite and nursing education program could overcome barriers. The hope was that hospitals and health systems with significant challenges in hiring new graduate nurses would support a program that provided a reasonable and predictable supply of RNs.

PLANNING AND IMPLEMENTING THE N2K PROGRAM

The design's purpose was to overcome the constraints and barriers identified, while still maintaining the integrity and uncompromised educational standards of traditional Associate Degree Nursing (ADN) programs. To realize this goal, the program operated as a unique cohort, separate from the proscribed schedule of traditional programs, while maintaining the identical educational content. This dictated that each cohort be structured so that it could support the cost of instruction independent of the traditional program structure.

Admission Criteria

Participants were selected based on multiple criteria. Each candidate was fully qualified for entry into the educational providers' nursing program. Standards in this regard were consistent with entry requirements into the educational providers' traditional program, and applicants were evaluated by college staff by their usual processes, that is, transcript review, and so on. Additionally, employers (in partnership with their unions when appropriate) evaluated applicants by their own human resource standards, and determined if the applicant earned good performance reviews in current positions, required letters of recommendations from current supervisors, and conducted interviews to gauge readiness, commitment, and strengths.

Curriculum Framework

The program worked in partnership with educational providers and participating employers to produce a time frame for each cohort that maximized efficiencies while accommodating participant and employer needs as much as possible. Weekly activities were compressed so that classroom and clinical activities occurred in four or four-and-a-half days to allow students to continue working on a limited basis (thus allowing employees to maintain health benefit coverage and some income). The typical 2-year nursing program with a summer break was generally compressed into six consecutive terms, allowing completion in 18 months. It is important to stress here that at no time were educational standards compromised in this process. All students received the same quality and quantity of classroom, lab, and clinical education as their counterparts in each participating college's traditional nursing program.

Classroom Instruction

Delivery models for classroom instruction varied among the eight cohorts. When practical, classes were held on-site on college campuses, or, at times in geographically convenient labs and classroom space leased for that purpose. Distance learning technology was used to some extent in several cohorts, and was used extensively for classroom delivery for one cohort composed exclusively of students from widely dispersed CAHs.

Clinical Instruction

When appropriate, clinical instruction was provided in the host hospitals that sponsored students. Qualified hospital nursing staff (many of whom had previous experience as clinical instructors) were selected, trained, and supervised by college faculty similar to arrangements used in traditional programs. Some clinical rotations required students to receive clinical instruction at larger, regional hospitals with appropriate specialty departments. It is significant to note the level of cooperation and support provided by participating hospitals and systems in this regard. Specific cooperative arrangements were developed to plan and implement clinical instruction activities. For example, in one term, a participating psychiatric hospital would host the entire cohort for their psychiatric rotation. In another term, another hospital partner would host the entire cohort for medical surgical rotations, and so on.

Student Support Services

Unlike traditional students who enter nursing programs as individuals, usually utilizing their own financial and other resources, these students were sponsored by employers who anticipated their return to employment as an RN on completion of the program. To maximize the potential of that success, a variety of student support services were purposefully included in this design. Hospitals were encouraged to sponsor at least two students in a cohort so that participants could study together, share travel expenses, and so on. Hospitals assigned experienced nursing staff to serve as informal mentors and morale boosters. College partners dedicated specific instructional staff to the cohort to ensure continuity and ongoing student support. Program staff maintained an active linkage between students, employers, and the educational provider so that all three parties could work together to resolve problems as they arose.

Budgetary Considerations

Each cohort was designed to be a stand-alone cost center. All educational expenses (tuition, books, instructor time, lab fees, college overhead, etc.) were itemized and accounted for in budget planning. Costs for student support, planning, design, and coordination services provided by the Oregon Health Career Center were included. Generally, the cost of hospital nursing staff who participated as clinical instructors was provided in-kind by participating hospitals. When the total costs were taken into consideration, the per-student cost was determined based on the number of students in each cohort (generally this ranged from 16 to 24 students). Subsequently, the cost "per-slot" was the financial cost a participating hospital was required to pay for each student they sponsored in that particular cohort.

As previously described, hospitals participating in the Nursing 2000 (N2K) program historically faced many challenges in recruiting and hiring nurses for their facilities. Those challenges translated into significant costs, such as advertising, recruiting, sign-on bonuses, relocation costs, and so on. In addition, many hospitals were forced to use interim (and expensive) "agency," or "traveler" nurses to temporarily fill critical positions. Many rural hospitals also reported anecdotally that nurses hired from outside their communities rarely stayed beyond the limits of their initial contract, thus requiring a renewal of recruitment and hiring challenges.

Almost universally, these hospitals were able to accurately quantify the cost to them of hiring a new nurse, which they could compare to the per-slot cost of sponsoring a student in the N2K program. Based on this comparison, hospitals generally reported a return on their sponsorship investment within 2 years of the student's employment as an RN. Since students already established relationships through prior employment, commitment to the community, employer, and special populations, a 2–3-year "loan repayment" service obligation was not a problem.

Faculty and Staff

The educational coordinator played the key educational role in the N2K model. This person was a specific faculty member of the educational partner who was released from other responsibilities to coordinate and oversee the educational service delivery of the program. In some cohorts, this was a full-time commitment with responsibilities for overseeing classroom, lab, and clinical activities. In other cohorts, two faculty members shared this responsibility with one overseeing classroom and the other lab and clinical activities. In many of the cohorts, these faculty members taught some courses and provided some lab and/or clinical instruction as appropriate. Due to the complexity and unique aspects of the N2K model, college partners typically assigned seasoned, experienced faculty to the project. The full time equivalency (FTE) of other faculty was increased, or temporary faculty members were at times hired to "backfill" during the N2K project time. As indicated earlier, the cost of these educational coordinators (as well as all other college faculty and support staff utilized in the cohort's education) was included in the overall and per-student cost rate for that cohort.

Cohort Composition

With one exception, cohorts were composed of students from multiple employers. (In that one exception, a single large health care system sponsored all the students in the cohort.) Students generally came from patient service positions in their hospitals, with most being either CMA or CNA. Hospitals required employees to have a work history with their employer of at least 2 years. In rare instances, a single student was sponsored by an employer. More typically, there were at least two and as many as six or more from one employer. Students generally received support and encouragement from their employers as they independently accrued their required prerequisites. However, in two iterations of the program, students entered the cohort and completed all their prerequisites as a group in a specially designed, accelerated program prior to their enrollment as a cohort in the nursing program.

PROGRAM EVALUATION AND OUTCOMES

Between 2002 and 2010, seven N2K cohorts were completed. Five Oregon community college Associate Degree Nursing programs participated in one or more of the cohorts as educational providers, ultimately generating student degrees. Twelve Oregon hospitals and health systems sponsored students in one or more cohorts, as did one Oregon Community Health Center. Among participating hospitals, six rural CAHs participated in the program. Four of those hospitals participated in two cohorts. There were nine graduates from the initial pilot cohort. Subsequent cohorts graduated as many as 23 students. Of 122 students who entered the cohorts, 111 (91%) completed, graduated, and successfully passed their RN licensure exams. All but one of those completers returned to their sponsoring hospital and were employed there as RNs. The individual cohorts included:

- *Chemeketa Cohort.* Educational program was provided by Chemeketa Community College, Salem, Oregon. Hospital partners included Salem Hospital, Salem, Oregon; Willamette Valley Medical Center, McMinnville, Oregon; and Oregon State Hospital, Portland and Salem, Oregon. Graduated nine students in June 2005.
- *Cascades East AHEC Cohort.* Educational program was provided by Central Oregon Community College, Bend, Oregon. Hospital partners included St. Charles Medical Center, Bend, Oregon; St. Charles Medical Center, Redmond, Oregon; Harney District Hospital, Burns, Oregon; Mt. View District Hospital, Madras, Oregon; Pioneer Memorial Hospital, Prineville, Oregon; and Lake District Hospital, Lakeview, Oregon. Graduated 16 students in December 2005. This cohort was operated by the Cascades East Area Health Education Center, Bend, Oregon.
- *Clackamas Cohort #1.* Educational program was provided by Clackamas Community College, Oregon City, Oregon. The single hospital partner was Kaiser Permanente Northwest, northwestern Oregon and Southwestern Washington. Graduated 23 students in December 2007.
- *Portland Cohort #1.* Educational program was provided by Portland Community College, Portland, Oregon. Hospital partners included Kaiser Permanente Northwest, northwestern Oregon, and southwestern Washington; Willamette Falls Hospital, Oregon City, Oregon; Oregon State Hospital, Portland and Salem, Oregon; and Tuality Healthcare, Hillsboro, Oregon. Graduated 16 students in December 2008.
- *Clackamas Cohort #2.* Education program was provided by Clackamas Community College, Oregon City, Oregon. Hospital partners

included Kaiser Permanente Northwest, northwestern Oregon, and southwestern Washington; Willamette Falls Hospital, Oregon City, Oregon; Oregon State Hospital, Portland and Salem, Oregon; and Virginia Garcia Memorial Health Center, Hillsboro, Oregon. Eighteen students graduated in December 2009.

■ *Mt. Hood Cohort.* Educational program was provided by Mt. Hood Community College, Gresham, Oregon. Additional educational services provided by Central Oregon Community College, Bend, Oregon. Hospital partners included Harney District Hospital, Burns, Oregon; Lake District Hospital, Lakeview, Oregon; Mt. View District Hospital, Madras, Oregon; Pioneer Memorial Hospital, Prineville, Oregon; and Blue Mt. District Hospital, John Day, Oregon. Graduated 14 students in March 2010.

■ *Portland Cohort #2.* Educational program was provided by Portland Community College, Portland, Oregon. Hospital partners included Kaiser Permanente Northwest, northwestern Oregon, and southwestern Washington; Willamette Falls Hospital, Oregon City, Oregon; Oregon State Hospital, Portland and Salem, Oregon; and Virginia Garcia Memorial Health Center, Hillsboro, Oregon. Fifteen students graduated in December 2010.

A major strength of the N2K model lies in the ability to address the nursing workforce needs of health care providers facing chronic recruitment barriers. Community Health Centers usually cannot offer salaries and benefits that are competitive with other health care employers. They also often require nurses who are bilingual, which creates an additional challenge. Providers who serve difficult populations, such as psychiatric hospitals, find it difficult to attract nurses interested in and committed to working with those populations. Small community hospitals in isolated rural communities have great difficulty in attracting nurses who are eager to relocate and make long-term commitments to rural practice.

Although changing economic conditions and other factors may ease the nursing workforce hiring needs of major employers, the recruitment and retention difficulties of the health care provider groups that we have identified here continue. The N2K model allows these employers to support and partner with current high-performing employees who have already proven to themselves and to their employer that they are dedicated to working with these populations in these health care environments. In isolated rural communities in particular, this model offers one of only a few limited opportunities to advance to a professional employment level without relocating for the necessary education.

Human Resource Officers and Nurse Managers also reported a significant impact on organizational culture. N2K provides a tangible public evidence of the employers' respect and commitment to their workforce. Nurses felt that the support impacted on morale and a sense of teamwork throughout the organization.

The advantages for participating community colleges are also clear. The N2K model allows them to increase the capacity of their nursing programs without further burdening their public tax base or student tuition. The partnering hospitals bring rich resources of clinical training sites and clinical instructors to the table to expand the capacity of nursing faculty. The N2K model also serves colleges, by helping them integrate features to increase the efficiency and effectiveness of their programming with innovations such as modified schedules and the use of distance learning technologies.

In summary, even though the N2K model helped to augment college faculty by utilizing qualified hospital nursing staff, it does not address the looming crisis in nursing education—the growing shortage of nurse educators. Advantages of the N2K model centers on the local and institutional support for an employee/student. Initiative and commitment are critical to successfully complete all the educational and employer mandates but there are other short- and long-term benefits for individual and institutional program participants. Throughout their educational experience, students experience a strong support system of supervisors, coworkers, and management. Moreover, graduates emerge debt-free from this educational experience and are guaranteed a position by an employer they want to work for. By completing the educational requirements to become a licensed nurse, the financial status of the individual and his or her family also improves and they become a valuable health care resource in their communities. Finally, the gratitude expressed by the participants, their employer, and the various Oregon communities is profound.

REFERENCES

Northwest Health Foundation. (April, 2001). *Oregon's nursing shortage: A public health crisis in the making.* Issue Brief No. 1. Retrieved from http://nwhf.org/images/files/Nursing_Shortage_-_Health_Crisis.pdf

Oregon Workforce Investment Board. (2002). *Health care sector employment initiative, initial draft report.*

18

Rural Preceptors' Concerns With Nursing Student Evaluation

Olive June Yonge, Florence Myrick, Linda Ferguson, and Quinn Grundy

The nature of the preceptor evaluation process for nursing students in rural practicums is the focus of a grounded theory study. The setting for the study was two Prairie Provinces in Canada with similar features to the intermountain regions of the United States. Rural settings provide students rich learning experiences and providers experience positive recruitment and retention opportunities. Barriers to adequate formative and summative evaluation processes reveal the need for an evaluation framework, preceptor education, and support. Clarifying evaluation expectations may improve preceptor and faculty relationships, evaluation effectiveness, and nursing practice outcomes.

In 2001, of the total number of Registered Nurses (RNs) employed in nursing in Canada, 18% worked in rural or small town areas, compared with 21% of the general population (Canadian Institute for Health Information, 2007). One strategy to increase the number of nurses seeking employment in rural areas is to expose them to the history, culture, landscape, and unique characteristics of what it means to work in rural health care facilities through the creation of rural-based preceptorship programs for student nurses. Increasingly, nursing faculty choose rural settings for student placements owing to the rich learning opportunities that are fostered by the nature of generalist practice (Schoenfelder & Valde, 2009; Sedgwick & Yonge, 2008). Thus, rural preceptorships can be a vehicle for the recruitment of nurses to underserved rural areas and doubly serve as an incentive for faculty and rural-based nurses alike to create and maintain preceptorship programs at these sites (Sedgwick & Yonge, 2008; Shannon et al., 2006).

Preceptorship programs offered in rural areas differ from those offered in urban areas, particularly those geographically closest to the university or college by which the program is physically supported. In rural areas, preceptors may feel a sense of professional isolation or lack of on-site support of a faculty contact person who in fact may not visit throughout the entire preceptorship program. Moreover, preceptors may be supported primarily by telephone calls, e-mail, or Skype. These resources, however, may prove to be insufficient, especially if there is a particular challenge in the nature of student performance.

When viewing preceptorship through a teaching–learning lens, an area that is particularly troublesome for preceptors and faculty alike is evaluation. Preceptors are required to formally evaluate students according to guidelines specified by the university. Some preceptors are comfortable in this role, while others are unprepared and find the evaluation process daunting (Dolan, 2003; McCarthy & Murphy, 2008; Seldomridge & Walsh, 2006; Yonge, Krahn, Trojan, & Reid, 1997). Ironically, this same process of evaluation is also a challenge for experienced educators whose major role is to teach and who, unlike preceptors, are not simultaneously responsible for a patient assignment at the same time. The researchers, therefore, selected evaluation and the rural setting as worthy of research, recognizing the challenges of rural nurses and appreciating the uniqueness of the setting for the preceptorship of nursing students. It was our assumption that there would be a need to enhance the formal preparation of rural preceptors as educators in this area. Furthermore, in preceptorships, nursing faculties rely heavily on clinical preceptors to provide accurate evaluations of student performance (Dibert & Goldenberg, 1995). To be effective, preceptors must be provided with an evaluation framework and appropriate tools that include formative and summative evaluation (Qualters, 1999). Thus, the researchers decided to ascertain the nature of the process involved in preceptor evaluation of fourth-year nursing students who had chosen a rural preceptored site for their final practicum.

BACKGROUND

Nurses who work in rural areas are described as autonomous expert generalists with the ability to be able to adapt nursing interventions to low-tech environments (Bushy, 2001, 2005), and frequently be able to extend their practice into the domain of other health professionals (Weinert & Long, 1989). Rural experience higher-than-average turnover rates, while those who remain in the setting frequently cite job satisfaction and teamwork as reasons for continuing in practice (Hegney, McCarthy, Rogers-Clark, & Gormann, 2002). Beatty (2001) notes that little has been done to investigate rural nurses' learning needs or the context of their practice setting. In addition, professional isolation prevents these nurses from networking with colleagues.

The research as to how preceptors engage in the evaluation process or how this process is assimilated into their role is limited. Furthermore, often they are not prepared to assume the evaluation role. In one of the first studies exploring the evaluation process in preceptorship, Ferguson and Calder (1993) examined the basis of preceptor evaluations and whether performance criteria were valued differently between preceptors and faculty. Their findings indicate that

> if faculty who have preparation in educational theory and practice have difficulties with the evaluation process, this problem must be even greater for nurse preceptors, many of whom have little or no preparation in clinical teaching and evaluation of students.
>
> *—Ferguson & Calder, 1993, p. 31*

Lack of consistency of ratings, instructor bias, concern about the reliability and validity of evaluation tools, and a general reluctance to document poor performance were noted (Ferguson & Calder, 1993). In 1997, Yonge et al. (1997) discovered the discrepancy between how little preceptors are prepared for the evaluative role and yet how frequently they are expected to fulfill that role. Preceptors often feel unprepared to use strategies such as reflection-on-practice and evaluation taxonomies and instead rely heavily on assessment of skills rather than on competencies, and lack the time for the evaluation process owing primarily to their clinical commitments (Dolan, 2003; McCarthy & Murphy, 2008; Seldomridge & Walsh, 2006).

Yonge et al. (1997) also differentiate between informal, ongoing evaluation and formal, documented evaluation. Informal or formative evaluation is a process of tracking, monitoring, adjusting, and regulating behavior through ongoing feedback. Daily, informal, immediate, "on-the-spot" feedback is most effective for student learning and least challenging for the preceptor (Clynes & Raftery, 2008; Glover, 2000; Lee, 2005; Qualters, 1999; Yonge et al., 1997). Ongoing feedback should be informative, specific, and focused on behavior the student can change (Glover, 2000; Lee, 2005). The "feedback sandwich" is recommended as a successful feedback approach and it comprises a *positive comment*, followed by *ideas for improvement*, followed by *another positive comment* (Glover, 2000).

Summative evaluation involves measuring, ranking, and formal grading. Preceptors report great difficulty with summative evaluation owing to unwieldy evaluation forms, the challenge of objectivity, time pressures, student challenges, and the need for additional data (Streubert & Carpenter, 1999; Yonge et al., 1997). Faculty need to assist preceptors in the summative evaluation process (Dolan, 2003; McCarthy & Murphy, 2008; Seldomridge & Walsh, 2006; Yonge et al., 1997). For rural preceptors, the assistance might be in the form of manuals or telephone calls; as we discovered in this research project, however, at times the best assistance emanated from the students, the very people who were to be evaluated.

METHOD

Owing to the lack of research in the area of preceptorship and evaluation, and viewing evaluation as a process, the researchers began with a grounded theory study as it afforded the researchers a firsthand opportunity to deal directly with *what was actually going on* in the preceptorship experience *and not what ought to have been going on*; "the grounded theory method tells it like it is" (Glaser, 1978, p. 14).

The settings for this project were rural sites in two western Canadian provinces. Statistics Canada (2009) defines a rural area as a place having a population of less than 1,000 and a density of less than 400 persons per square kilometer. In Canada, the term *rural* might be perceived as referring to areas where access to health care services is limited by distance and lack of qualified care providers, particularly physicians (Alberta Physicians Resources Planning Group, 1997). Rural is also described as anything that is not urban, implying health care delivered away from large urban centers. Rural placements in this project were located from one to ~16 hours driving distance from the urban center in which the universities were located. Ethical approval to undertake this study was obtained from the universities' health research ethics boards in the two provinces in which the research took place.

Twenty-six rural-based preceptors were interviewed. The university ethics committee requested that clinical placement coordinators provide the researchers with the names of students assigned rural placements. Fourth-year nursing students were then approached through visitation in class and given an information letter. Consenting students provided their assigned preceptor a letter of invitation that was followed by an introductory telephone call from a member of the research team. All participants were given a verbal explanation of the interview procedures and purpose of the study; they signed a written consent form, were apprised of their right to refuse to answer any question without fear of reprisal, and were advised that they were free to withdraw from the study at any point throughout the process.

Both university-based programs required the students to complete a structured preceptorship (one-to-one pairing of a student with an RN) in the final semester of their 4-year baccalaureate nursing program. One of the programs was a 9-week, full-time preceptorship in a setting of the student's choice during which the preceptor and student were visited ideally twice by a faculty member (distance permitting): at midterm and at the culmination of the preceptorship. If problems arose during the preceptorship, faculty might visit more frequently. Verbal and written evaluation took place at midterm and at the termination of the rotation. The preceptor and student each completed a student evaluation using a tool provided by the university that was based on the professional competencies outlined by the provincial regulatory body. The faculty member took these competencies into account and assigned a pass/fail grade on the clinical component. A letter grade was derived from written assignments. The second program was a 6-week preceptorship, 3 weeks spent in a community setting (with one preceptor) and 3 weeks in an acute care setting (with a second preceptor). For this program, faculty did not visit preceptors throughout the preceptorship. The formal evaluation was completed at the end of the rotation. Preceptors in both programs were prepared for the experience through optional preceptor courses, a preceptor manual, and were guided by the course outline and final evaluation form provided to them. Interactions with faculty via telephone or e-mail were also available on the initiative of the student, the preceptor, and/or the faculty member.

Preceptors worked in rural hospitals (including medical, surgical, and obstetrical nursing), public health clinics, and community health centers. Two preceptors were male and 24 preceptors were female. Preceptors ranged in age from 27.5 to 58.5 years, with a mean age of 42.3 years. Fourteen (53.8%) preceptors were baccalaureate prepared and 12 (46.1%) preceptors were diploma prepared. The preceptors ranged in experience from first-time precepting to having precepted over 10 students in a rural setting.

The data collected included demographics in the respective settings primarily through data obtained from the individual interviews and from the researcher's field notes. An interview guide consisting of open-ended questions such as "How would you describe the process that you go through in guiding nursing students during their preceptorship experience?" was used for initial interviews (90 min) with follow-up interviews guided by emerging categories (Strauss & Corbin, 1990). Nearly all interviews were completed face-to-face, although a few were carried out via telephone owing to the constraints of distance. All interviews took place near the final stage of the structured clinical preceptorship. Rigor in this qualitative study was addressed by establishing creditability, fittingness, auditability, and confirmability (Guba & Lincoln, 1989).

Data analysis occurred concurrently with data collection (Glaser, 1978; Stern, 1980). Data saturation transpired when only recurring themes emerged and further incidents did not help explain the emerging theory. The core variable that resulted from the study was "the challenge of formal evaluation." For preceptors, their lack of role clarity as evaluators, absence of a framework to conceptualize evaluation, and the need for greater support in this role function made the formal, or summative, evaluation an onerous task.

DISCUSSION OF FINDINGS

The experiences of rural preceptors told us that in their eyes, preceptorship is a tool of encouragement—encouragement in the choice of profession, development of self-confidence, and accessing opportunities to gain experience in the rural setting. They also viewed their role as providing confirmation to the university that the student has successfully completed another piece of a greater program. Many preceptors, however, struggled with the concept of a formal evaluation and found it difficult to incorporate systematic monitoring and evaluation into this supportive role. In other words, they were concerned with the process of evaluation, culminating in the formal evaluation. One preceptor explained: "the hardest thing I find is evaluating a student, and putting it down on paper and communicating it to them. I don't want to ever hurt somebody's feelings."

Nature of Their Work

While the researchers wanted to know about the process of evaluation, the preceptors also believed that the researchers should understand the context of rural nursing. It was important for them to describe the learning experiences afforded by students who chose rural preceptorships. Preceptors clearly indicated that they perceived rural practice to be unique with different challenges and needs than those of their urban counterparts. Preceptors identified their situation as uniquely "rural" or mentioned that rural preceptorship could serve as a recruitment strategy. Several preceptors characterized their rural practice as a "generalist practice." One preceptor expressed it as "we do everything ... so you work everywhere." Most preceptors' responsibilities included everything from maternity care to emergency care, to admitting, discharging, and patient education as well as involvement in a variety of committees. Emphasis was laid on psychological and family care together with an individual's physical health. It was suggested that a positive facet of rural preceptorship was the variety of experience to which a student would be exposed.

One of the emergent themes was understanding the nature of rural communities and working as professionals in a setting where "everyone knows everybody." This reality created an informal working environment and one predisposed to teamwork. Many preceptors, however, discussed the challenges of multiple role relationships, including knowing a student or a student's family, precepting a student related to a superior, and dealing with issues of sensitivity or confidentiality with the student. For example, students were discouraged from participating in Sexually Transmitted Diseases (STD) counseling or practicing in their home communities. On the other hand, preceptors realized the advantage of being a member of a small community and the trust and high quality of care multiple role relationships fostered in their practice.

Participants described the lack of resources in the rural setting when compared with an urban setting. One preceptor stated, "we don't have all the resources of the big hospitals ... we don't have the people. We don't have the specialties." Consequently, rural nurses experienced an increase in the breadth of their responsibilities (e.g., public health nurses had greater participation in community programming). Due to the lack of technology they also had a heavier paperwork load as rural facilities were frequently short of computers. When attempting to contact university instructors, dial-up internet and the lack of cell phones made communication challenging. One preceptor indicated the accessibility of telehealth and suggested it as a possible method of preceptor preparation and support.

Preceptors also commented on the variability of experience in rural practice, acknowledging that "not everybody's cut out" for rural practice. This perception was specific to extremely busy periods followed by "slow spells" that were largely weather and seasonally dependent. The demographics of an area (e.g., a large number of postnatals at one time) and adverse weather conditions (e.g., no-shows at clinics when the weather is $-40°C$) were the two contributors cited.

Preceptor as Teacher and Evaluator

Preceptors described their role as a teacher who provides knowledge and information, facilitates learning needs, supports the student, gives encouragement, acts as supervisor who monitors learning, serves as a guide, orients the student, provides the student with positive learning experiences, helps students reach their goals, acts as a role model, and provides students with alternate perspectives on clinical nursing practice. As one preceptor summarized: "I view my role as a preceptor to provide an encouraging and safe environment for a student to engage in advanced nursing student level practice, to provide optimum learning experiences and positive learning experiences for students—my student."

Preceptors acknowledged the necessity of setting out specific learning goals and objectives for the preceptorship experience. Most preceptors, however, did not do so and were unclear about the purpose of the placement and what had to be accomplished to constitute a "pass." Preceptors who were successful in setting out clear goals and objectives did so by familiarizing themselves with the formal evaluation tool prior to commencement of the preceptorship. Some used student self-evaluations to set individualized learning goals and to gauge "where we're starting from," creating learning plans and outlining expectations collaboratively with the student.

Each preceptor had a different set of behaviors that were used as indicators as to how a student would be rated at the final evaluation. One preceptor stated, "I do have in my mind definite things that I would like to see," yet for each preceptor these "definite things" were criteria based on behaviors that they personally valued. The following criteria were reported as being "the most important" a student must display during a rural preceptorship: ability to work as a colleague, attitude, critical thinking, enthusiasm for learning, medication knowledge, awareness, organizational abilities, proficiency, safety, adaptability, basic knowledge, caring, patient interactions, professionalism, confidence, and punctuality.

Preceptors were able to outline various strategies they used to evaluate students. The most commonly cited was the use of immediate, daily, honest, verbal feedback. As one preceptor described: "I'm honest and straightforward . . . I try and be specific." Preceptors described feedback as an informal, ongoing evaluation strategy that occurred spontaneously, in a variety of settings (anywhere from the bedside to in the car to during coffee breaks). Feedback was much easier to deliver than the formal written evaluation and was most successful when delivered as close, in time, to the event as possible. With reference to a student who had performed poorly, one preceptor explained: "You don't want to hear about it in two weeks. You want to hear about it now." Opportunities for feedback had to be actively created and, not surprisingly, feedback was more prevalent in community settings in which preceptors and students had built-in debriefing sessions in the car between appointments. Preceptors admitted that it was difficult to deliver negative feedback in a constructive manner and gauged the success of their feedback on the students' reactions. One preceptor emphasized the importance of constructive feedback saying: "But occasionally you have to be critical and constructive, cause ultimately, you have to imagine that this person could easily be your teammate ... what kind of nurse do you want to work with?" Other nursing staff and members of the health care team were used as sources of feedback during the rotation and for the final evaluation. Lastly, preceptors acknowledged the importance of documenting feedback along the way in order to create a basis for the final, formal evaluation.

Successful evaluation strategies also included questioning and supervision. Many preceptors employed questioning to determine the student's level of knowledge but most importantly to determine the student's perception of their own abilities. Preceptors were alert to the types of questions students posed, affording them insight into the student's critical thinking, attitudes toward learning, and the extent of their knowledge. One preceptor expressed that "a mixture of confidence/knowledge and questioning behaviors is the best" because it displays proficiency and yet a willingness to continue learning. It is a strategy that is described as helping students to "guide themselves." Such supervision ensured for accurate evaluation in which preceptors observed students intently, evaluating their level of practice, gradually allowing for greater independence. The preceptors identified two unsuccessful strategies: use of quizzes and written assignments to test a student's knowledge.

The final step in the evaluation process was the completion of the formal, written evaluation at the culmination of the preceptorship to be submitted to the nursing faculty. Preceptors were divided on their reactions to the evaluation tool; however, there was general consensus that the tool was the most difficult aspect of their preceptorship experience and they concurred as to why it may not work very well. One preceptor summarized her perception as follows:

At first, I guess, [the evaluation form is] a bit overwhelming; I mean, they're your standard professional jargon-type, nursing-type things. But if you read through the criteria that they give you, it becomes clearer ... but I think their real evaluation is just what I'm writing in-between. Like, the feedback I'm writing, I think that's where the real evaluation is.

Preceptors who were able to manage the formal evaluation process had documented their feedback throughout the experience and had familiarized themselves with the student's learning objectives at the start. Specific challenges preceptors cited regarding the formal tool were found to be too much work, tedious and wordy; too vague, lacking in guidelines as to what kinds of behavior constituted standards such as "acceptable," "exceeds acceptable," etc.; too constraining without enough room for writing comments; and inappropriate for community nursing, but better applied to acute care. In one case, the nature of the rural setting prevented an objective evaluation because the student was related to one of the preceptor's superiors. Conversely, one preceptor felt that it was effective in "that they actually get you to sit down with the person, like once a month we sit down with them."

Preceptors described the need to significantly adapt their evaluation strategies when faced with an unsafe student, a process described as a difficult and the most challenging type of student to evaluate. The term unsafe student refers to those students: (a) whose level of practice is questionable in the areas of safety or (b) with marked deficits in knowledge and psychomotor skills, motivation, or interpersonal skills (Scanlan, Care, & Gessler, 2001). The feedback strategy continued to be employed; however, it became time-consuming and did not guarantee positive results. Feedback had to be "gentle, but firm," immediate, positive, and ongoing. It was described as "unfair" if a student did not have the benefit of receiving quality feedback regarding poor performance. Preceptors had to rely much more heavily on teaching rather than evaluating. Subsequently, the role of the faculty surfaced to a much higher level of importance. One preceptor explained: "As a preceptor, I'm a guide and I'm an assistant, but I'm not a professor ... Personally, I would be in contact with their clinical instructor, identify the problem, and go from there." Many preceptors abandoned their typical evaluation strategies to rely heavily on faculty support for the management of unsafe student behaviors, which in turn created serious dilemmas for preceptors at rural sites in which faculty presence is typically diminished, if not absent.

Data revealed that students play an integral part in the evaluation process. Preceptors stated that typically "strong" students are generally sent to rural placements, which in turn impacted on the time and effort they spent on evaluation. They described the evaluation of strong students as being "easy." As the formal evaluation was difficult for many preceptors, however, it was often the student to whom they turned to guide them through the process, the student being familiar with the university's expectations and evaluation tools. Some preceptors used student self-evaluations to help with their final evaluation and viewed this approach as a more appropriate way of involving students in the evaluation process. Student self-evaluations were helpful in setting learning goals, ensuring accuracy of the preceptor's final evaluation, and providing the preceptor with feedback on the experience. While preceptors clearly outlined the functions of their role and nature of the rural Canadian setting, they did not include the role of the evaluator. They described in detail the evaluation process, commenting on successful strategies as well as what they would do differently in the future, such as the delineation of learning objectives at the commencement of the rotation.

Preceptors described the evaluation process as self-directed and identified areas in which they required greater support such as completing summative evaluation and evaluating the student with unsafe performance. The preceptors revealed strategies that were effective (informal feedback, ongoing documentation, and development of learning objectives) and areas in which they required considerably more support (formal evaluation, evaluation of a student with unsafe performance, and need for a framework for evaluation). There is considerable inconsistency reflected in the evaluation process undertaken by rural preceptors. This inconsistency is apparent in how the role of the preceptor is described, the variety of criteria on which evaluation is based, steps taken (or not) in the evaluation process, evaluation strategies employed, and the variable role of the student and instructor in the evaluation process.

First, not a single preceptor in this study acknowledged the function of preceptor as "evaluator" on behalf of the university or profession, although the other roles reported were consistent with those described in the literature for urban preceptors (Dibert & Goldenberg, 1995; Usher, Nolan, Reser, Owens, & Tollefson, 1999). The majority of preceptors in this sample were, at the very least, expected to give their student a pass or fail recommendation at the culmination of the preceptorship. Blum (2009) developed a preceptorship model derived from a participatory action research project that emphasizes the contributions of all stakeholders in student evaluation and in particular greater preceptor participation in evaluation. Formal recognition of the preceptor role could raise awareness of the responsibilities and preparation required to execute it.

Preceptors assumed multiple role relationships to the health care agency as recruiter, to the student as a mentor and guide, and to the faculty as an evaluator. These multiple roles may conflict; without recognition of this conflict, preceptors have little support with which to navigate such roles and responsibilities (Seldomridge & Walsh, 2006). In a rural setting, such conflict could be compounded by multiple role relationships and high visibility within the community (Yonge, 2007). Thus, it is important to characterize the evaluation process as the responsibility of the preceptorship triad: preceptor, student, and faculty member, and to clearly define the scope of each role throughout the preceptorship.

The evaluation process must include both a framework (to determine what is being observed) and a tool (a method to record what has been observed) (Qualters, 1999). In this study, it became apparent that preceptors lacked an evaluation framework and thus inconsistencies existed in "what is being observed." Preceptors recognized, in retrospect, the need for delineating learning objectives at the beginning of the placement (Glover, 2000; Kemper, Rainey, Sherrill, & Mayo, 2004). In the process of developing learning objectives, students could identify their learning needs and strengths and limitations, preceptors could begin to identify learning activities at the clinical site, and faculty could help to link learning objectives with outcome competencies. Seldomridge and Walsh (2006) discuss the faculty's role in translating broadly stated course objectives into meaningful learning experiences and student-centered learning goals. Preceptors in this study who perceived themselves successful in the evaluation process had familiarized themselves with the formal evaluation tool at the commencement of the preceptorship. A "working backwards" approach could be encouraged to make the preceptorship more comprehensive from initial learning goals through to evaluation.

The lack of a framework for evaluation in rural preceptorship has caused preceptors to be especially self-directed, given their professional isolation and decreased access to faculty support and professional development as compared to their urban counterparts (Beatty, 2001; Yonge, 2007). Preceptors explained that they had devised personal criteria for evaluation, and sought guidance from students and colleagues when navigating the evaluation process. This process, however, resulted in a lack of reliability in student evaluation. It also points to a lack of preceptor preparation for the evaluation role (McCarthy & Murphy, 2008; Yonge et al., 1997). Face-to-face workshops and other forms of preceptor preparation have been used successfully to encourage preceptor–faculty dialogue, to orient preceptors to the evaluation role and to furnish preceptors with strategies for evaluation (Hallin & Danielson, 2009; Riley-Doucet, 2008; Walsh, Seldomridge, & Badros, 2008).

As described, daily, informal, immediate, "on-the-spot" feedback is most effective for student learning and also least problematic for the preceptor (Clynes & Raftery, 2008; Glover, 2000; Lee, 2005; Yonge et al., 1997). Preceptors also reported the use of observation and questioning as successful strategies for evaluation. However, they were described as being more intuitive than conscious—activities that occurred automatically. Myrick and Yonge (2002), in an article on preceptor questioning and its impact on student critical thinking, explain that

> Preceptors are in a prime position to challenge the way preceptees think, encourage them to justify or clarify their assertions, promote the generation of original ideas, explanations, or solutions to patient problems, provide mental and emotional tools to help resolve dilemmas, and provide a more personal environment with the one-to-one relationship (p. 176).

IMPLICATIONS

The theory underlying questioning and the skill itself could be promoted through preceptor education and workshops. Effective questioning can help determine a student's knowledge base, the process involved in their clinical decision making, and their critical thinking skills ultimately providing the grounds for evaluation (Myrick & Yonge, 2002). The finding that the use of quizzes and written assignments was unsuccessful as a teaching strategy could be attributed to the fact they are ostensibly designed for a more didactic approach to teaching and learning and would not be particularly appropriate or useful in their application to the practical realm of teaching in preceptorship.

The concerns that preceptors reported regarding formal evaluation are consistent with those reported by urban preceptors in other studies (Seldomridge & Walsh, 2006). Strategies that ensured success included documentation of feedback throughout the preceptorship together with delineation of learning objectives at the outset. Interestingly, the rural setting itself created additional challenges as the multiple role relationships preceptors had within the rural community occasionally interfered with the objectivity of the final evaluation. Thus, preceptor preparation for the evaluation process that is specifically "rural" in content could be very beneficial for rural-based preceptors in dealing with the unique challenges of this setting.

It was interesting to note that strategies for evaluation and teaching were dramatically adapted when preceptors had to work with a student who had unsafe behaviors. In a study by Luhanga, Yonge, and Myrick (2008), preceptors reported that it is much easier to make critical decisions about a student's performance when ensured the support and guidance of a faculty member. Rural preceptors could greatly benefit from the integration of strategies to work with such students during preceptor orientation as they may not have the benefit of the physical presence of a faculty member during the experience. Additionally, faculty presence in the form of phone calls, e-mails, and site visits greatly influenced preceptor perception of faculty support (Luhanga et al., 2008), and thus faculty need to be encouraged to maintain an ongoing presence at the rural site through phone calls, Skype, and e-mails.

From another perspective, preceptors perceived that rural placements were generally the recipients of "strong" students and perceived the evaluation of such students to be "easy." This perception may be misguided inasmuch as the placements in these two particular programs are coordinated through a modified lottery system whereby students' choice of placement, home address, and grades are sometimes taken into account. This perception could lead to inflated evaluations if students are perceived as naturally "strong," or students may miss out on the benefits of feedback for growth in clinical practice if they are perceived as such. Even strong students need to be challenged in their practice, and thus preceptors could be taught strategies such as the questioning as previously discussed (Myrick & Yonge, 2002). Lastly, although preceptors perceived the evaluation of "strong" students to be easy, they often still relied on the student for guidance during the evaluation process. This approach suggests that the respective roles and responsibilities of the preceptorship triad may be poorly defined and require clarification so that appropriate teaching–learning boundaries can be maintained.

The Next Step

The findings of this study were used directly to collaborate with a small group of preceptors in a rural setting, the purpose of which was to develop a workshop that could be used to enhance the evaluation skills of preceptors. Three researchers and three rural preceptors met for one day in a rural setting and developed a framework for evaluation of students in a rural setting. This framework identifies a triad required to engage in the process of rural evaluation. This triad is the preceptee, faculty, and preceptor (the WHO). Next, is a discussion on the importance of goals and objectives for both the preceptor and the preceptee (the WHAT); bringing awareness to the times and settings where evaluation can be accomplished (the WHEN/WHERE); increasing the understanding of the value of evaluation in the preceptee rural learning experience (the WHY); and lastly discussing strategies for performing evaluation (the HOW) (see Figure 18.1).

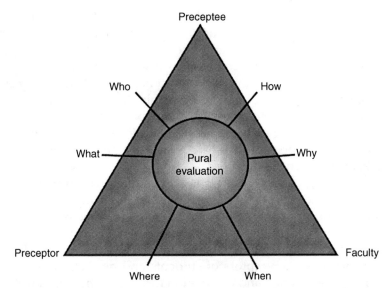

FIGURE 18.1   A framework for preceptor evaluation of student performance in rural settings

   This framework guided an intervention for rural preceptors in the form of a workshop. The workshop was piloted with three nurse preceptors at a rural hospital located within driving distance of one and one-half hours from the university. Based on feedback from these preceptors, the intervention was refined and subsequently yielded a 3-hour rural preceptor evaluation workshop. Workshops were then conducted in five rural settings, with 19 preceptors, over the course of 14 months. The feedback received reinforced the challenges preceptors encounter with evaluation. What they found as most valuable was the breakdown of the evaluation process into smaller units; the provision of "starting phrases" for student evaluations; the suggestion of journaling throughout the preceptorship experience as a form of documenting student behaviors; and the discussion of how to manage difficult or unsafe students.
   Follow-up telephone interviews were conducted with nine nurses who had attended the evaluation workshop. The telephone interviews indicated that the rural preceptors appreciated the organization of the workshop using the framework. The fact that the workshop focused on rural preceptors and used examples and strategies specific to their situation was also helpful. All the preceptors indicated that they believe in preceptorship for a variety of reasons. They did not mind precepting prior to the workshop; however, they did not always

agree to do so because they saw the formal evaluation as an onerous task. As a result of the workshop, they were able to see that with daily organization, evaluation and feedback could be less cumbersome. The presence of a faculty member at each workshop made preceptors feel that faculty were truly available and concerned with how they evaluated students throughout the preceptorship. Lastly, the material used in the workshop intervention has been incorporated into the University Preceptor Manual at one site so that these strategies can be implemented even prior to the arrival of the student at the rural site (see Yonge, Myrick, & Ferguson, 2011).

In summary, currently, students are guiding their preceptors as to how to complete the evaluation forms, that is, a faculty responsibility. It is important for faculty to be more systematic in the preparation of preceptors for such an important role as student evaluation and, even more important, to base this preparation on research evidence. In particular, rural-based preceptors of students and novice nurses require greater role clarification and recognition to support their responsibility as evaluators on behalf of an educational institution. The evaluation framework for the evaluation of nurse preceptors examined in this study needs to be applied in other sites aside from the two Prairie Provinces in Canada. The rural setting provides rich learning experiences with positive recruitment outcomes; thus, preceptor support and development could ensure sustainability of these valuable placements.

ACKNOWLEDGMENTS

Funding: The authors would like to thank the Social Sciences and Humanities Research Council (SSHRC) of Canada for their support of this research.

Participants: The authors would like to thank the health regions for permission to access rural sites, the nursing managers for access to staff participants, and lastly, nursing preceptors who took the time to share their thoughts on the experience of rural evaluation, and to attend and evaluate the workshop itself.

Project Staff: The authors would like to acknowledge Research Assistants Marke Ambard, Jan Scott, Judy McTavish, BScN, and Barb Neufeld, BScN for their work on this project.

REFERENCES

Alberta Physicians Resources Planning Group. (1997). *Alberta physicians planning group report.* Edmonton, Alberta: Author.

Beatty, R. M. (2001). Continuing professional education, organizational support, and professional competence: Dilemmas of rural nurses. *The Journal of Continuing Education in Nursing, 32*(5), 203–209.

Blum, C. A. (2009). Development of a clinical preceptor model. *Nurse Educator, 34*(1), 29–33.

Bushy, A. (2001). Critical access hospitals: Rural nursing issues. *The Journal of Nursing Administration, 31*(6), 301–310.

Bushy, A. (2005). Rural nursing practice and issues. *Nevada RN Information, 14*(2), 22–29.

Canadian Institute for Health Information (CIHI). (2007). *Distribution and internal migration of Canada's Registered Nurse workforce*. Ottawa, Ontario: CIHI.

Clynes, M. P., & Raftery, S. E. C. (2008). Feedback: An essential element of student learning in clinical practice. *Nurse Education in Practice, 8*(6), 405–411.

Dibert, C., & Goldenberg, D. (1995). Preceptors' perceptions of benefits, rewards, supports and commitment to the preceptor role. *Journal of Advanced Nursing, 21*, 1144–1151.

Dolan, G. (2003). Assessing student nurse clinical competency: Will we ever get it right? *Journal of Clinical Nursing, 12*, 132–141.

Ferguson, L. M., & Calder, B. L. (1993). A comparison of preceptor and educator valuing of nursing student clinical performance criteria. *Journal of Nursing Education, 32*(1), 30–36.

Glaser, B. G. (1978). *Theoretical sensitivity: Advances in the methodology of grounded theory*. Mill Valley, CA: Sociology Press.

Glover, P. A. (2000). 'Feedback. I listened, reflected and utilized': Third year nursing students' perceptions and use of feedback in the clinical setting. *International Journal of Nursing Practice, 6*, 247–252.

Guba, E. G., & Lincoln, Y. S. (1989). *Fourth generation evaluation*. Newbury Park, CA: Sage.

Hallin, K., & Danielson, E. (2009). Being a personal preceptor for nursing students: Registered Nurses' perceptions before and after introduction of a preceptor model. *Journal of Advanced Nursing, 65*(1), 161–174.

Hegney, D., McCarthy, A., Rogers-Clark, C., & Gormann, D. (2002). Retaining rural and remote area nurses: The Queensland, Australia experience. *The Journal of Nursing Administration, 32*(3), 128–135.

Kemper, K., Rainey, C., Sherrill, W., & Mayo, R. (2004). Guidelines for public health practitioners serving as student preceptors. *Health Promotion Practice, 5*(2), 160–173.

Lee, C. D. (2005). Rethinking the goals of your performance-management system. *Employment Relations Today, 32*(3), 53–60.

Luhanga, F., Yonge, O., & Myrick, F. (2008). Precepting an unsafe student: The role of the faculty. *Nurse Education Today, 28*, 227–231.

McCarthy, B., & Murphy, S. (2008). Assessing undergraduate nursing students in clinical practice: Do preceptors use assessment strategies? *Nurse Education Today, 28*, 301–313.

Myrick, F., & Yonge, O. (2002). Preceptorship questioning and student critical thinking. *Journal of Professional Nursing, 18*(3), 176–181.

Qualters, D. (1999). Observing students in a clinical setting. *Family Medicine, 31*(7), 461–462.

Riley-Doucet, C. (2008). A self-directed learning tool for nurses who precept student nurses. *Journal for Nurses in Staff Development, 24*(2), E7–E14.

Scanlan, J. M., Care, W. D., & Gessler, S. (2001). Dealing with unsafe students in clinical practice. *Nurse Educator, 26*(1), 23–27.

Schoenfelder, D., & Valde, J. (2009). Creative practicum leadership experiences in rural settings. *Nurse Educator, 34*(1), 38042.

Sedgwick, M., & Yonge, O. (2008). Undergraduate students' preparedness to "go rural." *Nurse Education Today, 28*(5), 620–626.

Seldomridge, L. A., & Walsh, C. M. (2006). Evaluating student performance in undergraduate preceptorships. *Journal of Nursing Education, 45*(5), 169–176.

Shannon, S. J., Walker-Jeffreys, M., Newbury, J. W., Cayetano, T., Brown, K., & Petkov, J. (2006). Rural clinician opinion on being a preceptor. *Rural and Remote Health, 6*(490). Retrieved 9/5/2011 from http://www.rrh.org.au/publishedarticles/article_print_490.pdf

Statistics Canada. (2009). *Population urban and rural, by province and territory.* Ottawa, ON: Government of Canada. Accessed on August 8, 2010 at http://www40.statcan.gc.ca/l01/cst01/demo62a-eng.htm

Stern, P. N. (1980). Grounded theory methodology: Its uses and processes. *IMAGE: The Journal of Nursing Scholarship, 12*(12), 20–30.

Strauss, A., & Corbin, J. (1990). *Basics of qualitative research: Grounded theory procedures and techniques.* Newbury Park, CA: Sage.

Streubert, H. J., & Carpenter, D. R. (1999). Qualitative research in nursing. In *Advancing the humanistic imperative* (2nd ed.). New York, NY: Lippincott.

Usher, K., Nolan, C., Reser, P., Owens, J., & Tollefson, J. (1999). An exploration of the preceptor role: Preceptors' perceptions of benefits, rewards, supports and commitment to the preceptor role. *Journal of Advanced Nursing, 29*(2), 506–514.

Walsh, C., Seldomridge, L., & Badros, K. (2008). Developing a practical evaluation tool for preceptor use. *Nurse Educator, 33*(3), 113–117.

Weinert, C., & Long, K. A. (1989). Rural nursing: Developing the theory base. *Scholarly Inquiry for Nursing Practice: An International Journal, 3*(2), 113–127.

Yonge, O. (2007). Preceptorship rural boundaries: Student perspective. *Online Journal of Rural Nursing and Health Care, 7*(1). Retrieved 9/5/2011 from http://www.rno.org/journal/index.php/online-journal/article/viewFile/7/176

Yonge, O., Krahn, H., Trojan, L., & Reid, D. (1997). Preceptors evaluating nursing students. *Canadian Journal of Nursing Administration, 10*(2), 77–95.

Yonge, O., Myrick, F., & Ferguson, L. (2011). The process of developing a framework to guide rural nurse preceptors in the evaluation of student performance. *Nurse Education in Practice, 11,* 76–80.

III

Program Development, Management, and Evaluation

Section three addresses the transition-to-practice program mainten-ance issues of development, management and evaluation. The appreciative inquiry model is presented in Chapter 20, by Crusoe, as a method for innovative development. Tieman offers business rationales for implementing nurse transition-to-practice (TTP) pro-grams in rural health care facilities. Chapter 21 includes an exemplar business plan to support nurse leaders during the development of a TTP program.

Chapter 22 consists of an interview with a director of nurses in a critical access hospital about leadership issues in Southeastern Idaho. Asay shares a personal journey and offers insights on strategies to improve the rural nurse quality of care. Molinari elaborates on an instructional design system to improve teaching outcomes in Chapter 23. This model was designed in a new residency to standardize professional nurses' instructional strategies in order to increase nurse competencies. In Chapter 24 Molinari examines philosophical and pro-gression issues in transition-to-practice curriculum.

Chapter 25 by Josephsen reviews distance education instructional tools. Distance education techniques can improve educational access so that nurses can maintain professional competence, pursue an advanced degree, and develop practice expertise. Bushy and Hewett follow in Chapter 26 with a discussion of simulation in continuing education. A review of simulation types and strategies for use in small rural health care facilities are offered. Finally, section three concludes with a concentration on varieties of program outcome evaluation by Molinari and Bushy. Using analytics to measure educational program outcomes is critical to refine and sustain a transition-to-practice initiative.

19

Appreciative Inquiry: A Model for Positive Change and Innovation

Kristen Crusoe

A successful nurse transition-to-practice program mandates the integration of a curriculum into an organizational culture. *This chapter introduces appreciative inquiry (AI) as one approach to planning and implementing professional development initiatives steeped in an organization's strengths. The AI philosophy and processes are explained and subsequently applied to designing and evaluating nurse transition-to-practice program in a rural context.*

Change is constant in a global society that is instantaneously connected with rapidly changing technology. Nurses also constantly must contend with change, such as modifying patient care practices that can lead to improved health outcomes; or, incorporating evidence-based practices to improve practice techniques; or, altering personal and professional issues. In fact, a significant role for the nurse is that of a change agent; that is, one who facilitates new approaches to existing conditions. Implementing and sustaining change are skills most novice nurses are not proficient in, and are usually learned over time with experience and support from experienced colleagues.

Change efforts often fail because of resistance or poor follow-through. When change is mandated from the top of the organizational hierarchy without engaging staff knowledge and wisdom, the outcomes can be less than satisfactory. Those impacted by change, or who have the most direct experience with the issue/topic, often fear the unknown, which is a primary cause of resistance. Nurses, particularly nurses who have demonstrated competency, may fear being seen as incompetent. Fear can lead to anger and increase resistance. The best way to lead and facilitate positive, collaborative change is to include everyone impacted by the change; or, who has knowledge about the issues to engage in the change process. Appreciative inquiry (AI) is a strength-based, inclusive, collaborative process for bringing about change that is sustainable, realistic, and is based on past successes so that fear of failure is not an issue.

AI: MANAGING CHANGE

One professional nurse core competency is related to managing change. The registered nurse (RN) is expected to use outcome data and to provide leadership in the modification of patient care and/or organizational issues toward identified outcomes. The RN also should be able to analyze issues, evaluate resources, and actively support change and innovation that can lead to improved outcomes. Leading and participating in change require knowledge about the change process along with skills in team building, collaboration, and effective communication. The American Organization of Nurse Executives (AONE) (2005) identifies understanding and managing change, and innovation as an essential leadership competency for nurses. Nurse leaders may perform a number of roles in the process of change (Huber, 2010). Whether an individual's role is a staff nurse implementing better practices, a nurse manager directing a unit-based innovation, or as a nurse leader championing an organizational initiative to improve the environmental culture, change requires knowledge, skills, and abilities to be an effective change agent.

Traditional problem-solving methods are most appropriate for linear, time-limited, mechanical, or functional problems that need to be fixed. Complex, human system issues and problems with a behavioral component require another approach. Patient safety, quality, and organizational culture issues require a positive, strength-based, inclusive, and collaborative program development method. Planning for change must be dynamic in nature and grounded in complex adaptive systems (CAS) (AONE, 2005). The AI model provides this approach. AI is both a philosophy and methodology for promoting sustainable positive organizational change. Outcomes include improved communication, collaboration, and nurse involvement in decision-making, enhanced cultural sensitivity, and awareness (Havens, Wood, & Leeman, 2006).

AI: SEEKING THE ROOT CAUSE OF SUCCESS

AI entails seeking out the *root cause of success*, and then, establishes action plans, systems, and processes to make the extraordinary become ordinary. As a methodology, AI is based on five underlying beliefs: Constructionist principle, principle of simultaneity, poetic principle, anticipatory principle, and the positive principle. A brief description of these five tenets follows.

The *constructionist principle* assumes that people cocreate reality through language and relationships. Change emerges from our behaviors and interactions. Humans choose to focus on positive, life-giving, collaborative relationships, and grounded in the language of possibilities and affirmation—or, we can choose to focus on negative, life-denying, destructionist language. These conversations take place within people during mental chatter; as well as, in moment-to-moment interactions with clients/patients, students, peers, colleagues, and in all relationships. Words do create worlds. Within the rich context of relationship, people find new ways of seeing and being together that enhances what is already working. Inquiry is inseparable from action. Its purpose is to create "generative theory." Rather than explaining yesterday's world, it articulates tomorrow's possibilities (Cooperrider & Whitney, 1999).

The *simultaneity principle* alludes to inquiry is a form of action research and, in this context, is an intervention. The questions asked are fateful because they determine the answers found. It is important to ask the best questions, the questions that will lead the group toward the most positive, purposeful, and life-affirming. Inquirers can ask, "What's wrong here? What's not working? Or, alternately ask," What is the best this person, this team, this group, this organization can offer? How can decision makers amplify or increase the frequency of positive actions and therefore, results? Groups moving positive directions encounter barriers. Focusing on "the positive" uncovers fresh, creative strategies for overcoming barriers. This method is not ignoring the problems in a Pollyanna fashion. Rather, the change agents are placing their energies on what has proven to be effective and successful—even if only to a small degree. The focus of inquiry is on an effective strategy, to amplify study, and learn how to generate action steps to make the extraordinary ordinary.

The *poetic principle* infers that "We can study whatever we choose." A program planner can study either problems or successes. Leaders can perform root cause analyses on everything that is wrong with work, patients, colleagues, systems, and selves, or perform root cause analyses on what brings a sense of joy, of accomplishment, and that connects the present to core values. Now, certainly, there will be times when root cause analysis of failure and sentinel events is needed, but once the weak points are identified, the program development process can change. Data systems can be established to construct baseline metrics for measuring improvements as well as failures. Determining effective outcomes emerges from the analysis of data. That is to say, seeking out positive exemplars and designing systems to reproduce successful outcomes, and, then integrating that approach into the institution's culture.

The *anticipatory principle* engages the power of imaging the future to guide present action. Individuals move in the direction of the future's image as determined by the institutional culture. The placebo effect, the Pygmalion dynamic, and the self-fulfilling prophecy all describe some aspects of this phenomena. For example, athletes' visions of performing well emerge from positive self-reflection and imagining that outcome. Likewise, optimism and anticipation of successful outcomes by the novice nurse evolve with mentors supporting a vision of successful performance as a professional.

The *positive principle* includes aspects of positive psychology. Affirming emotions such as caring, having a sense of purpose or meaning in one's life, hope, optimism, joy, resilience, and hardiness can counterbalance extensive life experiences that encourage helplessness, despair, and hopelessness.

AI VERSUS PROBLEM SOLVING

Several underlying assumptions differentiate AI from the more traditional problem-solving approach.

1. In every society, organization, or group, something is working.
2. What a person focuses on becomes his/her reality.
3. Reality for a person is created in the moment; and, within a group of individuals there also are multiple realities.
4. The act of asking questions of an organization or group influences the individual in some way.
5. A person has more confidence and comfort to journey into the future (the unknown) when he/she carries forward parts of the past (the known).
6. If one carries forward a part of the past, the person should be aware of what was best in the past.
7. It is important to value differences among individuals.
8. The language one uses creates an individual's reality.

When providers apply these assumptions to culture change within organizations, the importance of relationship and communication are appreciated. In traditional problem-solving approaches, change agents emphasize what is broken, what is not working, and what is wrong. The goal is to fix the problem, but not necessarily change or improve the overall culture. There is a place for this approach, especially in health care when correcting short-term, functional issues. The more complex, human system issues require different approaches. The method needs to be inclusive, collaborative, and strengths based.

AI includes two concepts. *Appreciation* means to recognize and value the contributions or attributes of things and people around us and *inquiry* means to explore and discover, in the spirit of seeking to better understand, and being open to new possibilities. Together, these concepts frame an approach to change and transform human systems that are grounded in appreciation and inquiry. AI is not a substitute for problem solving. There are times and situations when a linear, mechanical problem-solving approach is the best and only approach for time-limited, linear, mechanical problems such as a flat tire or other vehicular issue. Some human situations such as trauma and organ dysfunction require linear problem solving to determine if surgical procedures are required. But once the emergent situation has resolved, the AI approach reemphasizes health and vitality.

IMPLEMENTING AI PROCESSES

AI processes consists of discovery, dream, design, and destiny; or, the four "Ds." Each of these activities is different; yet, there is overlapping of all four activities.

Discovery entails asking positively oriented questions such as: When is ____at its best? What gives life to this person, team, or organization? Discovering the "best of what is.": What do organizations that retain nurses look like? The appreciative interview is used to drill into the core factors that contribute to nurse retention.

Dream entails envisioning the ideal. In turn, this requires asking a different type of question. "What might be?" Imaging what the "best of" might look like if it became the ordinary instead of extraordinary is a detailed process. Examining how to take the best and make it even better requires careful analysis of the ideal, and then adapting it to the local context. The next set of questions could ask: Imagine your facility as the best, most attractive work setting you have ever worked. What is happening? How does the team work together? What is staff development like? How is information shared? How do nurses advance? How are they recognized for achievement? How do they support one another during conflict? How does the team share information, engage each other in planning and problem solving, and celebrate successes?

Design entails planning and implementing a plan that includes key stakeholders. The plan should embed cultural values and aspirations as the change is put into place. The question of importance is; "What should be the ideal?" This "D" includes developing a plan. The details of creating and sustaining supports and teamwork are outlined. What are the three most important actions or behaviors that will enhance the team? Groups and individuals outline specific actions necessary for living the dream.

Destiny entails delivering the plan, or implementing the change or innovation so that it becomes reality, and can be sustained and adapted over time. This step takes the plan and makes it real in everyday life. Committing resources to the plan fashions reality. The team may ask questions like: What requests should be addressed first? How much time and effort is required for the specific outline? Who will supply the resources? How will success be recognized and reported?

The next step is to address the question: How does appreciative inquiry using the 4-D process apply to designing and implementing a nurse transition-to-practice program and improve retention in the nursing workforce? "More specifically, how can a small rural health care facility nourish, support, and retain recent graduates who are employed as a novice nurse?" "What are the contributing factors associated with poor retention?" What has the organization done incorrectly? Or could be doing better? Why can the facility not solve the problem? Why are new graduates not better prepared for practice?

The positive approach to improving practice can continuously apply this methodology to any questions. If the "positive topic" is not apparent, then reframe the issue from negative into positive terms. For instance, poor teamwork becomes winning teamwork; poor morale becomes high morale; lack of leadership becomes compelling leadership.

In summary, the philosophy of AI is to identify excellence in organizations and in individuals. In other words, seeking out best practices or models and building on these situations. A successful novice nurse transition-to-practice program fits within the organizational culture and builds on its strengths. Subsequently, successes are created, replicated, expanded, and celebrated. The process is all about asking the unconditional positive question. Finding small strategies or large values that keep the team engaged, ignited, and inspired to do their best, and to support others to do their best, is the secret to building positive cultures.

REFERENCES

AONE. (2005). *Guiding principles for the role of the nurse in future care delivery*. Healthful Practice/Work Environment.

Catalano, J. (2003). *Nursing now: Today's issues, tomorrow's trends* (3rd ed., Vol. 12, pp. 229–246). Philadelphia, PA: F. A. Davis.

Cooperrider, D. L., & Whitney, D. (1999). *Appreciative inquiry; Collaborating for change.* CA: Berrett-Koehler.

Havens, D., Wood, S., & Leeman, J. (2006). Improving nursing practice and patient care: Building capacity with appreciative inquiry. *Journal of Nursing Administration, 36*(10), 463–470.

Huber, D. (2010). *Leadership and nursing care management* (4th ed., Vol. 3, pp. 55–77). St Louis, MO: Elsevier.

BIBLIOGRAPHY

Hammond, S. (1998). *The thin book of appreciative inquiry.* Bend: Thin Book Publishing Company.

Institute of Medicine of the National Academies. (2010, August). *A summary of the February Forum on the Future of Nursing: Education.* Robert Wood Johnson Foundation.

Plsek, P., & Greenhalgh, T. (2001). Complexity science: The challenge of complexity in healthcare. *British Medical Journal, 323,* 625–628.

Shendell-Falik, N., Feinson, M., & Mohr, B. (2007). Enhancing patient safety: Improving the patient handoff process through appreciative inquiry. *Journal of Nursing Administration, 37*(2), 95–104.

Singhal, A., Buscell, P., & Lindberg, C. (2010). *Inviting everyone: Healing healthcare through positive deviance.* NJ: Plexus Press.

Stavros, J. (2003, March). *Cultivating a positive culture through appreciative inquiry.* MI: Lawrence Technological University.

Watkins, J., & Mohr, B. (2001). *Appreciative inquiry: Change at the speed of imagination.* San Francisco, CA: Jossey-Bass. Will add links to web sites

20

The Business Case for Rural Transition to Practice

Linda A. Tieman

This chapter highlights the rationale supporting the business case for implementing a nurse transition-to-practice (TTP) program within a health care institution, particularly in rural facilities. A business plan exemplar that can be used by the nurse administrator to support development of a TTP program for new nurses is included.

A new registered nurse (RN) enters the workforce with sound education, some clinical experience, high energy and ability to learn quickly, and the desire to build the competency of an expert professional. As with other professions, nurses also require a planned, well-managed, and evaluated program that can facilitate successful transition into the professional role. Sound financial analysis can validate the value of nurse transition programs as a wise investment for the health care organization. Facilitating the successful transition from new RN to novice professional has been discussed in the literature for decades. Earlier on, Kramer (1974) identified "reality shock" as a concern for nurses on first entering the workforce. Since then, a significant body of research exists on what is termed, "transition to practice" (TTP).

Nurse educators are told disturbing stories by recent graduates about harsh treatment and being hazed by experienced nurses. Graduates report that they receive minimal orientation and are assigned to responsibilities far beyond their neophyte capability. Some employers complain that new RNs are not prepared for the responsibilities of the role for which they are hired. Nurse administrators express frustration with the lack of preparation of recent graduates as well as the high costs associated with extended orientations and continual staff turnover. Additionally, more experienced nurses expect new RN graduates to possess a level skills to match that of their own. Seasoned nurses recall (erroneously or romantically) the ability to immediately step into the professional RN role and function independently on their own graduation. Whether fact or fiction, what is forgotten is how dramatically health care has changed over the years. Whether a rural or urban setting, unrealistic employer expectations create excessive stress and frustration for a new employee, resulting in job dissatisfaction and sometimes in the nurse leaving the profession. This outcome poses serious concerns for the profession as a whole and for an individual who senses failure and inability to be successful as a nurse. Additional questions about this loss of nurses center on the use of tax dollars to educate a nurse who subsequently leaves the workforce.

Health care facilities in rural settings have additional considerations relative to the sustainment of a stable nursing workforce. Not only do high RN vacancy and turnover rates negatively impact on the facility's overall financial status, but impact staff morale, quality of care, and patient satisfaction. When a rural community perceives that the local hospital is providing questionable care, residents often seek health care elsewhere. This further reduces revenues for a financially tenuous hospital and other business entities in the community. Doubts about the care provided by the local health care system also lead business owners to question whether or not employees and their families can receive adequate services locally. In turn, such doubts contribute to business relocation to more favorable communities. Essentially, availability of a reputable health care system plays a vital role in a small community's economic development and sustainability; and without a doubt, an adequate and stable nursing workforce is a critical element.

Administrators of rural health care facilities appreciate the value of maintaining a strong and stable nursing workforce. As for employees in these facilities, generally they are "place bound," associated with community roots, and not readily able to relocate to pursue educational opportunities offered in urban settings. Rural hospital executives report that their employees are loyal to the organization and prefer to continue to be employed in the facility. Yet, many of these individuals desire to purse the education to become an RN, and are frustrated by an inability to obtain the necessary education. Even more disconcerting for them is seeing RN vacancies filled with temporary high-cost traveling and agency nurses, who have little or no knowledge of the community, and limited loyalty to the local hospital.

Attracting and retaining RNs to rural settings has only recently received serious attention in the literature. Likewise the literature on developing and implementing an effective TTP program that fits the rural culture is sparse. Yet, the TTP program can be a successful strategy to ensure a stable and experienced nursing workforce that contributes to high-quality health care and the provision of critical nursing services.

PROJECTING COSTS

The value of reducing unnecessary turnover and increasing retention through TTP can be calculated by an employer using its own average RN salary and benefits calculations, its usual time to hire, and its known HR recruitment costs. For instance, the Washington (State) Department of Labor (WDOL) reports that the average base salary for an RN is $60,000 with ~35% more being customary for employee benefits, thus $81,000 annually. Turnover includes the departure, recruitment, and hiring of an employee from a business. The average cost to recruit and hire an RN to replace a nurse can be as much as 1.3 times the annual salary of an RN or about $105,000 in Washington State. Consequently, costs attributed to the turnover of an RN are greater than the annual salary for that position. Logically, retention of an experienced and loyal work force will be a cost-saving business strategy.

Monitoring Organizational Metrics

To build the case for TTP key factors, "organizational metrics," are needed. Monitoring select metrics over time can reveal trends, strengths, and opportunities for improvement for a single unit, department, or the institution as a whole—in this case nursing. Ideally, data for identified metrics are collected at the unit level, and then aggregated and compiled for the entire division of nursing. In small rural facilities such as Critical Access Hospitals (CAHs), metric data may need to be collected and analyzed for the entire facility. Metric data needed to establish the business care for a TTP program include:

- Average cost to the organization for annual salary and benefits paid to an RN (factor in differentials for education, experience, etc.).
- Costs to the employer of RNs (i.e., unemployment, payroll taxes, Labor & Industry (L&I), etc.).
- Average annual RN turnover rate (defined as exit/departure from the organization; does not include internal or lateral movement from one department to another).
- Cost of orientation for new RN employees (i.e., general orientation and work area-specific orientation).
- Average annual RN vacancy rate.

■ Annual cost of RN overtime.
■ Average length of time to fill a vacant RN position.
■ Average annual cost paid for agency or traveler RNs.
■ Average annual cost of education, vacation, sick time (sometimes called "nonproductive time").
■ Costs and expenses for recruitment of an RN (e.g., advertising, time associated with interviewing, travel expenditures, reference follow-up, etc.).
■ Average annual costs for Human Resource personnel to attend career fairs (costs for participation in events, lodging, travel, expenses, and compensation).

A detailed cost and financial analysis based on the organizational metrics follows and includes the following line items for the proposed TTP program.

■ Costs associated with educator(s) time for planning, delivery, and evaluation of program.
■ Costs for facility, technology, and supply for the TTP program specifically.
■ Hourly wage paid to participants while in the TTP residency (but, not providing direct patient care).
■ Salary and benefits paid to agency or traveler nurses and/or overtime paid to regular staff to supplement nursing coverage while a new hire is in the TTP program.
■ Differential salaries paid to nurse preceptors who mentor new hires in a TTP program.
■ Costs paid to consultants and outside speakers for the TTP program.
■ Costs incurred to partially supplement the new hire until one proficiently assumes a "full work load"; often "hidden" but nonetheless "real" costs, since the orienteer is not producing the revenue expected of an experienced individual in that particular position.
■ Costs for a new hire to travel to other facilities for education or meetings associated with the TTP program.

To argue the business case for the TTP program for new RNs, the nurse administrator must clearly articulate annual cost variances associated with (repeatedly) recruiting, hiring, and orientating new RNs in comparison with costs associated with a TTP program. One must offer supporting evidence that participants are more likely to remain in the organization and reduce staff turnover (i.e., higher retention rates).

Short term, it can be difficult to demonstrate the impact of TTP programs on quality of care and service outcomes, usually associated with staff experience and institutional memory. Longitudinally reviewing set data points and crucial incidents, one can demonstrate that experienced nurses having an understanding of an organization's culture, policy, and procedures can positively impact on patient care and satisfaction.

It also can be useful in making the case to have demographic data about the institution's nursing workforce, such as:

- Age distribution of RN employees (to project number and pattern of retirements and needed replacement).
- Education level of RN staff (to delineate pay differential).
- Tenure (years/months) of RNs in the organization (to delineate pay differential).
- RN workforce by full time equivalents (FTEs) (full time, part time).
- Certifications held by RNs (to identify areas of expertise; delineate pay differential).
- Data reflecting RNs participation in organizational committees, task forces, community service contributions, and so on.
- Other relevant information that provides a comprehensive picture of the nursing workforce within the institution and the value of contributions made within a small community.
- Patient profile of each work area (patient mix, case mix index, frequent diagnosis, Average length of stay (ALOS), etc.).
- Current and relevant clinical quality outcomes data.
- Current patient satisfaction data.

Business Plan Exemplars

Basic business plans are accessible on the Internet and business textbooks and can be adapted for TTP business plans. The business plan requires a brief introductory narrative describing the problem, and the available options with potential outcomes and financial analysis for each. The National Council of State Boards of Nursing (NCSBN) published online the *Business Plan Template for Employers*. www.ncsbn. org. Included is a list of hospitals that have used the NCSBN model, along with data that support the positive relationship of patient care quality and safety with the TTP program. The NCSBN has also developed a TTP model to test its theory that TTP can positively impact on quality-of-care outcomes, and will implement a pilot study of this model in several states. Information on the NCSBN model is discussed in Chapters 3 and 10 of this volume.

Another example is this Washington Center for Nursing template.

Why a Nursing Transition to Practice Program? Sample Community Hospital Cost/Benefit Analysis

(Organization or work unit/department)

Current costs

Current organizational or unit Annual RN turnover rate[1]	70%

(New grads left the organization within past year) 7 At Sample Community Hospital

New grads hired during the same time period) 10 at Sample Community Hospital

Time-to-fill a vacant RN position	20 weeks

Cost to replace 7 vacant RN positions

• Traveler or agency costs during vacancy for 1 RN	A. $48,000

40hrs/week × 5 weeks=800hrs at $60.00/hr to an agency

• Traveler or agency during vacancy for 7 RNs for 20 weeks	A[i]$336,000
• Recruitment costs	B. To be decided (Tbd) by organization
• Usual orientation costs	C. $ 32,300

40hrs/week × 4 weeks=160hrs at $$28.84/hr

• TTP program or other unique orientation costs	D. Tbd by organization
• Supplemental staff/OT during orientation costs	E. Tbd by organization
• Other costs	F. Tbd by organization

Total cost to fill vacant positions

Potential cost to replace 7 new grads for 20 weeks	$368,300 +
Using the customary national assumption that the cost of replacement of an RN is 1.3x the annual salary, a simpler method would indicate that the cost/RN in WA State is $81,000.[2] For 7 RN's it could be as much as	$567, 000 +

Why a Nursing Transition to Practice Program?	Current costs
Planning, designing, delivering, evaluating program[3]	
• Avg salary of faculty for program (1 educator FT@$90k/yr for 20 wks)	A. $41,538
Shared staff & resources in a rural TTP program, so costs could be	A $20,000
• Avg salary of participant for program (1 RN@$81k/yr for 20 wks)	B. $31,153
• Number of weeks of program	20
• Supply, food, equipment costs for program	C.$1,000
Total cost/participant for TTP program; total cost/# participants	D. $40,087
Total cost of TTP program (for 7 new RN grads)	
(A + B × 7 + C)	$280,609

Note: Costs may be overstated, depending on the Rural TTP model, the ability to share resources, and the pace at which each new RN graduate progresses.

---

[1]Turnover: annual RN exits from the organization, not moves within the organization
[2]$60,000 +35% for benefits = $81,000 per year, x1.3 + $105,300
[3]Assumes overhead is part of departmental expense
Source: Washington State Center for Nursing, www.WACenterforNurising.com

PRESENTING THE CASE FOR THE TTP PROGRAM

Program presenters must be prepared to respond to the following, oft-asked question; "Why invest more for each new RN who is hired in this institution along with the current costs for orienting new hires?" Improved retention rates, positive financial impact, and improved quality are three key answers.

Rationale for this response includes the following.

While completing the TTP program, the RN who has completed regular orientation would be caring for patients and thus become familiar with the professional RN role. The RN would be assimilating the organization's culture, learning its policies, processes, and patterns of communication, and over time, assuming a heavier workload. In turn, the mentoring of the new RN provides support as the individual develops critical thinking and nursing skills, which contributes to greater confidence and enhanced job satisfaction. All these factors are documented to increase retention rates.

Both sides of the RN workforce equation must be balanced. On the one hand, allocating resources for effective recruitment planning and programming is critical; on the other, effective approaches to retain staff and reduce turnover rates are also necessary. In a small facility reducing RN turnover rates and improving retention of nurse can yield cost savings within 3 or fewer years. The small margins realized by all hospitals, rural being no exception, demand clear data to support TTP.

Engaging Staff in Presenting the Case

Chief Nurse Executives (CNOs), regardless of their official title or setting, are considered to be among senior administration in the health care organization. In reality, persuasive argument in making the case must engage the broader organization. Support for the investment of organizational resources into a TTP program, particularly in a rural facility, must extend into all areas of the institution. For instance, welcoming new RN creates impacts on many employees in that facility. The current staff have a vested interest in ensuring a successful experience for every new employee and for that reason should be actively engaged in the planning, implementation, and evaluation of the TTP program. In a small rural hospital, experienced RNs who are engaged and committed to the TTP program are critical to the initiative's success. These experienced nurses are usually highly regarded, and in a position to explain the human impact of high turnover rates, the demands of repeatedly being asked to precept new hires and/or describe near misses and actual errors with patient care. Insights about patient dissatisfaction, clinical quality outcomes, and physician concerns about the nursing care within the institution are important to discuss. In a rural community, maintaining adequate and experienced nursing staff is critical to sustaining healthy communities. Both professional and ancillary personnel are in a position to make the most authentic arguments to administration for investing in a TTP program. If there is a Professional Practice or Staff Nurse committee, it can be pivotal to moving the TTP business proposal forward.

In summary, this chapter describes the business model for a TTP program. The health care system often is the largest employer in a rural area, and an essential aspect of a healthy and thriving community. Implementing TTP programs to retain new RN graduates in the local workforce serves the community as well as the health care institution that implements such programs.

REFERENCES

Kramer, M. (1974). *Reality shock: Why nurses leave nursing.* St. Louis: CV Mosby Company.

BIBLIOGRAPHY

Advisory Board Company. (2006). *Transitioning new graduates to hospital practice: Profiles of nurse residency program exemplars.* Washington, DC: Author.

Agency for Healthcare Research and Quality (AHRQ). (2000). *Medical errors: The scope of the problem.* Fact Sheet, Publication No. AHRQ 00-P037, Rockville, MD: Author.

American Health Care Association. (2008). *Report of findings: 2007 AHCA survey nursing staff vacancy and turnover in nursing facilities.* Accessed from http://www.ahcancal.org/research_data/staffing/Documents/Vacancy_Turnover_Survey2007.pdf

American Nurses Association. (2000). *Scope and standards of practice for nursing professional development.* New York, NY: Author.

Ashcraft, A. S. (2004). Differentiating between pre-arrest and failure-to-rescue. *Medsurg Nursing, 13*(4), 211–216.

Barton, A. J., Armstrong, G., Preheim, G., Gelmon, S. B., & Andrus, L. C. (2009). A national Delphi to determine developmental progression of quality and safety competencies in nursing education. *Nursing Outlook, 57,* 313–322.

Beecroft, P., Hernandez, A. M., & Reid, D. (2008). Team preceptorships: A new approach for precepting new nurses. *Journal for Nurses in Staff Development, 24*(4), 143–148.

Beecroft, P. C., Kunzman, L., & Krozek, C. (2001). RN internship: Outcomes of a one-year pilot program. *JONA, 31*(12), 575–582.

Benner, P. (2004). Using the Dreyfus model of skill acquisition to describe and interpret skill acquisition and clinical judgment in nursing practice and education.
Bulletin of Science, Technology & Society, 24(3), 188–199.

Benner, P., Sutphen, M., Leonard, V., & Day, L. (2010). *Educating nurses: A call for
radical transformation.* San Francisco, CA: Jossey-Bass.

Berens, M. J. (2000, September 10). Nursing mistakes kill, injure thousands: Cost-
cutting exacts toll on patients, hospital staffs series: Dangerous care: Nurses'
hidden role in medical error. First of three parts. *The Chicago Tribune,* 20.

Berkow, S., Virkstis, K., Stewart, J., & Conway, L. (2008). Assessing new graduate
nurse performance. *JONA, 38*(11), 468–474.

Beyea, S. C., von Reyn, L., & Slattery, M. J. (2007). A nurse residency program for
competency development using patient simulation. *Journal for Nurses in Staff
Development, 23*(2), 77–82.

Bjørk, I. T., & Kirkevold, M. (1999). Issues in nurses' practical skill development in
the clinical setting. *Journal of Nursing Care Quality, 14*(1), 72–84.

Board of Registration in Nursing, Division of Health Professions Licensure, Massachusetts Department of Public Health. (2007). *A study to identify evidence-based
strategies for the prevention of nursing errors.* MA: Author.

Clarke, S. P., & Cheung, R. B. (2008). The nursing shortage: Where we stand and
where we're going. *Nursing Management,* March, 22–28.

Cronenwett, L., Sherwood, G., Barnsteiner, J., Disch, J., Johnson, J., Mitchell, P.
et al. (2007). Quality and safety education for nurses. *Nursing Outlook, 55,* 122,
131.

Del Bueno, D. (2005). A crisis in critical thinking. *Nursing Education Perspectives,
26*(5), 278–282.

Diggle, P. J., Heagerty, P., Liang, K. Y., & Zeger, S. L. (2002). *The analysis of longitudinal data* (2nd ed.). Oxford: Oxford University Press.

Dracup, K., & Morris, P. E. (July 2007). Nursing residency programs: Preparing for
the next shift. *American Journal of Critical Care, 16*(4), 328–330.

Ebright, P. R., Urden, L., Patterson, E., & Chalko, B. (2004). Themes surrounding novice nurse near-miss and adverse-event situations. *JONA, 34*(11),
531–538.

Elfering, A., Semmer, N. K., & Grebner, S. (2006). Work stress and patient safety:
Observer-rated work stressors as predictors of characteristics of safety-related
events reported by young nurses. *Ergonomics, 49*(5–6), 457–469.

Fink, R., Krugman, M., Casey, K., & Goode, C. (2008). The graduate nurse experience: Qualitative residency program outcomes. *JONA, 38*(7/8), 341–348.

Flying start. (2010). Accessed from http://www.flyingstart.scot.nhs.uk

Goode, C. J., Lynn, M. R., Krsek, C., & Bednash, G. D. (2009). Nurse residency programs: An essential requirement for nursing. *Nursing Economics, 27*(3), 142–147.

Greiner, A. C., & Knebel, E. (Eds.). (2003). *Health professions education: A bridge to
quality.* Washington, DC: The National Academies Press.

Halfer, D. (2007). A magnetic strategy for new graduates. *Nursing Economics, 25*(1),
5–11.

Halfer, D., Graf, E., & Sullivan, C. (2008). The organizational impact of a new graduate pediatric mentoring program. *Nursing Economics, 26*(4), 243–249.

Hofler, L. D. (2008). Nursing education and transition to the work environment:
A synthesis of national reports. *Journal of Nursing Education, 47*(1), 5–12.

Johnstone, M. J., & Kanitsaki, O. (2006). Processes influencing the development of graduate nurse capabilities in clinical risk management: An Australian study. *Quality Management in Health Care, 15*(4), 268–278.

Johnstone, M. J., & Kanitsaki, O. (2008). Patient safety and the integration of graduate nurses into effective organizational clinical risk management systems and processes: An Australian study. *Quality Management in Health Care, 17*(2), 162–173.

Joint Commission White Paper. (2002). *Health care at the crossroads: Strategies for addressing the evolving nursing crisis.* Retrieved November 15, 2009, from http://www.jointcommission.org/NR/rdonlyres/5C138711-ED76-4D6F-909F-B06E0309F36D/0/health_care_at_the_crossroads.pdf

Jones, C. M. (2004). The costs of nurse turnover, Part 1. *JONA, 34*(12), 562–570.

Jones, C. M. (2005). The costs of nurse turnover, Part 2. *JONA, 35*(1), 41–49.

Jones, C. M., & Gates, M. (2007). The costs and benefits of nurse turnover: A business case for nurse retention. *OJIN, 12,* (3).

Kalisch, B. J. (2006). Missed nursing care: A qualitative study. *Journal of Nursing Quality Care, 21*(4), 306–313.

Keller, J. L., Meekins, K., & Summers, B. L. (2006). Pearls and pitfalls of a new graduate academic residency program. *JONA, 36*(12), 589–598.

Kentucky. (2010). Accessed from http://kbn.ky.gov/education/pon/entry/

Kohn, L., Corrigan, J., & Donaldson, M. (Eds.). (1999). *To err is human: Building a safer health system.* Washington, DC: The National Academies Press.

Kovner, C., & Djukic, M. (2009). The nursing career process through the first 2 years of employment. *Journal of Professional Nursing, 25*(4), 197–203.

McKay, C. A., & Crippen, L. (2008). Collaboration through clinical integration. *Nursing Administration, 32*(2), 109–116.

Mississippi. (2010). Accessed from http://www.monw.org/

My InnerView. (2008). *2008 National survey of consumer and workforce satisfaction in nursing homes.* Accessed from http://www.ahcancal.org/research_data/staffing/Documents/MIVConsumerWorkforceSatisfaction2008.pdf

Nadkarni, V. M., Larkin, G. L., Peberdy, M. A., Carey, S., Kaye, W., Mancini, M. et al. (2006). First documented rhythm and clinical outcome from in-hospital cardiac arrest among children and adults. *Journal of the American Medical Association, 295*(1), 50–57.

NCSBN. (2002). *Report of findings from the 2001 employers survey.* Chicago: Author.

NCSBN. (2004a). *Report of findings from the 2003 employers survey.* Chicago: Author.

NCSBN. (2004b). *Report of findings from the 2003 practice and professional issues survey: Spring 2003.* Chicago: Author.

NCSBN. (2005). *Working with others: A position paper.* Accessed from https://www.ncsbn.org/Working_with_Others.pdf

NCSBN. (2006a). *Evidence-based nursing education for regulation (EBNER).* Chicago: Author. Retrieved October 17, 2008, from https://www.ncsbn.org/Final_06_EBNER_Report.pdf

NCSBN. (2006b). *A national survey on elements of nursing education.* Chicago: Author.

NCSBN. (2006c). *Transition to practice: Newly licensed registered nurse (RN) and licensed/vocational nurse (LPN/VN) activities.* Chicago: Author.

NCSBN. (2007). *The impact of transition experience on practice of newly licensed registered nurse.* Data presented in February, 2007, Transition Forum, Chicago, IL.

NCSBN. (2009a). *An analysis of NURSYS® disciplinary data from 1996–2006.* Accessed from https://www.ncsbn.org/09_AnalysisofNursysData_Vol39_WEB.pdf

NCSBN. (2009b). *Post-entry competence study.* Accessed from https://www.ncsbn.org/09_PostEntryCompetenceStudy_Vol38_WEB_final_081909.pdf

NCSBN. (2009c). *2008 RN practice analysis: Linking the NCLEX®RN examination to practice.* Accessed from https://www.ncsbn.org/08_Linking_the_NCLEX_to_Practice_Vol36.pdf

NCSBN. (2010a). *2009 LPN/VN practice analysis: Linking the NCLEX®PN examination to practice.* Accessed from https://www.ncsbn.org/10_LPN_VN_PracticeAnalysis_Vol44_web.pdf

NCSBN. (2010b). *Transition to practice: A business plan template for employers.*

Nicol, P., & Young, M. (2007). Sail training: An innovative approach to graduate nurse preceptor development. *Journal for Nurses in Staff Development, 23*(6), 298–302.

O'Rourke, M. W. (2006). Beyond rhetoric to role accountability: A practical and professional model of practice. *Nurse Leader, 4*(3), p28–33, 44. Accessed from whttp://tinyurl.com/2g9rps3://tinyurl.com/2g9rps3

Orsolini-Hain, L., & Malone, R. E. (2007). Examining the impending gap in clinical nursing expertise. *Policy, Politics, & Nursing Practice, 8*(3), 158–169.

Phillips, J. M. (2006). Preparing preceptors through online education. *Journal for Nurses in Staff Development, 22*(3), 150–156.

Pine, R., & Tart, K. (2007). Return on investment: Benefits and challenges of a baccalaureate nurse residency program. *Nursing Economics, 25*(1), 13–18.

Roxburgh, M., Lauder, W., Topping, K., Holland, K., Johnson, M., & Watson, R. (2010). Early findings from an evaluation of a post-registration staff development programme: The Flying Start NHS Initiative in Scotland, UK. *Nurse Education in Practice, 10*(2), 76–81.

Scott, E. S., Engelke, M. K., & Swanson, M. (2008). New graduate transitioning: Necessary or nice? *Applied Nursing Research, 21,* 75–83.

TIGER. (2010). *The TIGER initiative.* Accessed from http://www.tigersummit.com/Home_Page.php

Townsend, L. B. (1931). Teaching the classes following the physician's lecture. *American Journal of Nursing, 31*(10), 1183–1186.

Vermont Nurses in Partnership (VNIP). (2010). Accessed from whttp://www.vnip.org/://www.vnip.org/

Wiggins, M. (2006). The partnership care delivery model. *JONA, 36*(7–8), 341–345.

Williams, C. A., Goode, C. J., Krsek, C., Bednash, G. D., & Lynn, M. R. (2007). Postbaccalaureate nurse residency 1-year outcomes. *The Journal of Nursing Administration, 37*(7/8), 357–365.

Wisconsin. (2010). Accessed from whttp://wnrp.org/:///wnrp.org/

Yonge, O., Hagler, P., Cox, C., & Drefs, S. (2008). Listening to preceptors. *Journal for Nurses in Staff Development, 24*(1), 21–26.

21

Conversation With a Rural Director of Nurses

Nancy Asay and Deana L. Molinari

A say, an expert rural nurse administrator, presents an interview of her personal experience as a rural nurse. She discusses the challenges and rewards of nursing management in a small hospital, reaffirming the benefits of nurse transition-to-practice initiatives tailored to meet local needs. Her story highlights strategies that could improve health care in rural settings.

Most often, the focus of nurse transition-to-practice programs is the new graduate or someone who wishes to "become" a specialist. For instance, in the literature we read how states and provinces address recruitment and retention through competencies (Bassendowski & Petrucka, 2010; Ramritu & Barnard, 2008). North Carolina, Vermont, and Mississippi focus on the rural nurse shortage by developing preceptor education (Smedley, Peter Morey, & Race, 2010). Other groups emphasize nurse residencies (Maxwell, 2011). However, little was documented about nurse administrators' needs even though studies indicate that supervisors are the key to residency success (Molinari, Monserud, & Hudzinski, 2008). How do nurse administrators recruit and retain nurses? What are their recruiting and retention needs? A longtime rural nurse from Southeastern Idaho was asked these questions. She tells her personal story and offers ideas to improve health care.

Nancy is the acute care director at Oneida County Hospital on the border of Utah and Idaho. She earned an Associate of Science degree in nursing (ADN) in 1975 and a Baccalaureate of Science in Nursing (BSN) degree in 2004. Asay is a long-time resident of Malad, Idaho. She was first hired as a staff nurse at Oneida County Hospital shortly after graduation. She held that position until 1994 when she became the director of nursing service in this rural hospital.

HOW DID YOU BECOME A CHIEF NURSING OFFICER
OF THE ONEIDA COUNTY HOSPITAL

My true love is patient care. Rural nursing can be very challenging and difficult at times, but people appreciate what you are doing for them. It is always special to take care of a patient and hear how wonderful you are. The newer generation doesn't express appreciation as much as the older patients used to do, but I still find it rewarding to help those who are ill.

My mother worked here as a nurse for many years. I followed in her footsteps. I enjoy my career and I am dedicated to this facility because this is where I live. Malad, Idaho is a good place to live.

My first encounter with our rural hospital was in the old building built in the 1930s. It an orange brick two-story building. The ER and Radiology were on the second floor and the lab was on the first floor. There were patient rooms on both floors. The nurse's station was on the top floor right at the top of the stairs. There was no elevator, just a very steep indoor ramp that was real fun for a 4-year-old to run up and down. My mother was one of the few Registered Nurses in the community and was in high demand to be at work despite being the mother of six girls still at home.

Many times I would go to work with her and play on the floors that to me looked like checkered squares. I would spend hours hopping on the squares. Sometimes I would help the janitor rake leaves. There were always a huge amount of leaves at this facility to be raked. He would give me a dime at the end of the day. One day when I was feeling ill, I went to work with my mom and she put me in one of the patient room beds. She made me a handkerchief doll out of a sheet. It was really big and was the neatest cloth doll I had ever seen. What a memory. One other memory was of all the other people who worked there. My nicknames were "curly top" and "cookie" and "Phoebe's little girl."

After graduating from college, I came to work at Oneida County Hospital, now located in a new building. The facility was an 11-bed acute care and an 18-bed LTC facility. I married a high school classmate the same weekend as my college graduation and pinning ceremony. We stayed in our hometown. I planned to work part time so I would have time for building a family. Working part time turned into full time more and more often. Over the years insurance benefit rules changed so only full time workers qualified. I became a full time nurse while trying to raise a family of two boys and one girl. My husband ran the family dairy farm so he did not have health insurance.

I worked nights because I was the youngest in seniority. The director was a full time floor duty nurse on the day shift as well as the director. She worked Monday through Friday which meant the rest of the nurses worked weekends, evenings and nights.

My mother retired and died of breast cancer. Several other nurses approached retirement. My responsibility was operating room supervisor and circulating nurse. I supervised a licensed practical nurse (LPN) as my only scrub tech. We also worked our shifts on the floor. We worked around 125 hours in a two-week period way too often. If we had an obstetric case come in, someone would have to work the extra hours. My longest stretch of hours, straight without a break, was 28. We needed more nurses.

When our director of nursing service (DNS) retired we were under the direction of a nurse who retired from another facility. Her ideas were very different and I found it hard to adjust. She stayed two years then our leader was a young woman who moved to Malad and quickly became frustrated. In those days we had a couple of physicians who were demanding and tough to please. She did not last long.

Staffing was difficult. There were not any RNs or LPNs to be found and everyone was working more hours than they wanted. Administration did not want to keep paying for overtime. We had a difficult time scheduling vacations and holidays. We hired a new Doctor whose wife was an RN and she became the DNS for both the Long Term Care and the Acute Care facilities. She recruited two Filipino RNs. They were wonderful, very polite, smart, and both wanted to work all the hours they could get. Later on we got a Lab Technologist from the Philippines as well. The two RNs stayed five years each and the Lab Tec. stayed four years. They left to work in California and Washington. Later on we tried to recruit two more RNs from the Philippines but could not complete the visa process. The events of September 11, 2001 made it more difficult to get the foreign nurses.

By 1994 we had survived three different DNSs. I debated within myself and finally mustered up the courage to apply for the position. I knew nursing was my profession and career not just a job to help pay the bills or insurance. My young family was partially raised and I felt I could learn the job. I asked the administrator for leadership training if I took the position.

There were no leadership courses to be found in our area. Where do you go for help if you are a floor duty nurse stepping up to a house supervisor or Director of Nursing position? The need is especially great in rural America. Hiring a hometown nurse to fill the DNS position is better for the facility because of the community involvement this person would have. Strategic planning and staff loyalty require a nurse with understanding of community issues and networking abilities.

I know what I do now, as the DNS is important. I have good staff to support me and I do all I can to support them. That is why I stay and keep smiling and stay true to my values.

TELL ME ABOUT YOUR STAFFING CHALLENGES?

The lack of available personnel and education are our main problems. Hiring new nurses is not easy. It is almost impossible to recruit nurses. Advertising is a waste of money. We have never had a response from a regional or national ad.

We had some good foreign nurses once but visas were a problem another time. Once we sent a nurse to Canada to look for recruitment possibilities. That didn't go anywhere. You need to grow your own nurses. When you grow your own from community people they will stay or you will not get anyone to stay. We tried travelers and found that most unrewarding. The nurse would not do the job and left the house in a mess. We had to re-carpet the living room when she left after a three-month stay. Basically we can't afford agency nurses, travelers or per diem nurses. The per diem nurses that come from nearby towns are a problem because they don't develop a loyalty for the facility. They don't come to staff meetings or make care plans. They do what has to be done, but no extras.

I know four nurses who live in our little valley but work in larger facilities an hour away. Three of them rented an apartment together in the distant city so they don't have to travel so much each day. Even with paying for the apartment, the nurses felt the increased salary and better health insurance was worth the cost of traveling and rent.

Larger hospitals provide better health insurance because they qualify for a different risk pool. I keep hoping a collaborative group can get better rates, but not so far. We are competitive with retirement benefits but not health insurance. Another difference is "low [patient] census." Every hospital has to send nurses home if census is too low, but I think smaller hospitals must do it more often.

Education issues begin in high school. There are no easy solutions. In 1994 one male high school graduate announced plans to go to a Utah school to become a Registered Nurse. Giggles and snickers were heard throughout the gym. I was angry. We love the few male RNs and LPNs that we have in our facility. I wondered how we could overcome the prejudice. Eventually, a program to introduce nursing as a career was to be taken by every 6th grader. Public announcements were put on several of the TV stations throughout the State. Soon after this the Johnson and Johnson Company advertisements and posters "Be a Nurse" were seen. I have used these posters a lot.

We use LPNs for staffing the Long Term Care portion of the facility. Helping people become educated as a nurse is a problem for the rural hospitals. We try to take advantage of any classes in our area. There was an outreach LPN class once that some of our certified nurse assistants (CNAs) attended. Several small rural hospitals participated. There was another LPN class where we sent eight CNAs. After they graduated, one of them took a self-study, associate degree registered nurse (ADRN) program. After a couple of years she graduated and became an RN. One of the other LPN graduates went to school in Salt Lake City, Utah, which is about two hours away. She traveled a lot of miles over that year's time. Taking a four year program is not an option for a working mother. There is no light at the end of the tunnel by going the baccalaureate route.

The nearest college to us is 60 miles away but only had a four-year program. The Vocational Technology (Vo-tech) portion of the college furnished us with the LPN classes. A problem occurred due to their Vo-tech status. None of the LPN credits counted toward the BSN program. The graduates did not want to attend another four years of school requiring them to start from the very beginning. The anatomy and physiology (A & P) class was totally different for Vo-Tech LPNs than the BSN class. We desperately needed nurses, but there was nowhere to send Malad residents for school.

I was asked to serve on the Idaho Commission of Nursing and Nursing Educators representing small rural hospitals of Southeast Idaho. The meetings were held quarterly in Boise, Idaho; which for me was 300 miles away. I enjoyed the drive because I would listen to books on tape as I drove. The long trip became a mini vacation. I served on this board for 9 years. They asked me what we needed in our area. I told them about the following issues:

■ Why can't LPNs from a Vo-tech program get into the 4-year BSN program without having to start over? The nursing school (at the same college) does not recognize any of the Vo-Tech credits and do not award credit for working as an LPN. The competition is so fierce applicants need a 4.0 grade-point average to get into the BSN program. The program requires full time schooling. There is nothing in our area to help anyone from my hospital or community to become an RN. Traveling 60 miles each way to school for four years is just not possible for people. Most women need to work and care [for] families. Some are single parents.

We can contribute to the education process. We can do clinical rotations at our facility. Rural Nursing is something all nurses should have an opportunity to experience as part of their clinical experience. Rural nursing is very different from any other nursing specialty. You learn a lot of leadership skills in the rural setting. Why are the schools not requiring a rural facility rotation?

▩ LPNs were completing their basic education programs without being IV certified and without leadership education. We understood that there needed to be an orientation period, yet legally they could not work the long-term care shifts. They needed a charge nurse course to do so. We couldn't find classes to certify them for intravenous care and insertion so they can take patients on the acute care side. The LPN schools added 3 months to their programs and incorporated the IV skills and the Charge Nurse modules into their programs.

▩ We needed more associate degree in nursing programs. We have to travel 150 miles for an Idaho school or 80 miles to a Utah school and then pay out of state tuition. All the small rural facilities in Southeastern Idaho have this same concern. There are 12 of these small hospitals in our area screaming for help. One Senator from Idaho wants only BSN programs and BSN nurses in the state. He wants to do away with all the ADRN programs. I told the group that I would never survive without my ADRN employees. I can't get enough BSN nurses. I have nowhere to send staff to school for this. The ADRN programs in the state are producing more licensed nurses than the BSN programs. There just needs to be a better way for the ADRNs to obtain their BSN as part of a seamless educational ladder process. If the nursing educators want more educators there needs to be a way for ADRNs to obtain more education. Accreditation meetings held with all school directors worked to find solutions to this dilemma. Some advances were accomplished. For instance, schools now accept more credits from other schools, academic A&P classes in the Vo-Tech setting, and an educational ladder program was developed. Not all schools joined in this effort.

▩ Students could not transfer credits from one school to another and yet the schools are all Idaho schools and should have the same accreditation rules. They receive funding from the same state government. Class requirements are not the same from school to school. If you have an employee who moves to Malad form Northern Idaho or from Utah, they cannot go to the nearest University and pick up where they left off. Their credits just don't measure up to the University in Southeast Idaho. There is one college in our area that is a private school and the credits don't count at the Idaho Universities at all. The educational support for returning to nursing after a hiatus is missing. The Idaho Association of Leaders in Nursing started publicizing a refresher course throughout the State of Idaho and all surrounding states. This is a self-study course with some clinical hours to help older nurses to come back into the workforce.

■ I wondered if schools were really taking all the students they possibly could. Are the graduates staying to work in the State of Idaho? We lacked data. A task workforce was developed by ICNNE and is now housed with Idaho Association of Leaders in Nursing, to collect information to answer this question and many more.

■ We need easier access to leadership courses for new supervising nurses. One of the nurse educators in the group wrote a leadership course that was offered at all the colleges. I took it and loved it. I really learned a lot. I had been out of school for 20 years and could not remember having a leadership education. I brought the course back to my facility. We taught 8 classes to the staff of our facility. Several staff members wrote mission statements. We played some fun games. It was great to introduce some new ideas of leadership into our facility.

Other ICNNE members had similar issues. The problems did not belong to just my community and hospital. A lot was accomplished from the grants and efforts of this group. I could see more acceptance of nursing as a career for males and females. I could see the need for more nurse educators. The data collection provided good information to the nursing schools, healthcare facilities and to the legislature. The threat of having only BSN schools in the State of Idaho calmed down. But from all these efforts, we still did not have a nursing program in our part of the state that LPNs could go to so they could become RNs. They all have 5, 10, and even 15 years experience as a rural LPN but nowhere to go to get their RN. The self-study courses were trying to sell their programs and we tried to start a support group of our own but it was expensive and would not have transferable credits to a University in our area if you wanted to switch over or to later go on for your Masters degree. The self-study programs were just a very unsure way of going back to school. I was not able to support the self-study programs because I had not been that route myself.

In our Southeastern corner of the State of Idaho, a support group was formed, a co-op of fourteen hospitals in the area. Dues were paid. The purpose of the group was to gain buying power, provide support groups, education and leadership training, recruitment opportunities, legislative support, idea sharing, grant proposal opportunities and other activities. The Acute Care DNS support group meets and shares ideas.

A Vo-Tech [vocational technical] school In Idaho Falls, started their own ADRN program as an outreach program specifically for a small rural facility nearby. The students were able to do their clinical experiences at their own facility. A lot of their classes were online classes or on a tele-conferencing device. The students had to be an LPN and go to school for 12 months. Wow! We wanted this program for our facility. This Vo-Tech school said that they would do what they could to help us.

Well—guess what! The schools in the State of Idaho have territorial rights. We could not have the other school help us and the school nearest to us was not interested. We told the director of The Hospital Co-op of our dilemma. All the CEOs of The Hospital Co-op agreed that we needed someone to start a program for our area that would help all of us to advance our LPNs to RNs with allowing them to do clinical rotations at their own sites. The Vo-Tech part of the University nearest to us took on the challenge and hired a nursing educator to start this program for them. She followed every rule. She came to every facility to check on her students. She would call to make sure her students showed up and on time. Care plans were graded with a finetooth comb. Intensives were held weekly. Not all clinical experiences were held at one facility because everyone needed all types of patients but at least some of your clinical experiences were at your own facility and some of the classes were online. Some were still at the college. We finally had a program that would fit the needs of our LPNs who wanted to become RNs. This program started in 2006. They gave credit for the acceptance of the LPN student process for the following: LPN experience, credit for the Tees test, credit for GPA, letter of support from a medical facility. Because they are a State University they cannot give extra points for being from a rural facility. Now that the program has shown its success and that it has a stepladder for ADRN to BSN to MSN, students from the larger communities are applying. The rural hospitals are concerned that their students will not always get in. They take 30 students each year and half are from the bigger communities and the other half are from the rural supporting facilities.

This program was really needed in our area of the state. We do have employees who are going on for their BSN. We have had several of our LPNs advance to an RN. We have had more go for their LPN knowing that they can get their RN from this route of schooling. Right now we are fully staffed. We do not have traveler nurses. All of our current staff nurses are employees from our community.

HOW DO YOU RETAIN EMPLOYEES IN YOUR HOSPITAL?

We do our best to make people happy and encourage them to stay. Of course you have to hire the right kind of nurse to begin with. As I said before the only lasting solution is to grow your own nurse. So we give people every opportunity to further their education. We also hire mature people because the young ones tend to marry and then move.

We also give people responsibilities with special recognition. Everyone has a specialty they can share with others. There are a few managerial positions, but everyone can do something for the facility. We help people certify to teach classes. We have an operating room manager, a gastrointestinal lab manager, an obstetrics and nursery manager who teaches prenatal classes, a diabetic educator and support group leader, a wound committee leader, a bowel and bladder manager, and a psych-mental health specialist. All of these people also work [with] regular medical surgical patients, recovery and emergency room as well.

In summary, rural nursing is a specialty. We have unique problems, a special way of approaching practice, and we need special solutions to solve recruitment and retention issues.

REFERENCES

Bassendowski, S., & Petrucka, P. (2010). Perceptions of select registered nurses of the continuing competence program of the Saskatchewan Registered Nurses' Association. *Journal of Continuing Education in Nursing, 41*(9), 408–412.

Maxwell, K. L. (2011). The implementation of the UHC/AACN new graduate nurse residency program in a community hospital. *Nursing Clinics of North America, 46*(1), 27–33.

Molinari, D. L., Monserud, M. A., & Hudzinski, D. (2008). Rural nurse job satisfaction. *Rural and Remote Health 8* (online), 1055. Available from: http://www.rrh. org.au

Ramritu, P. L., & Barnard, A. (2008). New nurse graduates' understanding of competence. *International Nursing Review, 48*(1), 47–57. doi: 10.1046/j.1466-7657.2001.00048.x

Smedley, A., Peter Morey, P., & Race, P. (2010). Enhancing the knowledge, attitudes, and skills of preceptors: An Australian perspective. *Journal of Continuing Education in Nursing, 41*(10), 451–461.

22

Professional Clinical Education Model: An Instructional Design

Deana L. Molinari

This chapter describes an instructional design method called the Professional Clinical Education Model (PCEM). The theoretical foundations, processes, and implications are detailed. PCEM was developed for the Northwest Rural Nurse Residency (NWRNR) to enhance student learning outcomes and skill competencies. The new instructional design model was successfully piloted in a rural nurse transition-to-practice project, academic courses, and nursing continuing education classes.

Nursing education confronts an escalating dilemma. That is, content is ever increasing while clinical practice time is declining. The challenge suggests that the basics of nursing education require change. This chapter suggests the need for an instructional design that supports a new type of teaching, which includes clinical practice in theoretical settings. The model supports nursing science, nursing roles, and competency measurement to assure the quality of nursing care.

Nursing is a complex profession requiring the gathering and management of disparate data, planning care, implementing interventions, and evaluating outcomes (Molinari & Dupler, 2005). The educator's challenge is to find instructional designs that encourage patient care. Few instructional designs fully support health care practice in the classroom.

BACKGROUND

Instructional design is the systematic development of instruction to ensure quality. The purpose of an instructional design model is to guide teachers through an analysis and implementation of the entire instructional process. The instructional design process entails assessment of learners' needs and environment, identification of learning goals, implementation of an intervention, mastery of a delivery system, and outcome evaluation (Reigeluth, 1983; Amsden, 2008). There are numerous instructional design models, and each is based on learning theory and specific educational goals. Instructional designers often use technologies to facilitate the delivery and enhance learning outcomes. Essentially, instructional design systems order development tasks, convey content, and then evaluate outcomes.

Instructors in traditional higher-education programs are often based on the instructor's past learning experiences. Consequently, the nursing profession has historically been slow to change pedagogy practices. Novice instructors repeat teaching methods from the past. The systematic application of an instructional design model enables instructors to develop curriculum based on best practices rather than personal preferences. Scholars can compare the value of education methodologies, experiment with instructional tools, and measure competencies.

The Professional Clinical Education Model (PCEM) was developed in response to a need to standardize many teachers' online instruction methods and to increase nurse outcome competencies. The new instructional design was developed as part of an innovative rural transition-to-practice project. A participatory-action research methodology using appreciative inquiry and positive deviance was employed to solve several issues in the distance-based nurse residency (Susman, 1983).

The expert teachers in the PCEM study were from 22 from the United States. Some of the 63 teachers possessed advanced degrees and taught nursing subspecialties such as obstetrics, pediatrics, complementary health, informatics, geriatrics, pharmacology, trauma, and so on. The common desire among the participating nursing faculty was to improve the quality of patient care. Students' common desire were to understand teacher expectations and then to achieve class success. The Northwest Rural Nurse Residency (NWRNR) project developers' goal was to develop a teaching system that maximized learning outcomes of nurses in the innovative online program. The purpose of the transition-to-practice program was to provide professional experiences requiring application of both role and scientific principles. On approval from the Institutional Review Board (IRB) committee for protection of human subjects, data were gathered from teachers ($n = 63$) and students ($N = 260$) who were enrolled in the NWRNR program.

The teachers' challenges to deliver the professional development program for new graduates included having short instructional periods, requiring a limited number of clinical experiences, and using strategies that facilitated knowledge-transfer didactic classroom content to clinical practice (Schaefer & Zygmont, 2003). The issues are the same as those that academic instructors experience. There is little time to teach an ever-expanding content in an already highly intense and overloaded curriculum. At the same time, the need to measure nurse practice outcomes under realistic conditions increases. The public and the nursing profession demand quality and safety (Quality and Safety Education for Nurses, 2005). Unfortunately, the extra time needed to teach more complex principles has not been provided.

Traditionally, educators introduce theoretical principles sequentially: First, in the lecture hall and then in clinical settings for practice tasks and roles. Different teachers are used in each setting with different goals and teaching strategies. Separating nursing knowledge by location (classroom or clinical) increases students' difficulties in relating scientific principles (didactic content) to activities that occur at the patient's bedside.

Traditional learning objectives of clinical instructors and the theoretical teachers are also different (Boyle, Popkess-Vawter, & Taunton, 1996; Cleary, 1988). Traditional classroom teaching stresses theory and concept development. Some instructors believe that the content determines the selection of objectives used and the required outcomes. The layering of student expectations from simple to complex also presents learning difficulties.

An issue is the failure of theoretical instructors' objectives to write higher-order thinking strategies as defined by *Revised Bloom's Taxonomy* (Anderson & Krathwohl, 2001). Objectives that include verbs such as "identify," "describe," "discuss," and "apply" are insufficient for quality patient care. Bedside nursing care requires nurses to practice higher-order thinking processes such as "analyze," "evaluate," and "create."

The problem is further complicated by a paper-based professional entry exam and fewer clinical experiences (Tanner, 2005, 2006). The resulting educational outcome of traditional instruction is ineffective professional role tasks such as prioritization, problem solving, interdisciplinary communication, delegation, and clinical reasoning (Pine & Tart, 2007). To solve the complex education issues, educators and staff developers seek strategies that teach more content effectively and meet employers' demands for safe clinical practice (Tanner, 2007, 2009).

Teaching effectiveness is not a new issue. Dewey stated; "The belief that all genuine education comes about through experience does not mean that all experiences are genuinely or equally educative" (Dewey, 1938, pp. 25–26). A nursing student's aim is not to memorize knowledge but to practice safe patient care (Knowles, 1984; Tanner, 2007). Traditional classroom teaching strategies such as lectures and testing fail to integrate the complex thinking skills required for clinical practice (Benner, 2006). Combining classroom strategies with clinical experiences can be more efficient than teaching theory and clinical experiences separately.

Most learning theories focus on a particular issue such as stage of life, technology use, or student learning preferences (Kearsley, 2011). Learning theories discuss how people learn. Psychologists apply biological functions to the learning task.

The PCEM approach combines the strengths of several learning theories and focuses on health care providers' content needs. Designers reviewed organizational mission and vision, basic educational goals, nurse competencies, and professional standards as well as the literature about instructional design and learning theory. The developer's goal was to teach nursing practice skills in conjunction with nursing science. A search of learning theories reported in nursing articles identified several common elements (Banning, 2005).

Narrative pedagogy is a learning theory authored by Aristotle while others give Fisher the credit for the interpretive approach (1987). The strategy encourages relating patient care narratives so that students can recognize decision-making elements. The literature states that students experience increased interpretation, critical thinking, and concept analysis (Diekelmann, 2001). Reading stories of success, crisis, and misfortune provide recognition opportunities, but does not provide nursing practice.

Simulation is a strategy that encourages narrative pedagogy in realistic settings, that is, students "act or carry out the nursing role under patient safe conditions. Students are expected to physically and verbally respond to situations that are typical for the job, such as assessment, following protocols, and patient intervention management" (Notarianni, Curry-Lourenco, Barham, & Palmer, 2009). Simulation is a "meta" educational system. In other words, systems within systems must be managed. Fidelity is a measure of the closeness to reality the simulation provides. Low fidelity is less like a real situation than high fidelity. For instance, static doll-like-mannequins are less comparable to "real" humans than computerized mannequins or actors (i.e., standardized patients). Dramatic role playing by teachers and students aid participants in overcoming anxiety and fears as well as learning how to apply nursing science within the nursing role (Buxton, 2011). Simulation requires participants to practice bedside skills and provides deeper learning than listening to stories (Jeffries & Rizzolo, 2006).

Both simulation and narrative instructional models are helpful but have limited usefulness in the classroom. First, the addition of stories in a theory class provides opportunities to recognize principles and analyze components, but fails to place the student in the active providers' decision-making role (Brown, Kirkpatrick, Mangum, & Avery, 2008). Second, simulation places students in active nurse roles, but often requires clinical experience and/or special equipment. Classroom teachers need strategies to produce the highest levels of professional decision making within classroom.

DEVELOPMENT OF THE PCEM

The web-based NWRNR program, funded by the Health Resources and Services Administration (HRSA), targeted educating rural nurses. The first students were from Alaska, Washington, Idaho, Montana, and Wyoming. The program employed instructors to teach a single topic due to their rural crisis assessment and management expertise. Instructors did not meet one another or interact with the whole curriculum. Students did not physically gather in a room except during online class discussions. The social and geographical distance challenged program managers to design education that improved competence and confidence. A study of the residency's effectiveness commenced.

PCEM Philosophy and Guiding Principles

The PCEM instructional design system grew out of concepts from engagement (Kearsley & Schneiderman, 1999) and transformational (Mezirow, 1997) learning theories and the instructional design systems by Dick and Carey (1996) and Reigeluth (1992) (ADDIE) and Reigeluth (Elaboration). The framework provides the development and theoretical processes for combining classroom and clinical teaching strategies. Participants integrate new scientific content within clinical scenarios in safe classroom settings. Theory is taught in combination with clinical role skills using patient experiences.

Instructional design models order curricula processes and materials in a progressive manner. Instructional designers introduce simple concepts before teaching complex topics. The PCEM system does not separate theoretical topics from clinical topics and introduces complexity within patient care situations. Concepts are integrated in a biological-like system; for instance, a holistic wellness course progresses from simple pathophysiology to complex multiple morbidities. The PCEM orders the complexity of principles for the whole course and then goes a step further. Students are introduced to new concepts as they appear within a patient care setting with all of its complexity. This instructional design principle situates learning with patient care and does not permit a theoretical concept to be a class goal.

The traditional ADDIE instructional design consists of developmental phases: Analysis, design, development, implementation, and evaluation (Dick & Carey, 1996). The PCEM adds pre/postoutcome analysis, case study development, and competency measurement to the well-described process.

The Elaboration design theory's instructional design process encourages presenting simple concepts before complex concepts. The PCEM alters the Elaboration process in one area. Students experience a complex patient scenario at the beginning of class. Distractors from the class's objectives are encouraged if they relate to real patient care interactions. The initial scene presentation demonstrates the integration of science and role content in natural settings. Students use the initial scenario to self-assess personal knowledge, skills, and attitudes. The activity serves as a preassessment and as a learner readiness activity. The class ends with the same sort of complex scenario, this time for teacher assessment of learning outcomes.

PCEM Development Process

In 2009, the new residency program began evaluating teacher needs during the need assessment processes. Staff analyzed the teaching process using the appreciative inquiry–participatory-action research methods to provide evidence for the fast-paced continual improvement process (MacIssac, 1995). Instructors of previous distance-based professional staff development and academic programs were interviewed about program supports needed. Other distance-based residencies were investigated. The NWRNR provided the first instructors with orientation materials including: A description of the innovative project, program purpose, expected outcomes, media delivery instructions, continuing education standards, online supports, and basic instructional design counsel. Results of pre/post instructor interviews were combined with meeting minutes, observations, student interviews, chief nurse officer interviews, participant satisfaction, and knowledge surveys. Teacher processes and outcomes were analyzed using objectives, teaching strategies, personalities, and presentations. Staff conducted literature searches; reviewed nursing education standards; analyzed surveys; and interviewed key informants during each stage of the project's development.

Program evaluation
The program staff identified ideal goals and areas for development. All participants described role perceptions and needed supports to reach ideal outcomes.

- Residents expressed strong opinions about learning preferences. Residents recently passed the National Council Licensure Examination (NCLEX)—Registered Nurses. The novice professional nurses stated that they did not want lectures, tests, or passive "academic" teaching strategies. Participants desired best practice information, resources, procedures, and references. Interviewees believed that they possessed sufficient foundational knowledge for practice, but wanted more crisis assessment and management information. Their preference for increasing patient care task skills sometimes conflicted with the employers' request for role management skills (Lea & Cruickshank, 2007; Parker, Plank, & Hegney, 2003). Chief nursing officers and the literature reported that novices needed more practice communicating, thinking critically, prioritizing, and managing time and resources (Molinari, Monserud, & Hudzinski, 2008).
- Several nurses stated that their supervisors enrolled them in the course and residency participation was not their preference. Residents expressed widely varying class satisfaction opinions. Courses using clinical teaching strategies such as case studies and scenarios received higher-satisfaction scores. Achievement scores were higher after experiencing authentic case studies. Observation of the residents' learning process reported increased student engagement as evidenced by more student discussion and action.
- Residents produced lower-than-expected skill achievement ratings in lecture-style classes.
- Clinical and academic instructors were chosen for the first cohort of students. Analysis indicated that academic teachers designed different goals and presentations than did staff developers. Academic instructors set goals based on theoretical foundations and designed courses to reach knowledge, skill, and attitude goals. Staff developers began with standards and quality outcomes and designed backward, looking for tasks and procedures that would ensure the ideal practice.

▓ Teachers requested more information about teaching competencies with telemedicine and video web-based technologies for people they may not see.
▓ Project staff analyzed data and felt the need to create of a new type of instructional model based on teacher and resident needs. Teacher and student satisfaction and achievement scores were important for the program's success because lower-satisfaction scores could result in lower residency completion numbers.

Program developers felt that supporting both teachers and students was necessary to achieve relevance and success. The staff performed a best practices literature search, consulted with an instructional psychologist, employers, residents, and teachers, and studied national residency standards. There were no residency instructional design standards. Little online instructional design information was found in the literature, although teaching guidelines were available (Billings & Halstead, 2009). Tanner and Benner suggest the importance of student exposure to complex health care delivery to learn nursing skills (Benner, 1984; Tanner, 2009). The lack of supportive instructional designs and the acceptance of Tanner and Benner's work about educating nurses resulted in the development of an instructional design model called the Professional Clinical Education Model (PCEM). The PCEM was tested with the next six online resident cohorts (about 300 participants), academic classes, and other staff development courses. Use of the model produced immediate improvement in the NWRNR participant knowledge and satisfaction survey scores.

Outcomes

Program staff created uniform teaching guidelines and an instructional design methodology. Instructional design support was provided for instructors to work their way through the new methods. Continual interviews and outcome analysis after each class provided data for the fast-paced change process.

Pilot testing instructors reported altering past teaching processes. One instructor said, "This is fun. I feel more like a nurse when I bring hospital experiences into my class." Instructors reported that their purpose of teaching changed from delivering content to improving practice. Instructors spent more time developing pre/post tests, case studies, and simulations. Teachers required students to apply skills and create decisions "on the spot." Instructors reported a need to be prepared for a variety of possibilities. They developed flexible lesson plans dependent on student activities and needs. Preassessments provided foundational information required for teaching. Assessment was used more frequently for teacher decision making than in previous classes. Assessment became a teaching tool as well as an outcome measure.

Thinking backward

Teachers use outcome analysis and content analysis during the development process as well as during and after the class. The ADDIE instructional design system suggests that designers identify learning problems, develop goals and objectives, investigate learner needs, link to existing knowledge, consider the learning environment, and list delivery issues and the timeline. This is a forward-thinking process. The first step supports the next and so on.

The PCEM requires instructors to think backward through the design process. The goal of safe patient care is designed first. An analysis of professional practice expectations is required before other analyses begin. Practice and academic experts work together on curricular outcomes (IOM, 2010). The designer creates a list of patient care competencies first. The backward-thinking process requires teachers to analyze outcome measurement next. Teachers may refer to quality standards, evidence, and best practices. Instructors will also interview nurse leaders, look at previous testing results, and decide what is necessary for the new class. Once the practice and science competencies are identified, the scientific and practice content is determined. At this point, global and specific objectives are written. Each theoretical and scientific principle is linked to a professional competency.

Designing PCEM begins with identifying quality standards, expected student outcomes, methods of measuring quality achievement, ordering content needed to achieve competency, and then finalizing objectives. All this occurs during the analysis step of ADDIE. The analysis process permits a more relevant approach to objectives design. The new goal of writing objectives is to clearly state the student's expected quality practice achievement. If educators expect students to achieve only scientific knowledge, then participants are unprepared for bedside practice. Enveloping scientific achievements within practice achievements combines the two interdependent types of learning into one learning setting and requires demonstration of nursing practice outcomes achievement. Science supports and justifies practice and so the science content should not be the goal of any nursing educational course. Science is merely a tool for healing. The goal of learning is professional caring.

Designing relevant objectives requires understanding of *Blooms Revised Taxonomy* (Anderson & Krathwohl, 2001) and critical thinking. Critical thinking is a series of skills used to support clinical decision making (DeBono, 1991). *Blooms Revised Taxonomy* supports the design of objectives that can be linked to teaching strategies and measuring professional nurse outcomes. For instance, Anderson and Krathwohl (2001) describe lower-order thinking objectives requiring remembering, understanding, and applying teaching activities. Higher-order thinking involves analyzing, evaluating, and creating experiences. The highest-order thinking occurs in the creating category of activities and includes all other lower-order thinking skills. This fact is important for both fundamental and advanced practice topics. Lower-order thinking is never appropriate for nursing practice. Even the most novice nurse can exercise higher-order thinking when teachers use the PCEM design model. Consider, for example, the differences between objectives found in a medical terminology course.

■ Describe the fundamental word elements used to build medical terms.
■ Document care using fundamental word elements.

The first example requires students to regurgitate the text content while the second example requires the same principles but requires students to create terms and place them within the clinical context. Dictionaries and spell-check tools will enable students to verify their answers. The expected outcome for both objectives is the ability to use medical terminology. If the learning activity or outcome measure is a simulated patient chart, the student will quickly realize the importance of mastering word elements. The first example requires memorization; the second requires thinking on the spot-which is the goal of nursing education.

Another example of a simple objective is: *Students will differentiate types of hypertensive medications.* The objective calls for mastery of a cognitive skill and demands higher-order thinking. The PCEM suggests that cognitive skills objectives should be accomplished within clinical contexts. An objective such as *Differentiate clients' hypertensive medications by types* includes scientific knowledge objectives within clinical performance expectations. The difference between the two objectives is the patient. Nurses practice patient care rather than answer scientific multiple-choice questions.

Objectives that do not include patient care goals are insufficient for professional practice. A traditional objective about pharmacy content may require higher-order thinking activities as suggested by Anderson and Krathwohl, but still be insufficient for professional practice. For example, students will *compare the benefits and actions of calcium channel blockers, Angiotensin-converting enzyme (ACE) inhibitor, Angiotensin II receptor blockers, and beta-blockers.* Without patient assessment and management activities, the individual is not prepared for new graduate practice. Nursing education requires the integration of several scientific principles within a caring environment. Teachers who fail to include nursing practice principles are teaching a different discipline—for instance, pharmaceutical science.

The PCEM development matrix demonstrates the stages of instructional design. In summary, the backward-thinking process requires teachers to first address outcome measurement. Teachers refer to standards and evidence, interview nurse leaders, look at previous testing results, and decide what is necessary for the new class. Once the practice and science competencies are identified, the scientific facts and processes along with the practice roles and skills are linked into objectives.

The next phase requires instructors to "chunk" the content into smaller sections of simple to complex principles. Each chunk contains scientific and role principles to support patient care. A chunk is a class section that supports an objective.

Instructors begin each section with a specific or "pointed" patient care scenario and an assessment question. The narrative introduces the importance of the section, combines the care process with the scientific principles, and provides opportunity for student and teacher assessment. If the teacher determines that the section needs to be taught, the expected outcomes, content, and achievement measurement are delivered. This order in each section provides student control and proof of knowledge, skills, and attitude achievement. Teachers prepare a flexible lesson plan based on student feedback. Students control content presentation in each chunk through feedback about the initial patient care scenario. Each class consists of several sections. At the end of the class period, student achievement is measured within a complex patient care setting similar to the initial scene at the beginning of class (Table 22.1).

The PCEM requires applying an appropriate level of complexity to each class. That means matching clinical and role task complexity to scientific content complexity. Most scientific knowledge and skills are leveled in higher education. Sophomores are expected to master less complex content than seniors. For instance; schools may order physical assessment skills to begin wellness before disease-related assessment. Communication skills commence with terminology, and by graduation include team leading and civility issues. A problem occurs when not all nursing skills are leveled by complexity. Some instructors insert

TABLE 22.1
PCEM Instructional Design Matrix

PROCESS	MEASUREMENT	SCIENTIFIC KNOWLEDGE	PROFESSIONAL NURSING PRACTICE
Analyze	Standards, competencies	Facts, processes	Roles, skills, attitudes
Design	Discussion, testing, projects, simulation	Higher-order thinking, objectives, outcomes	Practice outcomes
Develop	Tests, knowledge, skills, attitudes tools	Chunk content, order content, apply leveled nursing science and roles	Simulations, cases, learning aids, and environment
Implement	Student interventions of clinical situations using scientific content	Educational interventions: leveled from simple to complex	Patient responses clinical roles/tasks leveled from simple to complex
Evaluate	Processes, achievement, satisfaction compared with standards. Case analysis, employer satisfaction	Chunk and class formative and summative tool analysis	Practice and decision-making formative and summative decision making

concepts such as cultural diversity or informatics into one class as an all or nothing topic rather than as a developing skill. The profession needs to level all nursing skills and then to teach them with increasing complexity over the curriculum. Skills in topics such as clinical decision making, patient teaching, evidence-based practice, quality improvement, and leadership can be improved through repeated exposure and achievement measurement.

Designing Tasks

The design tasks to be completed in all instructional systems include analysis, design, development, implementation, and evaluation. Each of the tasks contains many components.

Analysis

■ Analysis pertains to gathering previous course evaluation or need assessment data and evaluating the importance to the future project. The thinking process examines expected nursing outcomes and clarifies the design process elements. During analysis, the designer identifies the professional patient care quality elements, role and scientific outcomes, learner characteristics/needs/

experience/expectations, curriculum goals, environment strengths and constraints, media delivery options, and resources.

Design

■ Once professional and scientific outcomes have been outlined, global and specific objectives are specified. Other class/module/aids are also designed. This phase identifies the strengths and weaknesses of particular media for delivering the authentic patient care situations. Simulations and graphic scenarios are designed to meet the objective and outcome needs. Content and measurement are determined.

Development

■ Instructors create the simulations, graphics, tests, and other learning materials in this phase. Pilot studies of the materials are conducted.

Implementation

■ The plan is put into action. Teachers study the process and outcomes and journal findings. A scholarly approach enables fast changes before the next iteration. Simulations and teaching aids are tested with a real class and feedback data collected.

Evaluation

■ Evaluation began during the analysis phase, continued through development, and culminates in this phase before preparation for the next iteration of the course. There are several topics studied: instructional design process, teacher and student process, and satisfaction and achievement. Formative evaluation consists of measures of processes and achievement in each of the instructional design phases. Formative evaluation ties the design process together and keeps the phases from being separate entities. Summative evaluation can be defined in many ways. Some designers deny the existence of an "end" to the design or education process. For instance, achievement measures are designed for "chunks," classes, and courses. Population achievement can be self-assessed, criterion-related, or normative. The end is defined by the teacher who may wish to study several classes before totaling data and comparing with educational or professional standards. Analysis of the data begins the revisions process.

In summary, PCEM integrates classroom and clinical instructional strategies that reflect actual nursing practice. Content delivery approaches combine role and technical skills in representations of clinical practice. Participatory-action research was useful in developing and evaluating the instructional design model. NWRNR students and instructors expressed satisfaction with the design approach and delivery.

REFERENCES

Amsden, D. (2008). *Self-assessment: Students "know" better.* Retrieved from http://www.daveamsden.com/

Anderson, L. W., & Krathwohl, D. R. (2001). *A taxonomy for learning, teaching and assessing: A revision of Bloom's Taxonomy of educational objectives.* New York, NY: Longman.

Banning, M. (2005). Approaches to teaching: Current opinions and related research. *Nurse Education Today, 25*(7), 502–508.

Benner, P. (1984). *From novice to expert: Excellence and power in clinical nursing practice* (pp. 13–34). Menlo Park: Addison-Wesley.

Benner, P. (2006). *The use of nursing narratives for reflecting on ethical and clinical judgment.* Upper Saddle River, NJ: Prentice-Hall Publishers.

Billings, D. M., & Halstead, J. A. (2009). *Teaching and nursing: A guide for faculty* (3rd ed.). Philadelphia, PA: Elsevier Saunders.

Boyle, D. K., Popkess-Vawter, S., & Taunton, R. L. (1996). Socialization of new graduate nurses in critical care. *Heart Lung, 25*(2), 141–54.

Brown, S. T., Kirkpatrick, M. K., Mangum, D., & Avery, J. (2008). A review of narrative pedagogy strategies to transform traditional nursing education. *Journal of Nursing Education, 47*(6), 283–286.

Buxton, B. K. (2011). Interaction, unscripted. *Journal of Psychosocial Nursing and Mental Health Services, 49*(5), 28–32.

Cleary, M. J. (1988). Thinking styles of supervisors and implications for student teaching. *Teacher Educator, 24*(1), 16–23.

DeBono, E. (1991). *Teaching thinking.* London: Penquin Books.

Dewey, J. (1938). *Experience and education.* Indianapolis, Indiana: Kappa Delta Pi.

Dick, W., & Carey, L. (1996). *The Systematic Design of Instruction* (4th ed.). New York, NY: Harper Collins College Publishers.

Diekelmann, N. (2001). Narrative pedagogy: Heideggerian hermeneutical analyses of lived experiences of students, teachers, and clinicians. *Advances in Nursing Science, 23*(3), 53–71.

Fisher, W. R. (1987). *Human communication as a narration: Toward a philosophy of reason, value, and action.* Columbia, SC: University of South Carolina Press.

Institute of Medicine. (2010). *The future of nursing: Leading change, advancing health.* Washington, D.C.: National Academies Press.

Jeffries, P. R., & Rizzolo, M. A. (2006). Designing and implementing models for the innovative use of simulation to teach nursing care of ill adults and children: A national, multi-site, multi-method study. *National League of Nursing.* Retrieved from: http://www.nln.org/research/LaerdalReport.pdf

Kearsley, G. (2011). The theory into practice database. Retrieved from http://tip. psychology.org

Kearsley, G., & Shneiderman, M. (1999). Engagement theory: A framework for technology-based teaching and learning. Retrieved July 18, 2009, from http://home. sprynet.com/~gkearsley/engage.htm

Knowles, M. (1984). *Andragogy in action: Applying modern principles of adult education.* San Francisco, CA: Jossey Bass.

Lea, J., & Cruickshank, M. T. (2007). The experience of new graduate nurses in rural practice in New South Wales. *The Electronic Journal of Rural and Remote Health Research, Education, Practice and Policy, 7,* 814.

MacIsaac, D. (1995). *An introduction to action research.* Retrieved from: http://www. phy.nau.edu/~danmac/actionrsch.html

Mezirow, J. (1997). Transformative learning: Theory to practice. *New Directions for Adult and Continuing Education, 74,* 5–12.

Molinari, D. L., & Dupler, A. (2005). Online critical thinking in problem-solving groups. In G. Berg (Ed.) *Encyclopedia of international computer-based learning.* Hershey, Pennsylvania: Idea Group, Inc.

Molinari, D. L., Monserud, M., & Hudzinski, D. (2008). The rural nurse internship: A new type of nurse residency. *Journal of Continuing Education in Nursing, 39*(1), 42–46.

Notarianni, M. A., Curry-Lourenco, K., Barham, P., & Palmer, K. (2009). Engaging learners across generations: The progressive professional development model. *Journal of Continuing Education in Nursing, 40*(6), 261–266.

Parker, V., Plank, A., & Hegney, D. (2003). Adequacy of support for new graduates during their transition into the workplace: A Queensland, Australia study. *International Journal of Nursing Practice, 9,* 300–305.

Pine, R., & Tart, K. (2007). Return on investment: Benefits and challenges of a baccalaureate nurse residency program. *Nursing Economics, 21*(5), 13–18, 39.

Reigeluth, C. (1992). Elaborating the elaboration theory. *Educational Technology Research & Development, 40*(3), 80–86.

Reigeluth, C. M. (1983). *Instructional-design theories and models* (Vol. I). Mahwah, NJ: Lawrence Erlbaum Associates.

Robert Wood Johnson Foundation. (2005). Press release November 2005 phase I. Retrieved from http://www.qsen.org/overview.php

Schaefer, K., & Zygmont, D. (2003). Analyzing the teaching style of nursing faculty. *Nurse Education Perspectives, 24*(5), 238–245.

Susman, G. I. (1983). *Action research: A sociotechnical systems perspective.* London: Sage Publications.

Tanner, C. (2005). The art and science of clinical teaching. *Journal of Nursing Education, 44*(4), 151–152.

Tanner, C. (2006). Thinking like a nurse: A research based model of clinical-judgment in nursing. *Journal of Nursing Education, 45*(6), 204–211.

Tanner, C. (2007). Curriculum revolution revisited. *Journal of Nursing Education, 46*(2), 51–52.

Tanner, C. (2009). The case for cases: A pedagogy for developing habits of thought. *Journal of Nursing Education, 49*(6), 299–300.

23

To Be or to Do?

Deana L. Molinari

Educators debate on where, what, and how to teach the next generation of nurses. Creating a transition-to-practice curriculum requires answering philosophical, experiential, budgeting, and resource questions. Comparisons of orientation and residency programs are outlined. A discussion of commonly encountered transition-to-practice issues as well as instructional design processes for rural practice and educational topics are presented. The suggestion of promoting an ecosystem of rural educators and providers to answer transition-to-practice questions is promoted.

There are several philosophical tensions in nursing education. Academicians and employers often disagree about "what" and "how" to teach potential nurses. Rural educators even ponder "where" to teach nurses.

The "where" debate often revolves around resources because if urban and rural locations or academic and profession sites possessed equal resources, most employers would prefer teaching at the local bedside. The "where" question arises when there is a lack of local education expertise. Rural hospitals often lack nurses with advanced educator status. Without an experienced staff developer, managers must decide whether or not to spend scarce resources on sending a person to an urban educational setting. The decision also involves answering the question of whether or not the urban training is effective for rural practice needs (Molinari, Monserud, & Hudzinski, 2008).

The "what" discussion poses a philosophical question. "Do I teach students 'to be a nurse' or 'to do patient care'?" Answers influence instructional design issues such as the educational topics chosen, the order of presentation, which teaching strategies to use, and the types of evaluation that are appropriate. Answering the question determines the student's skills at graduation and influences the profession. If an instructor values the "being" a nurse alternative, then the topics chosen emphasize nursing role skills. The teaching strategies involve reflection and management of complex patient scenarios. An instructor, who values "doing" patient care, chooses technical skills and teaches with skill demonstrations emphasizing efficiency.

Since both types of thinking are necessary, some say that there is no debate. The profession calls on a person's character or "being" to support the practice or "doing" of nursing. The patients' preferences and the new graduates' goals are safe practice (Hillman & Foster, 2011). In other words, a nurse's action, or the "doing" of nursing, is an expression of the nurse's "being."

The philosophical question subsumes another tension involving the progression to expertise. Students grow through stages of development from novice to expert (Benner, 1984). The tension is heightened during the transition-to-practice period because experts teach novices. New graduates and novices in new roles understand practice in concrete terms, while expert teachers view practice as an integration of complex principles and probabilities (Molinari & Monserud, 2009). For example, new graduates are anxious to follow the rules and make decisions based on clear policies and procedures. On the other hand, the expert is more likely to consider logic and patient preferences. According to Benner, an experienced nurse's clinical knowledge becomes a blend of practical knowledge and theory (1984). That is to say, "Expertise develops as the clinician tests and modifies principle based expectations in the actual situation" (Alligood & Tomey, 2010, p. 141). So, is the "to be" or "to do" question a curriculum design or experiential issue? In traditional teaching, technical skills are often taught before role skills.

Educational research indicates that student thinking patterns begin developing from initial exposures to professional practice and progress throughout the education process (McMullen & McMullen, 2009). Students are socialized into their roles from the first days of "becoming" a nurse. Therefore, if a lesson plan focuses on task completion (doing), the student will learn to value performing tasks well. Employers complain that new graduates often lack role skills such as clinical reasoning, prioritizing, and relating interprofessionally which enable an individual to "be" a nurse (Molinari et al., 2008). Employers require more than technical skill proficiency; so traditional teaching methods are questioned and health care providers provide education.

Transition-to-practice programs assist graduates in becoming safe nurses. "Being" a safe nurse demands the integration of a plethora of complex role skills. Clinical educators do not plan lessons that progress through a list of technical tasks. Clinical educators role-model nursing while filling in the new employee's practice gaps. Their curriculum planning questions are not "what" to teach, but rather "how" to teach nursing. Since repetitive experience encourages expertise, the transition-to-practice (TTP) period is an excellent time to teach "being" and "doing" at the same time.

TRANSITION-TO-PRACTICE PROGRAMS

The clinical educator balances additional tensions. One involves the diverse roles of educational programs. There is a difference between orientation and residencies or preceptorships. Orientation programs are short educational presentations offered at the beginning of employment with the purpose of assisting new employees to find their way in the organization. Educators:

- Share the organization's philosophy.
- Explain benefits, policies, and procedures.
- Introduce the documentation system for financial support and patient care.
- List resources supporting nursing practice.
- Discuss professional development requirements.
- Provide information management resources.
- Outline hierarchal authority lines and communication expectations.
- List task competencies and check-off methods.

The main difference between a residency and an orientation is the program's purpose. Residencies occur after orientation and often last longer. The purpose is to improve patient care rather than ease organizational operations. Residencies provide clinical supervision and role competencies (e.g., leader, communicator, team member, patient care provider, teacher) rather than the orientation's task competencies (blood-transfusion protocols, ventilator management, electronic health record documentation, hemodynamics, and reading electrocardiogram (EKG) strips). Both types of support are necessary for professional development (Dyess & Sherman, 2009).

Patient care education (see Table 23.1) uses different educational strategies from orientation programs. Some patient education programs are competency based while others are experientially based. Both approaches include a formal education process that is conducted in the employment setting and uses application learning (Beyea, von Reyn, & Slattery, 2007; Carryer, Boddy, & Budge, 2011; Chunta &

TABLE 23.1
Residency Curriculum Content

SKILL COMPETENCIES	KNOWLEDGE TOPICS
Communication	Documentation, listening, interprofessional transitions/problem solving/handoffs, leadership gradients, civility, patient, cultural, relationship building, instructing, motivating, feedback, boundaries, conflict resolution, clarity, perspective seeking, and sensitivity
Patient-centered care	Priority setting, time management, leadership, cultural sensitivity, lifespan developmental issues, discomfort assessment and management, crisis assessment and management, patient/family/community decision making, integration of care processes and system, clinical reasoning, decision justification, interpersonal sensitivity, relationship centered, value appreciation, health beliefs, and expectations
Teamwork and collaboration	Clarifying accountabilities, scopes of practice, consistency, increase use of bedside technologies to reduce memory reliance, collaborative/lateral/creative/critical thinking processes, and case management
Evidence-based practice	Evaluating literature, applying literature to appropriate context, methods, data gathering, analysis of large databases and local data, system analysis, integrate knowledge in care plans and problem solving, question formation/answering, and integrate and rate several types of evidence for each issue
Career management	Self-care, resume preparation, types of nursing positions interviewing, self-protection: malpractice issues and insurance, delegation, basic legalities, bioethical issues, professional development planning, self-care, stress management, self-reflection/assessment and quality improvement of daily practice, value based practice, and time management
Quality improvement	Understanding of improvement processes, participation/creation/evaluation of patient care/workforce/facility improvement, creating/understanding/evaluating measurement outcomes, reduce hazards and potential risks, and use and measurement of best practices
Information management	Understand the importance and local methods of information management, gather and analyze data from local databases pertaining to patient care/workforce/facility issues, clarifying/analyzing/evaluating data meanings, communicate findings, ethical issues, and documentation
Leadership	Abilities to assess, plan, act, and improve systems, personnel, and patient care, resource management for safe care, professional development, patient/professional teaching principles, administrative versus patient priority balancing, socialization within the rural and health care communities, policy development, and the basic abilities to work and to work with others

Source: Yonge, O. (2009). Meaning of boundaries to rural perceptions. *Journal of Rural Nursing and Health Care, 9*, 15–23; Issel, L. M. (2009). *Health program planning and evaluation* (2nd ed.) Jones and Bartlett Publishers; Goode, C. J., Lynn, M. R., & Bedash, G. D. (2009). Nurse residency programs: An essential requirement for nursing. *Nursing Economics, 27*(3), 142–159.

Katrancha, 2010; Guhde, 2010; Krugman et al., 2006; Sherman, 2010). The choice between experiential education or competence measurement reflects the educator's values and answer the "to be" and "to do" debate. According to education literature, the choice also depends on the way the teacher learned as a student (Falk, 1994). Few rural staff developers have knowledge of learner development and learning theory. Few clinical educators begin with learning assessments or can alter strategies to meet student learning preferences (Fanutti, 1993).

Clinical Teachers

The clinical educators' role is to link a new nurse's critical thinking processes with clinical reasoning frameworks and then to integrate evidence with practice decision-making. These skills are mastered through repetitive active learning strategies in a patient care context.

During professional development years, experienced nurses rather than academic educators facilitate novice development. At this level of education, students are expected to be nurses who practice safely. Developmentally, the new graduate ranges between a novice and an advanced beginner. Clinical educators are not expected to teach basic nursing principles or tasks but report anecdotally that time is spent doing so.

Bedside educators can be called staff developer, mentor, coach, or preceptor. Requiring nurses to function in educator roles without advanced training minimizes the role's importance. Bedside educators need preparation and ongoing support (Chapter 11). Table 23.2 contains an example of preceptor education topics.

Healthcare facilities sometimes fail to value bedside educators. Preceptors may possess the least education about teaching and learning. Many clinical educators state they need more support than is available. For instance, a traveler nurse may be hired to manage a critical care position if the organization lacks the expertise. One rarely hears of a traveling staff developer, yet the role impacts on patient safety and the organization's budget. Sometimes the manager approaches the role as if any experienced nurse could manage the assignment. The rural clinical educator role could be enriched with more support and collaboration. More levels of education could be provided if small rural facilities collaborated with larger ones or with an educational organization specializing in rural education.

Other managers consider educator expertise as well as clinical experience. The first bedside instructor requires specialized personality characteristics due to the role's professional modeling and counselor requirements. Emotional intelligence and self-control are as necessary

TABLE 23.2
Preceptor Educational Support

CATEGORIES	EDUCATION TOPICS
Foundational topics	Measuring critical thinking, applying rural nurse theory to practice, minimizing reality shock, preceptor as a team member, motivation, socialization and professional development stages, art of knowing, knowledge integration, emotional competence/intelligence, cultural issues, ethics, generational differences, professionalism, and team building
Roles	Assessor, socializer, teacher, organizer, supervisor, role model, communicator, coach/facilitator, manager, priority setter, and time manager
Teaching principles	Working with diverse learning and personality styles, clinical teaching models, lesson planning, information exchange, teaching strategies, and goal and objective setting
Competency measurement	Methods and strategies, standards, remediation, basics of evidence-based practice
Self-improvement	Journal keeping, goal setting, career management, preceptor competencies, quality improvement, prioritization, delegation, and liabilities
Communication	Facilitation, promoting the organization, generational differences, conflict management, and networking

to the role as clinical expertise. Chapter 5 indicates that lateral violence is related to nurse turnover; therefore, preceptor interaction skills are closely observed (Jones, 2004). Chapman et al. (2010) report new employees on small nursing staffs experience more difficulty managing violence than those in urban centers. The employee's inability to hide from incivility results in increased levels of absenteeism, staff turnover, or even permanent exit from the profession. The risk of choosing the wrong person as a clinical coach or teacher results in expensive organizational outcomes.

The new employee's preceptor requires support. North Carolina leaders state that nurses need at least a baccalaureate degree to be chosen for the advanced training (Chapter 13). The educational preparation in various preceptor education programs may be four hours or a master's degree depending on the organization's perceived importance of the role. Initial education is not enough. Ongoing support for novice preceptors includes workshops, conferences, articles, journal clubs, discussion boards, mentors, and listservs.

Supporter

Some residency programs provide an additional support person besides the preceptor. The supporter is not considered a teacher and does not perform as a supervisor, an administrator, or even as a unit peer. The support person's role is to listen and facilitate self-reflection. The resident's supporter addresses general employment barriers to growth and development. For example, the Las Vegas model gathers residents once a month with a trained facilitator who asks questions as well as listens to issues (Kowalski & Cross, 2010).

The Northwest Rural Nurse Residency uses peers via an online discussion board for this purpose (Chapter 11). The Rural Nurse Internship (Molinari & Monserud, 2008) used volunteers from other hospitals who communicated via email or phone calls. The supporter did not judge or write progress reports. Rather, the purpose is to provide positive insights in a nonthreatening manner.

TEACHING TOPICS AND STRATEGIES

Educators can use developmental strategies to lead a new employee from relying on concrete rules to thinking in general principles. When approaching education using developmental methods, educators teach principle frameworks rather than tasks at every developmental stage of development.

Benner suggests that novices favor "to do" checklists. Orientation programs fit the need by providing concrete procedural task lists. Orientation programs ease novices into the organizational processes and lists standardize team processes, but both are insufficient to produce safe clinical reasoning.

Residencies focus on frameworks and processes. Frameworks are abstract relationship lists or graphics that enable recent graduates to remember practice roles and responsibilities. Consider discharge planning frameworks. The discharge planning process might address learner readiness, patient expectations, network resources, basic principles, goal setting, evaluation methods, and accountability reports.

Frameworks remind the nurse of clinical reasoning points while task lists dictate behaviors. Providing a novice nurse with a task list for the discharge planning process outlined above could be laborious and inflexible. Computerized charting employs task lists. Computers are well suited to numerous tasks such as listing all the assessments necessary for the six-item discharge planning framework. A task list suggests standardization rather than customization of general principles. Since no two patients are alike, standardization of discharge interventions is impossible. The patients' knowledge, experience, support network, and health conditions force management diversity.

Competency

Determining where a nurse is on the continuum from novice to expert requires measurement. Unfortunately, most competence measurement considers a safety dichotomy rather than a developmental progression. Benner suggests that advanced beginners think in terms of general rules as opposed to the novice's "right" versus "wrong" decisions. Competent nurses think in terms of principles. Benner suggests that the novice-to-expert progression lasts for years. Factors contributing to the speed of development are not yet understood.

Consider some of the limitations of competence measurement. Using a polar scale of yes/no fails to consider complexity. The checklist approach to measuring competence is inherently dishonest. Like the novice's thinking, dualistic measures are too simplistic and do not consider context diversity. Consider the vital-sign task list. A clinical educator is forced to report whether or not a nurse collects the data. There is compliance or there is no compliance. Expert nurses know that not all vital signs are "vital" in every context. A polar measurement reduces nursing to a series of tasks without demonstrating relationships or the concept's importance to clinical reasoning. Since the meaning of the vital signs outcomes varies with age and context, competence should consider diversity of context. Using a rubric based on Benner's stages of growth with space for comments can provide more information.

Teaching Styles

Philosophic and progression questions dictate teaching styles and strategies and the speed with which learning occurs. There are two basic educator types. The *preacher* provides lectures with entertainment, graphics, spoken, and written words. The preacher specializes in data, tasks, protocols, and information transfer. Conversely, the *teacher* designs a safe learning environment and encourages experimentation to facilitate knowledge, skill, and attitude growth. Both educator types are respected; however, each has benefits and pitfalls.

A preacher's problem becomes evident when the graduate enters the employment arena. Preachers can produce graduates who are successful on examinations but have difficulty practicing independently. While the preacher imparts facts and details, the style fails to empower students to think for themselves (Institute of Medicine, 2009). Task masters read effectively, pass competence exams, follow directions, and "apply" principles. Vulnerable patients, however, require the creation solutions. Generating quality care requires independent problem solving based on principles. Even though a preacher's outcome (the graduate) speaks the nursing language, there is no guarantee that they can "be" nurses.

Nurses are information managers, decision makers, and care integrators (Sherman, 2010). Nurses assess disparate options, anticipate the future, create plans, and evaluate the past. Nursing processes require combining scientifically based principles with protocols; that is, the integration of processes with task skills. Nursing *is* a complex profession and novice nurses must practice *being* while learning to *do* complex tasks.

STANDARDS

The philosophic and progression issues are discussed in practice standards. *The Future of Nursing* (Institute of Medicine [IOM], 2010) asserts that education should be organized around care coordination activities such as respiratory care rather than focusing on medical specialties such as pediatrics. The IOM also suggests that the curriculum is taught in a seamless transition from the academic setting to the point of care suggesting a developmental approach to the philosophic and progression issues. Health care providers and nurse educators are encouraged to collaborate on at least a year of postgraduation professional development. Additionally, nurses are urged to continue lifelong learning rather than viewing degree attainment as a terminal goal.

Care Competencies

Quality and Safety for Education in Nursing (QSEN) provides six nursing competencies for entry-level practice: patient/family-centered care, teamwork and collaboration, safety, evidence-based practice, quality improvement, and informatics (QSEN, 2010). These competencies integrate a multitude of complex processes and principles based on the "to be" philosophy and progression steps can be measured. TTP programs can use the QSEN framework to design curriculum. An adaptation of the QSEN new graduate competencies is found in the appendix and the QSEN new graduate competencies are available on www.QSEN.org.

Each level of transition-to-practice from certified nursing assistant to nurse practitioner publishes standards of care (Carryer et al., 2011; Sullivan-Bentz et al., 2010). Each nursing specialty requires more education (Sherman, 2010; Thompson & Lulham, 2007). It is unlikely that one standardized transition-to-practice experience can be developed or is even desired, but utilizing QSEN competencies provides structure for TTP.

Nursing education and standards lack a seamless progression. There is a lack of progression based on education and a lack of progression from academic setting to professional practice. If academic and professional settings considered themselves similar to an ecosystem, a more accurate definition of developmental growth could be created.

There would be many benefits to an ecosystem organization. A collaboration among professional and academic educators could address answers to the "to be" or "to do" question at all nursing development levels. Basing developmental progression on professional practice standards such as the QSEN competencies could form a curricular skeleton and evaluation resources while preserving individual teacher creativity. Collaboration among professional organizations, nursing schools, and providers increases educational effectiveness, quality, and practice time while reducing administrative costs (Hillman & Foster, 2011).

Consider the differences in nursing education that would occur if students were taught "to be" from the first day of school. Educators would teach students "to be a nurse" and include task completion within role framework instructional designs. Complex simulation scenarios would test competence. There could be less regurgitation of textual concepts because nursing science supports patient care. Simple tasks would be tested within nursing role and patient care contexts. The reduction in a linear progression from "to do" to "to be" would be replaced by a combination of the two teaching strategies. Academic learning flows into professional development rather than requiring different thinking strategies. Teachers would bring the bedside into the classroom more often challenging students to integrate roles and tasks like nurses. Clinical reasoning would be introduced at the most elementary academic levels. Content duplications could be reduced over the course of nurse development. Clinical educators in transition-to-practice programs could then extend knowledge in specialty content areas.

GENERAL TTP TEACHING GUIDELINES

Once basic philosophical and progression questions are decided, TTP teachers consider other curriculum design issues. The following tips may facilitate the preparation process.

Designing Issues

- A transition-to-practice program requires analysis of the agency's mission and vision.
- Novices require time and experience to become experts; therefore, the highest impact and most frequent patient occurrences are chosen as educational topics.
- Classes are a continuation of the academic program and do not repeat basic nursing principles. Registered nurses are considered competent in basic principles of safe care. Teachers approach lesson planning as if speaking to experienced nurses who want to know more about a topic.

Environmental Issues

Feeling safe is necessary to learn according to the retention literature (Chapter 5) and transition researchers (Bernabeo, Holtman, Ginsburg, Rosenbaum, & Holmboe, 2011). Curriculum design therefore includes more than ordering the presentation of learning events. Nurturing environments address learning experiences as well as personnel. Bernabeo et al. state that rotating among facility units can produce both positive and negative impacts. New employees develop flexibility and insecurities. Employers need to decide whether avoiding critical situations, shortened documentation, and hiding information are worth the need for improved organization and triage skills. Perhaps more support during transitions among units can avoid negative reactions to new environments.

Learning in clinical settings requires designing a learner-centered environment where participants experience caregiving while making mistakes. Reflecting on experiences deepens learning. If the environment is punishing, reflection produces self-protection rather than patient protection. Clinical learning environments also provide opportunities for iteration and integration of complex practice principles. Since patient protection is the goal of health care, consideration of how to develop new graduate expertise while protecting patients is considered during curriculum planning.

There are various levels of learning safety and professional nurses may need to experience several before competence is achieved. Listening to experts talk about clinical tasks is insufficient education, but perhaps the most common strategy for teaching professional nurses. Mentors/coaches/facilitators need instruction about how to safely teach novices.

Consider one of the safest teaching strategies: the case scenario. The new nurse is exposed to a patient care challenge and mentored through the thinking process (Stanton & Dunkin, 2009). This provides the highest level of safety and the lowest levels of professional accountability. New nurses are particularly fond of mentor's stories of past experience because these are case scenarios where an answer is already available. The new nurse then evaluates the expert nurse's management of the situation.

- Critiquing another nurse's practice provides safety, reflection, and thinking without accountability. This level of experience is still insufficient for learning safe patient care. Patients need practitioners who can create solutions, not just evaluate someone else's solution.
- Simulation provides a totally safe setting but forfeits some reality during the learning process. The higher the realism level the more authentic the experience.
- Shadowing expert clinical nurses ensures more reality than simulation and still provides patient safety but fails to ensure accountability.
- Assigning novices to a small caseload provides reality and accountability with fewer responsibilities and less stress than expected of experts.
- Mentoring novices who manage regular caseloads by providing debriefing periods at the end of each shift provides a greater level of responsibility and accountability. Discussion on real patient care challenges offers authenticity and the benefits of problem-based learning. Since the nurse was accountable for the care, the highest levels of responsibility are expected. Mentoring novice reflection provides the clinical complexity that is often difficult to replicate with safer teaching strategies.

Mentoring also demonstrates a commitment to professional development. The practice is caring, objective, and empathetic. There are several types of mentoring. Journaling provides self-assessment and gives an individual the opportunity to mentor oneself by looking at past actions and feelings and then changing goals. Topics that surface in journal keeping are time management, difficult personalities, scarcity of resources, fears, prioritization, and management of emotional situations like end of life/palliative care trauma. These topics may need further discussion and strategizing with an expert mentor.

Expert nurse mentors act as positive role models by showing professional initiative, personal attitude responsibilities, and the ability to explore options.

■ Using authentic cases provides real examples of leadership, patient outcomes, and professional roles; these cases are integrated with specific evidence-based journal reviews and the residents' own personal experiences. This type of strategy combines safety and realism and is often used in conjunction with practice in new roles.

Technology

Informatics is the required content for transition-to-practice programs. It is the management of information. Practice demands managing diverse information. Informatics includes computerized charting as well as all types of documentation. Information sharing is not limited to data entry. Decision support and electronic client health care push nurses to understand more than how to operate a computer.

The methods of teaching informatics principles depend on local context. A facility with electronic charting will teach differently than one without computerized records. Academic informatics education is different from professional development. A nurse may learn to use online library databases to support evidence-based practice during school and find that rural facilities lack internet subscriptions. In basic education programs, students learn to create simple databases but a bedside nurse creates systems to gather data that answer patient care questions.

Some forecasters believe that a phone with health care applications will replace the computer. Many rural hospitals do not allow cell phones although urban facilities require nurses to carry phones. Use of mobile devices with nursing software enables just-in-time information at the point of care. A mobile device is perhaps the best way to ensure that a novice asks evidence-based questions of reliable resources for policies, protocols, procedures, standards, and evidence. Wireless mobile devices can decrease peer-based questions, keep employees tied to a constant stream of "truth," and reduce the number of practice errors. The device encourages critical thinking by providing examples, lists of symptoms and diagnoses, alternatives, access to virtual classrooms, apps for patient supervision, clinical shadowing, connections with supervisors, committees, social integration, journal clubs, and other professional resources. The devices also enhance communication among health care providers.

Simulation and Learning Laboratories

Simulation can be an effective strategy for developing competence, confidence, and entry-into-practice if the teacher is versed in instructional design. Simulation strengthens assessment, clinical reasoning, and clinical skills when performed with reflection or debriefing (Guhde, 2010). Simulation can be used in orientation programs with particular tasks according to Beyea et al. (2007). Computerized mannequins for human patient simulation are expensive and require a lot of specialized support, making it difficult for small rural facilities. Since many learning content topics depend on realistic settings such as critical thinking, human factors engineering, interprofessional processes, and patient safety, cheaper solutions are necessary. Cheaper simulation tools include static mannequins, standardized patients, role playing, and case studies. Simulation is also used to replicate clinical practice, teach skills, and evaluate practices and outcomes while giving repeated practice opportunities.

Measuring Progress

Competencies define skills as well as define expectations for practice. Competencies are considered higher levels of clinical practice skills representing care management mastery. At the same time, competencies provide a foundation for decision-making skills under a variety of clinical situations across all care settings. Competency testing demonstrates:

- Critical judgment
- Evidence-based practice
- Relationship-centered care
- Interprofessional collaboration and teamwork
- Leadership
- Assisting in self-care practices
- Teaching
- Delegation
- Supervision of caregivers
- Genetics and genomics
- Cultural sensitivity
- Practice across the lifespan
- End-of-life care
- Professionalism

Performance-based measurement requires a structured evaluation and is most often the weakest point of simulation and competence measurement. The study of rubrics can quickly reveal performance levels when used in conjunction with goals, objectives, and outcomes. Performance-based competence measurement requires teachers to design the learning process backward.

RURAL CURRICULUM DEVELOPMENT PROCESS

Curriculum development involves an iterative analysis process. Topics such as customer needs, professional standards, goals and objectives, and measurement standards are repeatedly referred to as a course is constructed. Sifting through the initial analyses reveals items necessary for the curricula decisions. If an agency experiences several head traumas and few baby deliveries, a teacher focuses on neuro assessment rather than obstetric assessment. Standards for neurological care are then identified and methods of measuring standard achievement are designed. At that point, goals and objectives are created. The content needed to be mastered to achieve the goals are listed and finally learning strategies are designed. The process seems backward from the intuitive one used by experienced nurses. Rather than saying that we need to teach the Glascow scale, instructors begin with professional standards of care and work backward through the development process to reach the question of whether or not to teach the Glascow scale.

New educators begin instruction development with seeking out what the public wants. Health consumers indicate a desire for nurses who demonstrate the following characteristics:

- Are responsive to their needs
- Are congenial in their interactions
- Are competent
- Provide education

Rural nurses are familiar with community residents. Nurses often understand the environmental, sociopolitical, and economic issues, which may underlay client presentation for health services (Molinari et al., 2008). Therefore, meeting consumer needs is a common practice. Researchers maintain rural nurses:

- Know the community
- Are tightly networked with professionals, relatives, and friends
- Lack anonymity
- Are isolated from support services
- Possess a broad range of skills and knowledge

Rural educational programs encourage nursing practice that monitors the health of individuals, groups, and communities (Bushy, 2000). This knowledge is used during assessment, planning, and evaluation of interventions. Bushy asserts that rural nurses think, see, and experience their practice differently than other nurses. Dunkin also contends (2000) that the rural nurse's style of practice requires an intimate knowledge of the community and of individuals within the community and concentrates on interpersonal skills.

Evaluation

Programs determine the usefulness of a curriculum by collecting data. Data from national and regional areas construct the initial curriculum. Once the program is developed, local data are needed for revisions. Gathering data about program costs, outcomes, and its acceptance is necessary to prove relevance. Small changes adapt programming to institutional needs. Adaptations can increase participant satisfaction. Data also provide a record of personal growth. Competence measurement, personnel records, incident reports, and patient satisfaction surveys yield information for performance and program analysis.

Generational Issues

Not all new graduates are of the same age. Differing generational issues challenge clinical educators. The youngest generation's values of self-care are in conflict with the oldest generation's values for sacrifice and agency loyalty. Agencies must plan to value diversity because perceptions impact on peer communication, work habit expectations, and educational performance standards (Altier & Krsek, 2006).

As mentioned previously, feeling safe is important to learning rural nursing principles according to retention (Chapter 5) and transition researchers (Bernabeo et al., 2011). Curriculum design therefore includes more than ordering learning events. According to Bernabeo et al., rotating among facility departments can have both positive and negative impacts. New employees develop flexibility and insecurity. Employers need to decide whether avoiding critical situations, shortened documentation, and hiding information are worth the need for improved organization and triage skills. Perhaps more support during the changes can avoid negative reactions to new environments.

Content Topics

Clinical content titles may or may not sound like academic topics. We know that the design process may be similar but the purposes and teaching strategies will probably differ. Since new graduates are excited to achieve professional nurse status, they often resist learning as if they are still in school, so naming clinical courses is not an insignificant matter (Chapter 5).

Providing a list of competencies can ease new nurses into understanding the need for professional development (Barnsteiner, 2010). QSEN competencies can structure continuing education (CE) topics. As the profession develops, nurses are required to learn new content as well as basic care principles. For example, informatics is recognized as a professional competence while genetics was recently added to the list of suggested professional competencies. Academic programs teach the science of genetics/genomics while CE classes focus on the application of the principles. The QSEN new graduate competencies are available on www.QSEN.org.

The IOM suggests designing courses around caregiving rather than medical disciplines. The IOM recently addressed CE in Redesigning Continuing Education in the Health Professions (2009) suggesting competence evaluation at the bedside. Learning patient care does not mean presentation of protocols and measuring task skills. Professional development evaluation is asked to stress interprofessional and principled care assessment and management. The report also calls for more contextual studies about the science of CE to increase the amount of best practices data. This means the literature will publish more program development and evaluation reports.

CONCLUSION

Designing curricula remains a challenge for professional developers. There are many aspects to consider when molding the careers of individuals and a profession. As we enter what Michael Bleich, chair of the IOM's nursing committee, calls the "golden age" of nursing, designers want to seriously debate the philosophical and developmental progression questions. If a nurse says "I am a nurse," shouldn't teachers create "to be" lesson plans? Measurement achievement during patient care scenarios that integrate role expectations, clinical tasks, nursing science, and interprofessional communication will demonstrate confident nurses creating complex process "to do" lists.

Clinical educational content and processes differ from academic settings and yet the forming of a nursing education ecosystem consisting of staff developers and theoretical teachers could revolutionize education processes improving patient care outcomes. Collaboration is the key to successful education. Data provide the answers to key program development questions when rural educators collaborate with academic educators to create new transition-to-practice programs.

REFERENCES

Alligood, M. R., & Tomey, A. M. (2010). *Nurse theorists and their work* (7th ed.). Maryland Heights Missouri: Mosby Elsevier. ISBN 978-0-323-05641-0.

Altier, M. E., & Krsek, C. A. (2006). Effects of a 1-year residency program on job satisfaction and retention of new graduate nurses. *Journal for Nurses in Staff Development*, 22(2), 70–77.

Barnsteiner, J. H. (2010). *Quality and safety education in nursing: Enhancing faculty capacity*. San Antonio, Texas: QSEN Faculty Development Institute.

Benner, P. (1984). *From novice to expert: Excellence and power in clinical nursing practice*. MeMo Park, CA: Addison-Wesley.

Bernabeo, E. C., Holtman, M. C., Ginsburg, S., Rosenbaum, J. R., & Holmboe, E. S. (2011). Lost in transition: The experience and impact of frequent changes in the inpatient learning environment. *Academic Medicine*, 86(5), 591–598.

Beyea, S. C., von Reyn, L., & Slattery, M. J. (2007). A nurse residency program for competency development using human patient simulation. *Journal for Nurses in Staff Development*, 23(2), 77–82.

Bratt, M. M. (2009). Retaining the next generation of: The Wisconsin nurse residency program provides a continuum of support. *The Journal of Continuing Education in Nursing*, 40(9), 416–425.

Bushy, A. (2000). Special and at-risk populations. In A. Bushy (Ed.), *Orientation to nursing in the rural community* (pp. 73–85). Thousand Oaks, CA: Sage.

Carryer, J., Boddy, J., & Budge, C. (2011). Rural nurse to nurse practitioner: An ad hoc process. *Journal of Primary Health Care*, 3(1), 23–28.

Chapman, R., Styles, I., Perry, L., & Combs, S. (2010). Examining the characteristics of workplace violence in one non-tertiary hospital. *Journal of Clinical Nursing*, 19, 479–488.

Chunta, K. S., & Katrancha, E. D. (2010). Using problem-based learning in staff development: Strategies for teaching registered nurses and new graduate nurses. *Journal of Continuing Education in Nursing*, 41(12), 557–564.

Dunkin, J. W. (2000). A framework for rural nursing interventions. In A. Bushy (Ed.), *Orientation to nursing in the rural community* (pp. 61–72). Thousand Oaks, CA: Sage Publications, Inc.

Dyess, S. M., & Sherman, R. O. (2009). The first year of practice: New graduate nurses' transition and learning needs. *The Journal of Continuing Education in Nursing*, 40(9), 403–410.

Falk, B. (1994). *Teaching the way children learn*. National Center for Restructuring Education, Schools, and Teaching. Retrieved from http://coe.winthrop.edu/tepc/research/Articles/FALKARTICLE.HTM

Fanutti, C. A. (1993). *How nurse educators in associate degree programs learn to teach*. Higher Education—Dissertations and Theses. Paper 41. http://surface.syr.edu/he_etd/41

Goode, C. J., Lynn, M. R., & Bedash, G. D. (2009). Nurse residency programs: An essential requirement for nursing. *Nursing Economics*, 27(3), 142–159.

Guhde, J. (2010). Using online exercises and patient simulation to improve students' clinical decision-making. *Nurse Educator's Perspective*, 31(6), 387–389.

Hillman, L., & Foster, R. R. (2011). The impact of a nursing transitions program on retention and cost savings. *Journal of Nursing Management*, 19(1), 50–56. doi: 10.1111/j.1365-2834.2010.01187.x

Institute of Medicine (IOM). (2009). *Redesigning continuing education in the health professions.* Washington, DC: National Academies Press.

Committee on the Robert Wood Johnson Foundation Initiative on the Future of Nursing at the Institute of Medicine (IOM). (2010). *The future of nursing: Leading change, advancing health.* Washington, DC: National Academies Press.

Issel, L. M. (2009). *Health program planning and evaluation* (2nd ed.). Boston: Jones and Bartlett Publishers, ISBN: 0763753343.

Jones, C. B. (2004). The costs of nurse turnover, Part 1: An economic perspective. *Journal of Nursing Administration, 34*(12), 562–570.

Kowakski, S., & Cross, C. L. (2010). Preliminary outcomes of a local residency programme for new graduate registered nurses. *Journal of Nursing Management, 18*(1), 96–104. doi: 10.1111/j.1365-2834.2009.01056.x

Krugman, M., Bretschneider, J., Horn, P. B., Krsek, C. A., Moutafis, R. A., & Smith, M. O. (2006). The national post-baccalaureate graduate nurse residency program: A model for excellence in transition to practice. *Journal for Nurses in Staff Development, 22*(4), 196–205.

McMullen, M. A., & McMullen, W. F. (2009). Examining patterns of change in the critical thinking skills of graduate nursing students. *Journal of Continuing Education, 48*(6), 308–310.

Molinari, D. L., Monserud, M., & Hudzinski, D. (2008). The rural nurse internship: A new type of nurse residency. *Journal of Continuing Education in Nursing, 39*(1), 42–46.

Molinari, D. L., & Monserud, M. A. (2008). Rural nurse job satisfaction. *Rural and Remote Health, 8*(4), 949. Available from www.rrh.org.au

Molinari, D. L., & Monserud, M. A. (2009). Rural nurse cultural self-efficacy and job satisfaction. *Journal of Transcultural Nursing, 20*(2), 211–218.

Robert Wood Johnson Foundation. (2010). *Quality and safety competencies.* Retrieved from http://www.qsen.org/competencies.php.

Sherman, R. O. (2010). Lessons in innovation: Role transition experiences of clinical nurse leaders. *Journal of Nursing Administration, 40*(12), 547–554.

Stanton, M., & Dunkin, J. (2009). A review of case management functions related to transitions of care at a rural nurse managed clinic. *Professional Case Management, 14*(6), 321–327.

Sullivan-Bentz, M., Humbert, J., Cragg, B., Legault, F., Laflamme, C., Bailey, P. H. et al. (2010). Supporting primary health care nurse practitioners' transition to practice. *Canadian Family Physician, 56*(11), 1176–1182.

Thompson, P., & Lulham, K. (2007). Clinical nurse leader and clinical nurse specialist role delineation in the acute care setting. *Journal of Nursing Administration, 37*(10), 429–431.

Yonge, O. (2009). Meaning of boundaries to rural perceptions. *Journal of Rural Nursing and Health Care, 9*, 15–23.

24

Rural Distance Education Delivery and Design

Jayne Josephsen

Innovative educational strategies and initiatives are needed to address the learning needs and preferences of rural nurses. Recruiting and retaining nurses in geographically remote regions is often highly dependent on access to continuing professional education. Geographical, financial, and technological constraints are associated with limited access to continuing educational opportunities. This chapter focuses on distance educational infrastructures and instructional techniques used in transition-to-practice programs for supporting rural nurses' learning needs, maintaining professional competence, and developing expertise.

Communication technologies led to the advent of distance education, enabling universities and medical centers to offer professional learning opportunities to adults located in remote locations. In its most general form, distance education refers to any educational offering that is not delivered in the traditional face-to-face classroom setting (Guri-Rosenblit, 2005). That is to say, the on-site instructor and the off-site students are not in the same room. The separation between teachers and students can be as close as another part of the building or as far as the opposite side of the globe.

A myriad of distance technologies are available to meet the learning needs of geographically bound nurses. Among others, current electronic and communication distance education technologies include interactive web-based audio and video capabilities, telephonic conferencing, webinar offerings that include the use of whiteboards, Powerpoint presentations, document editing, Wikis that allow for group problem solving, blogs, electronic file sharing, online testing, and polling software, along with the remote control of off-site learners' computers.

Increasingly, rural health care facilities collaborate with universities, medical centers, and other rural health care providers to establish distance education networks and infrastructures to meet the growing demand for education (Bushy, 2006; Francis, Bowman, & Redgrave, 2001; Lloyd & Bristol, 2006). Distance education offerings benefit rural nurses who feel isolated or lack supervisory support. Indeed, nurses with these perceptions report intent to leave employment; therefore, access to distant education can contribute to retention (Molinari, Jaiswal, & Hollinger-Forrest, 2011). Ultimately, rural-focused educational partnerships enhance patient care quality and client safety by encouraging the use of best practices.

BARRIERS TO RURAL DISTANCE EDUCATION

Offering successful distance education programs requires planners to address rural-specific issues during curriculum development and course delivery. Teaching strategies must be tailored to fit the learning needs and preferences of the distance (off-site) learner. Offerings can be delivered synchronously (in real time) or asynchronously (available to learners for a designated period of time). Most distance education courses for nurses are delivered via the Internet, using synchronous video and interactive discussions. The presentations can be archived so that nurses working in other shifts can participate in asynchronous discussions. Instructors may employ graphics, audio, and interactivity to engage the distance learner; however, some distant learners encounter difficulties with "large electronic files." High-speed Internet connectivity is necessary for video and large graphic files. Many rural communities, especially those in frontier regions of the nation, do not have cable television or DSL telephonic capability. DSL stands for "Digital Subscriber Line." It is a medium for transferring data over regular phone lines and can be used to connect people to the Internet. However, like a cable modem, a DSL circuit is faster than a regular phone connection.

Residents in remote communities may need to use satellite phone or dial-up telephone connections. In some communities, connecting to the Internet involves long-distance telephone charges. Few rural residents connect to the World Wide Web with broadband or high-speed Internet connections. Increasingly, broadband Internet services are being installed in rural communities; however, the public utility service may only be available to residents within the town's limit. For those who live immediately outside of that boundary, broadband services may not be available or may be cost prohibitive (Cejda, 2007; Horrigan & Murray, 2006).

There are other barriers to consider when planning rural distance education. What are the learners' computer accessibility and level of computer literacy? Individual computer ownership among rural residents varies greatly (Day, Janus, & Davis, 2005). Consequently, distance learners experiencing these limitations often may become frustrated and discouraged because they are not able to access course materials and unable to fully participate in the classroom experience. Instructors who are cognizant of rural student logistical realities are more likely to make instructional design accommodations. A variety of teaching techniques permit all distance learners to successfully participate in course offerings.

Correctly matching technologies, teaching strategies, and learner abilities will manage the rural distance learning challenges. Instructors can combine web-based content with telephone calls for advisement or consultation activities. The postal service and telephonic facsimile (FAX) can facilitate the transfer of materials and written correspondence. Other communication and electronic technologies that may already exist in a community can often be accessed for educational purposes. For example, telemedicine and telehealth technologies were developed to provide health care access. When not being used for consultation purposes, the tools can be used for educational presentations, case studies, or simulation exercises. Other less complex technologies can also be used for educational purposes such as video, DVD and audio recordings, smart phones, radio and television broadcasting, and personal data assistants (PDAs). In other words, educators in conjunction with their off-site educational partners and learners need to use the technologies and tools available in specific communities. Instructor creativity in adapting modalities to learning outcomes is basic to distance education.

In light of technology limitations, some university educators and program planners espouse that rural nurses would greatly benefit by attending conferences and classes offered in urban areas. Regional meetings are thought to overcome feelings of isolation. However, attendance may not be a feasible option. Small hospitals employ small nursing staffs. In fact, administrators struggle to cover all shifts and sending nurses to conferences complicates an already difficult task. Travel produces a nurse shortage and the hospital must budget for a replacement as well as paying for per diem, registration, and travel. Another problem with urban teachers or conferences is the unseen bias associated with the fact that nurses who are employed in larger institutions tend to specialize in one practice area (Montour, Baumann, Blythe, & Hunsberger, 2009).

The scope of nursing practice is similar regardless of the setting, be it rural or urban. However, nurses in rural settings are expected to possess a broad generalist knowledge base, specialist knowledge in crisis assessment, and management in all nursing subspecialties. Consequently, a nurse who is employed in a small facility may find the information he or she is exposed to in a course or workshop offered in the urban context is difficult to relate to the rural setting where resources, technology support, and problem-solving processes are different (Molinari, Monserud, & Hudzinski, 2008).

Patient care and nursing processes vary associated with contextual influences as well as rural residents' beliefs and values. For example, compared to those in more populated regions, patients in rural and frontier areas may define health differently and have unique expectations of their providers. In turn, these culturally based preferences impact the delivery of nursing care (Lee & Winters, 2006). Distant educators must consider these issues when adapting course designs and delivery methods. Ultimately, finding and implementing instructional techniques that produce optimal outcomes is the goal of distance education, regardless of the context or the program.

DISTANCE EDUCATION INFRASTRUCTURES

Partnerships are formed to address instructional challenges and prudently use resources. Partnerships among educational entities, health care facilities, and rural communities can turn negative perceptions of isolation and a lack of support into thriving continual professional development. The partners design and implement educational opportunities that integrate a multimodal technology within a theoretical framework that is relevant for rural nurses. Best practices for distance education identify the need to provide learner collaborative practice, promote membership in a learning community, require interactive learning, and integrate problem-based learning strategies (Beldarrain, 2006). Educational best practices complement health care administrators' desire that nurses within their facility meet competency objectives rather than teacher-centered objectives.

Core nursing competencies include interactive skills, including communication, assessment, problem solving, leadership, resource management, and teaching. In turn, distance education offerings should emphasize opportunities for learners to work with others to practice these skills and facilitate integration into their nursing practice. For example, didactic and interactive content can be followed by a competency measurement session to validate the degree to which the learner is able to connect these with practice; thereby, support mastery of the stated competency objectives.

Many nursing skills are intrapersonal in nature requiring practice for proficiency; for instance, critical thinking, emotional intelligence, and knowledge integration. Adult learning theory supports mastery of intrapersonal competencies. For instance, educational best practices for adults allow for construction and integration of knowledge based on "real-life" experiences, collaboration, and discussion with other learners (Guri-Rosenblit, 2005; Klein & Fowles, 2009; Lenburg, 1999; Topping, 2008).

Distance education programs that provide opportunities for learner interaction with educators, colleagues, peers, and experts can facilitate knowledge construction within a learning community. Interpersonal and educational interaction expands a learner's (i.e., rural nurses) network and reduces one's sense of professional isolation. Instructional techniques such as synchronous discussion, chat room conversations, and narrative storytelling are useful approaches to enhance the formation of a "cyber learning community." These strategies vicariously contribute to successful knowledge construction among distance learners. Essentially, these cyber-based techniques replace traditional face-to-face networking activities such as formal study groups, in-class discussions, and informal social interactions that occur outside the classroom.

The role of the distance educator includes creating an environment that supports the development of a "cyber learning community" through facilitation of participants' learning role (Beldarrain, 2006; Imel, 1998; Merriam & Caffarella, 1999). To reiterate, adult learners, in this case nurses in rural practice settings, bring unique perspectives to a class. As individuals they contribute to the development and sense of a learning community, facilitated by the educator who engages and encourages learners to share personal experiences and perceptions. When individuals interact and share experiences and knowledge, they add to the course content. Subsequently, this information makes the content applicable and relevant to learners' life and work. The instructor is also part of the learning community, and therefore expected to share one's perspectives and experiences. The instructor also role-models skills of interaction as well as professional behaviors such as the use of evidence-based practice and patterns of critical thinking.

RURAL DISTANCE EDUCATION INSTRUCTIONAL PRACTICES

Technology can be employed to deliver education and reduce social distance between teachers and students (Molinari, 2004). Implicit in distance education is the reality that the instructor and learners are separated geographically. For this reason, consideration of adult learning needs and preferences such as social meaning and knowledge construction become important. Learning platforms that facilitate peer interaction so that learners can share professional experiences lead to decreased professional isolation and overcome the sense of social distance. Social distance describes differences in groups of society as opposed to geographical difference. Social distance refers to affective difference which is a measure of the amount of sympathy individuals have for one another. The term may also refer to the "norms" accepted in one group over another. Another definition is the amount and intensity of interactivity experienced among group members. Social distance is known to reduce engagement and learning (Molinari, 2004). Therefore, distance educators consider social presence during course design. Social presence is the practice of projecting personal characteristics into the learning community, thereby presenting oneself as a real person.

Current technologies available that may address this issue of social distance include the use of Podcasting, social networking, and Blogging. Podcasting is similar to webcasting, but is a nonstreaming audio or video file that can be downloaded to digital music players, and repeated by the learner at later times. Podcasting, in particular, can create personal connections between teachers and learners or among the learners. Videos of practice skills along with narrative are called vodcasting and can bring nurses closer together. In contrast, podcasting and vodcasting can separate learners by substituting for interactions. Free open-source podcasting software is readily accessible and can be a valuable addition to an educator's instructional repertoire.

There is ongoing discussion among educators as to the value of social networking and blogging. When viewing these technological tools through the lens of distance education, advantages can be noted. For instance, social networking sites and blogs provide a central place for learners to "chat" and "discuss" ideas, share personal information, pictures, and solidify the "cyber learning community." Internet-based social networking tools become excellent venues for impromptu connections and relationship building among learners.

When available, social networking systems diminish social distance. The rural limitation is that social networking tools rely on Internet connections that may not be available to rural participants. If Internet access is limited, educators can increase the amount of vocal and audio participation via conference calls. Another strategy is to provide content-laden DVDs or CDs and have learners participate in exercises related to the content via telehealth connections or teleconferences.

Alternately, when telephonic dial-up is the only way to access the Internet, educators can modify electronic files as "text only" and ensure that the electronic file size is less than 50k. Text files, in turn, could be enhanced with DVD and/or CD graphics that are sent to the student via the postal service. If such parameters are integrated into the course design, distance learners most likely will be able to upload and download files and also participate in asynchronous discussion using dial-up connection to access the Internet.

Creating and connecting with the "cyber learning community" is the foundation for effective distance education and knowledge construction by a learner. After knowledge is constructed, it must be transitioned and internalized into personal meaning. This can be a challenging outcome for distance learners when the instructor is not immediately accessible in a face-to-face classroom. Thus, the instructor is not able to assess whether or not the translation of knowledge to practice is actually occurring. Strategies to remedy this situation could be through journaling, using hardcopy paper that is mailed to the instructor in a digital blog paper format, or an asynchronous online discussion assignment. These strategies are an effective way to facilitate learner self-reflection that can promote professional growth, emotional intelligence, and knowledge integration.

Focused questions encourage students to reflect. Open-ended questions should be designed to elicit learner's emotional responses and knowledge level. Questions also evaluate what went right in situations or what could be improved.

For example, if an educator is focusing on the competency of communication, one or more of the following reflective questions could be asked of learners:

- How did you give feedback to a colleague?
- What feedback elements were constructive?
- Describe the nonverbal communication signals you observed.
- Describe the emotions that you experienced during the interaction.
- How might you improve your communication techniques next time?

After a learner reflects on the questions, one's responses are shared in the designated discussion site with the "cyber learning community." Subsequently, other members of the learning community have an opportunity to reflect on, identify with, and comment on their experiences via the blog. Written assignments can contribute to individual learner's written communication skills, knowledge construction, and critical thinking skill development. The ability to interact with other learners and share personal experiences also allows a venue for learners to reflect on their own experiences and construct meaning related to the experience. Blogging facilitates sharing of knowledge and information for the benefit of all involved and allows expansion of learners' nursing practice repertoire. Ultimately, use of blogs as a journaling and collaborative tool engages learners in reflection and critical self-analysis related to situational outcomes (Josephsen, 2011, January).

Adult education goals are often based on revealing the student's unseen or unknown situational responses. Such reactions serve to direct nursing care and the effectiveness of the critical thinking process that guides that care. Effective instructional strategies in distance education that support the journey of guided discovery include a variety of self-reflective and problem-based practices such as simulation and debriefing, role playing, and the use of case studies or scenarios (Masters, 2005). These educational interventions encourage critical examination of issues and have been shown to enhance nursing confidence and decision-making abilities (Smith, 2007). The tools promote personal integration of knowledge into practice. Case studies centering on nursing issues such as delegation can be delivered as a power point presentation or in a narrative document format, with the inclusion of focused discussion questions related to the case scenario. Open-ended questions can instigate critical analysis and reflection; for example: What went wrong in the case study? What was done correctly? How did the roles of the various team members affect the outcome of the case study?

Distance learners find "big picture" case studies helpful in understanding the value of nursing competency and the impact of collaborative practice (Josephsen, 2011, April). Problem-based instructional strategies are also useful for teaching the value of evidence-based practice and support the development of rural nursing as a specialty practice, that being "expert generalist."

By virtue of the education, expertise, and public visibility, nurses often hold leadership roles in rural communities. Skills foundational to community roles are related to providing leadership and resource management. Distance educators can facilitate development of these competencies through learner self-assessment, use of online resources focusing on leadership and management skills, collaborative assignments via asynchronous discussion or Wiki participation, and projects that integrate didactic content with community needs.

A Wiki is a technological tool, much like the discussion board, in which several learners work together to develop and complete a group project such as developing an organizational policy or a relevant educational presentation. As with Podcasts, there are free open-source resources that provide Wiki sites for educational purposes and could be used by distance educators. Initially, the Wiki can be used as a file repository and a site for learners to connect with other class members. Essentially, the Wiki is a framework that allows learners to contribute individually on a group project, thereby exercising leadership, relational, and program development skills. Again, these instructional tools are not an option if an Internet connection is not available or may be somewhat limited with to a dial-up connection.

To reiterate, individual and group assignments can be developed for asynchronous learner activity and are especially useful if high-speed Internet connection is not available as well as for the convenience of the adult learners who have multiple roles and responsibilities. Participation via a conference call is another resource that can be used for group activities and problem solving. Regardless of the instructional strategy, the distance educators must become comfortable in using the tools to effectively facilitate learner collaboration and leadership competencies.

Rural nurses benefit from collaboration and sharing experiences and knowledge with their colleagues (Jerome-D'Emilla, Merwin, & Stern, 2010). Specific instructional techniques that offer problem-based learning and collaborative practice, along with the development of critical thinking and leadership competencies, are not limited to group projects, scenarios, or role playing. Depending on the available technology, some or all of these strategies may not be feasible options of instruction for some distance educational programs. Other teaching strategies a distance educator may want to consider include multiple-choice items or fill-in-the-blank questions related to a case scenario, use of concept-mapping tools, and designing activities that elicit personal assumptions and biases that may affect nursing care. Regardless of the strategy, the ultimate goal is to engage learners in the process of gathering information, developing alternatives, testing hypotheses, predicting outcomes, applying resources, and then evaluating interventions.

Robust distance educational systems are needed to meet the continuing educational needs of rural nurses. Evolving telecommunication technology, in particular, holds great promise in reaching and creating "cyber learning communities" in which learners can connect with other rural nurses and construct knowledge that can be applied to and improve rural nursing practice. Use of educational technologies can ease the geographic and financial limitations rural nurses face when considering the pursuit of advanced degrees or maintaining professional development and competence.

In summary, distance education faculty may be challenged to become proficient in planning and implementing distance educational offerings that fit cultural preferences and nursing practice in the rural context. Distance educational programs, if properly designed, provide a productive, collaborative, and flexible system of education that can be accessed by rural nurses and their communities (Morgan et al., 2006). Relevant distance continuing educational opportunities for rural nurses is essential to the growth of rural nursing best practices as well as recruiting and retaining nurses in underserved regions of the nation.

REFERENCES

Beldarrain, Y. (2006). Distance education trends: Integrating new technologies to foster student interaction and collaboration. *Distance Education, 27*(2), 139–153.

Bushy, A. (2006). Nursing in rural and frontier areas: Issues, challenges, and opportunities. *Harvard Health Policy Review, 7*(1), 17–27.

Cejda, B. D. (2007). Distance education in rural community colleges. *Community College Journal of Research and Practice, 31*, 291–303.

Day, J. C., Janus, A., & Davis, J. (2005). *Computer and Internet Use in the United States: 2003*. Washington, DC: U.S. Census Bureau.

Francis, K., Bowman, S., & Redgrave, M. (2001). *Rural nurses: Knowledge and skills required to meet the challenges of a changing work environment in the 21st century: A review of the literature*. Canberra, Australia: National Library of Australia.

Guri-Rosenblit, S. (2005). 'Distance education' and 'e-learning': Not the same thing. *Higher Education, 49*, 467–493.

Horrigan, J., & Murray, K. (2006). *Rural broadband Internet uses*. Washington, DC: Pew Internet and American Life Project.

Imel, S. (1998). *Transformative learning in adulthood* (Report No. EDO-CE-98-200). Columbus, OH: Adult, Career, and Vocational Education (ERIC Document Reproduction Service No. ED423426).

Jerome-D'Emillia, B., Merwin, E., & Stern, S. (2010). Feasibility of using technology to disseminate evidence to rural nurses and improves patient outcomes. *The Journal of Continuing Education in Nursing, 41*(1), 25–32.

Josephsen, J. (2011, January). *Utilizing blogblogs to facilitate meaning and knowledge construction in a preceptorship course*. Poster presented at the annual Mosby's Faculty Development Conference, Orlando, FL.

Josephsen, J. (2011, April). *Teaching delegation online: A multi-modal instructional strategy*. Poster presented at the annual WIN Communicating Nursing Research Conference, Las Vegas, NV.

Klein, C. J., & Fowles, E. R. (2009). An investigation of nursing competence and the competency outcomes performance assessment curricular approach: Senior students' self-reported perceptions. *Journal of Professional Nursing, 25*(2), 109–121.

Lee, H. J., & Winters, C. A. (2006). *Rural nursing: Concepts, theory, and practice* (2nd ed.). New York, NY: Springer Publishing Company.

Lenburg, C. B. (1999). The framework, concepts and methods of the competency outcomes performance assessment (COPA) model. *The Online Journal of Issues in Nursing, 4*(2), 1–13.

Lloyd, S., & Bristol, S. (2006). Modeling mentorship and collaboration for BSN and MSN students in a community clinical practicum. *Journal of Nursing Education, 45*(4), 129–132.

Masters, K. (2005). *Role development in professional nursing practice.* Sudbury, MA: Jones and Bartlett Publishers.

Merriam, S. B., & Caffarella, R. S. (1999). *Learning in adulthood: A comprehensive guide* (2nd ed.). San Francisco, CA: Jossey-Bass.

Molinari, D. (2004). The role of social comments in problem-solving groups in an online class. *American Journal of Distance Education, 18*(2), 89–101.

Molinari, D. L., Jaiswal, A., & Hollinger-Forrest, T. (Dec, 2011). Rural nurses: Lifestyle preferences and educational perceptions. *Online Journal of Rural Nursing and Health Care*, Retrieved from www.rno.org.

Molinari, D., Monserud, M., & Hudzinski, D. (2008). A new type of rural nurse residency. *The Journal of Continuing Education in Nursing, 39*(1), 42–46.

Montour, A., Baumann, A., Blythe, J., & Hunsberger, M. (2009). The changing nature of nursing work in rural and small community hospitals in southern Ontario, Canada. *Rural and Remote Health, 9*(1), 1089.

Morgan, J., Rawlinson, M., & Weaver, M. (2006). Facilitating online reflective learning for health and social care professionals. *Open Learning, 21*(2), 167–176.

Smith, M. E. (2007). From student to practicing nurse. *American Journal of Nursing, 107*(7), 72A–72D.

Topping, A. (2008). From learning outcomes to competencies: What are they and do they reflect practice? *Cancer Nurse Newsletter, Fall*, 4–6.

25

Simulation in Nursing Continuing Education: The Wherefore's and When-to's

Angeline Bushy and Beverly J. Hewett

*S*imulation in nursing education includes a continuum of approaches ranging from simple discussions of case studies to the complex care of multiple actors or computerized mannequins representing patients or employees. Simulation is used for multiple purposes such as teaching content, refining skills, and assessing competence. To effectively use simulation instructors need to be knowledgeable about simulation instructional methods and how to increase thinking skills; as well as equipment operation and use. Simulation is an excellent resource in a transition-to-practice initiative. This chapter describes simulation types and examines rural considerations. An annotated bibliography lists select publications related to simulation.

All types of simulation from role playing to sophisticated experiences delivered by telecommunication grow common across all domains of education and industry. This holds true for nursing as well. Distance learning innovations, as discussed in Chapter 23, make education more accessible in settings for nurses where, heretofore, learning opportunities were limited or nonexistent. Simulation, in particular is becoming more popular as a means to facilitate understanding didactic content and developing an array of skills. Simulated experiences provide the learner (i.e., novice nurses in rural practice settings) with experiences they may otherwise not be exposed to in the clinical setting (e.g., limited numbers of patients; in labor and postpartum, neonates, pediatrics, cardiac conditions, complex medical–surgical diagnoses, behavioral/mental health conditions, etc.). In other words, in some rural health care facilities, there may be few patient situations with low frequency and high impacts. Some patient care events may rarely be experienced or nurses may require periodic practice to remain safe and proficient in this type of patient care. Coupled with distance learning strategies, simulation exercises can be used to develop, sustain, and evaluate nursing skills in a variety of health care facilities located in more remote settings.

Simulated learning experiences have been used by educators in long-term care facilities to teach a variety of skills, including conflict resolution among staff and with supervisors, implementing novel evidence-based practices, and rehearsing motivational interviewing techniques, among others. Most situations that entail repeated exposure can be taught using simulation. Simulation offers an avenue to assess clinical judgment and critical thinking without jeopardizing patient safety. A simulated experience allows nurses to self-reflect actions or the failure to act, on personal skill sets and clinical reasoning. For rural health care facilities, simulation offers opportunities to critique and learn from the clinical decisions and practices of others without having to travel long distances to an urban-based institution. Additionally, the simulated experience is more likely to be relevant to the rural cultural context (Jefferies, 2007).

BACKGROUND

According to *Webster's New World Dictionary* (2003), the term *simulate* is defined as "to look or act like." In the broadest sense, simulation in nursing includes playacting, pretending with mock equipment, mechanical/task simulators, role playing scenarios, case studies and unfolding case studies, standardized patients, and virtual or computer situations. Considering Webster's definition, it becomes obvious that simulation in nursing education has been used for some time, be it using an orange to practice intramuscular and subcutaneous injections, practicing cardio-pulmonary resuscitation on a manikin, inserting Foley catheters in a static anatomical model, as well as role playing mental health disorders and communication techniques. All of these examples are simulations of one type or another. What these experiences have in common is that all occur in an artificial setting, and so the nurse or staff member will be able to carry out the procedure safely in the clinical setting with an "actual" patient.

More specifically, *simulation in nursing* involves carefully planned and orchestrated educational processes designed to imitate the workplace or a clinical environment. Simulation often incorporates technology and devices such as a computer-enhanced mannequin (Li, 2007).

Simulation can be viewed on a continuum. The one extreme of the continuum does not involve the use of any type of technology, for instance, role playing communication techniques, rehearsing a patient care event, scheduling an unanticipated fire drill, or even a pencil and paper disaster planning exercise. The opposing end of the simulation continuum is exercises that are technology driven with computerized software that parallels human physiological responses to a particular scenario. Several types of simulation are used for nursing education in both academic and clinical settings. The next section defines commonly used terms relative to simulation and simulated learning experiences. *Fidelity* is a term that refers to the degree of realism that the simulation provides, ranging from low (fidelity) to high (fidelity). Types of simulation include the following (Decker, Sportsman, Puetz, & Billings, 2008; Florida Center for Nursing, 2010):

- *Task trainer—anatomical* model to practice or demonstrate competency in a specific skill. For example, it is not unusual for the staff developer in a small hospital to use a training arm of insertion of an intravenous (IV) catheter, or a torso for practicing wound care.
- *Haptic system*—simulator that incorporates virtual reality with a mannequin to provide visual and touch feedback. Providing feedback is what differentiates this device from a task trainer, for example, the use of an IV insertion simulator that provides realistic visual cues and sensations of actually inserting an IV catheter.
- *Static mannequin (low fidelity)*—mannequin (e.g., doll) designed for practice of skills that does not have a computer interface. Historically, even in the smallest facility, "Mrs Chase" mannequins have been used for practicing insertion of tubes, performing personal hygiene, or demonstrating medication delivery techniques.
- *Human patient simulator (medium-to-high fidelity)*—mannequin that uses computer technology to provide physiological data to learners, such as heart rate, blood pressure, pulse, and respirations. Computer software can be programmed to demonstrate specific clinical conditions or diagnosis such as childbirth or shock. High-fidelity simulators respond to interventions that are delivered during the simulation exercise, such as medication or oxygen administration. Mannequins are available to represent the lifespan, including premature infants, neonates, children, pregnant women, and the elderly. This technology can be quite costly, quickly be outdated, and may need to be routinely upgraded.
- *Computer simulation*—software designed to allow the learner to gain knowledge, make decisions, and provide feedback. An example is simulation exercise that is designed for a nurse or a team to manage

a patient having a cardiac arrest. Some of these simulations are online web-based programs, and in other instances and institutions, license is purchased to make the program available to nurses within the facility. When using web-based simulations, similar challenges can present as described with distance education in the previous chapter.

■ *Virtual reality*—a computer-generated environment that offers multi-sensory experiences for the learner; it immerses the learner in a simulated environment. For example, virtual online hospitals and communities have been developed in which "nurse" avatars can interact in real time with "patient" avatars. Virtual reality can be designed for the nurse to realistically experience conditions such as decreased vision or impaired mobility and hearing. Virtual reality can also be used for skill development and refinement. Some nursing educators use a combination of video clips and unfolding case studies that allow simulations with a sense of realism, or real time. This strategy lends itself to distance education and does not require costly equipment or technological support, and thus, can be tailored to the skills and learning needs of nurses in a particular rural healthcare facility, such as a hospital, long-term care setting, or a public health agency.

■ *Standardized patients*—individuals trained to act out various situations and scenarios that allow for interaction of the learner with an actual patient. Standardized patients could be used in a variety of learning activities, including practicing interviewing techniques, physical examination skills, or to implement community-wide disaster preparedness that uses nursing students for "victims" in a particular emergency scenario.

Increasingly, simulation is used in nursing education programs and in clinical settings to provide realistic scenarios or situations for learners, including nursing students, nurses, as well as individuals in other disciplines who make up the health care team. Simulation in a critical access hospital, for example, may be used to teach basic and advanced health assessment skills, to develop critical thinking abilities, and to develop team collaboration. In other words, simulation can be used to depict any health condition or diagnoses; it can use low- or high-fidelity modalities, or combinations of the two. Essentially, the learning opportunities offered by a simulation will depend on the abilities of the staff who plan and conduct the simulated experiences.

In the Institute of Medicine (IOM, 2000) report, *To err is human: Building a safer health care system: A report to the Committee on Quality of*

Health Care in America, simulation training is recommended as one strategy that can be used to prevent errors in clinical settings. The *Report* states that, "... health care organizations and teaching institutions should participate in the development and use of simulation for training novice practitioners, problem solving, and crisis management, especially when new and potentially hazardous procedures and equipment are introduced" (IOM, 2000, p. 179). Use of simulation as a teaching strategy can contribute to patient safety and optimize outcomes of care. Simulations can provide opportunities for novice nurses to experience scenarios and intervene in clinical situations within a safe, supervised setting without posing a risk to the patient (Fowler-Durham & Alden, 2008).

While the uses of simulation are broad ranging, it is not a panacea that can be implemented in any place or at any time in an educational program, be it in a university or for a nurse transition-to-practice program. Careful thought must be given in selecting, designing, and implementing a patient simulation as the instructional method of choice should meet particular learning objectives.

When planning any educational activity, the purpose must first be determined. Subsequently, the most appropriate teaching strategy should be selected. Finally, the instructor determines the most appropriate tool (i.e., low fidelity, high fidelity) that is most appropriate to effectively teach the task. It is not the level of fidelity that determines the effectiveness of an educational tool. Rather, it is the knowledge and expertise of the faculty who design the experience. Simulation is a multidimensional exercise that requires the educator to examine the environment, the potential learning challenges, and the psychological perceptions of the learner as well as the equipment that best suits the situation (Fowler-Durham & Alden, 2008).

One cannot overstate that patient simulation is only as effective as the faculty member using it. Educators need to have at least a basic understanding of teaching–learning theories. Concepts from adult learning theories often serve as bases for the implementation of distance education programs and continuing education offerings for nurses. The creativity, clinical knowledge, teaching expertise, and technological abilities of the faculty are highly influential in effective use of simulations that promote meaningful learning. Patient simulation is a learner-centered instructional strategy, and the primary role of a faculty is that of a facilitator. The faculty role will vary depending on whether the simulation exercise is used for learning or evaluation of the learner's performance or competency with a set of skills. Thus, faculty require professional development before use of simulation.

BARRIERS AND DISADVANTAGES

Although simulation has many advantages, the disadvantages and barriers also need to be considered (Decker et al., 2008; Florida Center for Nursing, 2010) (Table 25.1). Foremost, simulation is not real—and the realism of a simulation will vary depending on the fidelity of the exercise. Even when "schooled" actors or standardized patients are used, with authentic props (e.g., clothing, equipment, moulage) in the simulation, it can be difficult to replicate all of the "real or actual" physical and emotional responses. Likewise, the learner may not fully participate or not take the experience seriously. Since simulation is not "real," it is difficult to replicate communication responses as well. Another concern is when instructors use simulation to teach "protocols" rather than critical thinking or clinical reasoning for a given event.

Associated with purchasing and maintaining high(er)-fidelity technology and simulation laboratories are high costs and beyond the budgets of most rural health care facilities. For example, the latest models of high-fidelity mannequins can range from $30,000 to more than $100,000 depending on the equipment features and warranties that are purchased with the equipment. High-fidelity simulators also require maintenance of the hardware and software, along with a temperature-regulated room for storage. Renovating space to establish a center for simulation is also costly. Costs will vary depending on the physical facilities in which the simulation lab will be housed. Simulation equipment may have a limited lifespan and regular maintenance of the equipment, hardware, and software is critical. Equipment and software may become obsolete and outdated, or there may be additional costs for upgrading. For these reasons, nurse educators in rural facilities are creative in designing simulation exercises for staff continuing education within their institution.

Adequate teaching personnel, technical support, and faculty and staff development are essential for effective simulation experiences. Often, these elements are overlooked when planning to develop simulation resources in a health care institution. Faculty training on the appropriate use of simulation as an instructional strategy, writing and editing scenarios, and then implementing the simulated scenario is often lacking, especially in small rural institutions where there are few nursing staff. Administrative support may also be lacking and this too is a barrier to this instructional modality, in particular, simulation that uses high-fidelity technology. Feedback and debriefing are critical with the learner as well as with faculty facilitators to address incorrect as well as appropriate actions. For this kind of exchange to

TABLE 25.1
Simulation in Nursing: Advantages and Disadvantages/Barriers

Advantages	-Allows learners to attain knowledge/skills in a safe/controlled environment
	-Provides opportunity to learn from experience, make mistakes without risk(s) to patients
	-Increase speed of learning skills/developing competence
	-Assures similar learning experience for each nurse for a given scenario; reduces variability in teaching/learning processes
	-Offers experience opportunities for high-risk clinical situations that may occur infrequently in the facility such as emergency childbirth, cardiac arrest, and care for pediatric patients
	-Allows for immediate feedback related to performance; debriefing an opportunity for review and reflection on the scenario processes
	-Permits flexibility in scheduling clinical experiences for a variety of learners/scenarios
	-Promotes patient safety and prevention of medical errors
	-Allows for quick (and oftentimes easy) implementation to educate in best practice procedure or remediate skills
	-Uses more realistic approach to patient care management; and for multidisciplinary team training opportunities
Disadvantages	-Realism of a situation varies depending on fidelity of the equipment/technology
	-Learner may not take the activity seriously and/or not be actively engaged
	-Difficult to replicate psychological, emotional, and physical responses in a given clinical situation of the patient/caregiver
	-Costs associated with purchasing, maintaining, upgrading hardware/software, and storing equipment, mannequin, technology
	-Costs associated with staff development to effectively use the technology as a teaching strategy
	-Resources required to develop and edit meaningful and appropriate scenarios
	- Lifespan of the equipment may be limited
	-Most effective with small groups of students followed by debriefing; simulation can be resource and labor intensive
	-Faculty and administrative support may be lacking
	-Without formal debriefing negative learning outcomes can occur

occur and be meaningful, there is a need for a capacity-building model that is supportive for all involved.

Most small rural hospitals do not have the resources for mid- to high-fidelity technology. Increasingly, smaller hospitals are establishing partnerships with tertiary facilities as well as institutions of higher learning that have a simulation lab. Idaho State University, for example, has a "traveling sim[ulatin] lab" with high-fidelity technology that is used in conjunction with nursing distance education offerings in rural outreach communities. Other rural-based nursing staff developers are creatively using less low-fidelity technology and "standardized" patients to design simulation scenarios for novice as well as experienced nurses.

IMPLEMENTING SIMULATION EXERCISES

Selecting, designing, implementing, and evaluating a simulation learning experience require forethought and careful planning. Fowler-Durham and Alden (2008) propose three phases: presimulation, intrasimulation, and postsimulation. Each of these will be briefly discussed in the subsequent sections. Table 25.2 summarizes presimulation, intrasimulation, and postsimulation activities for the learner and the instructor/evaluator and the learner (Fowler-Durham & Alden, 2008).

PRESIMULATION ACTIVITIES

Prior to using the simulation exercise with students, the instructor must be prepared to facilitate the learning experience. This includes being comfortable in using the equipment and familiarity with the scenarios to be used in the exercises. All who will be involved with the exercise should be provided a script of the scenario at least several days before the activity to allow adequate time to prepare and effectively facilitate the activity. Letting faculty members first participate as students (i.e., pilot testing) can be very effective to increase their comfort level with the simulated exercise. Using clinical faculty or more experienced nurses as facilitators of simulated scenarios can be a highly effective teaching strategy. Idaho State University has successfully used the expertise of retired nurses for the facilitator role. This approach provides an opportunity for clinical personnel to gain insights into how the novice nurse functions as a team member; as well as identify leadership qualities, assess communication skills and critical thinking abilities, and evaluate skill performance or competency. The simulation exercise is an opportunity for the clinician to assess how a novice reacts under pressure should a critical situation occur.

INTRASIMULATION ACTIVITIES

The actual scenario exercise should begin when the learner enters the simulation room. If this is the learner's first encounter with simulation activities, he/she may initially require assistance, coaching, and encouragement from the instructor or facilitator. When the simulation activity is for the purpose of evaluating skills or competency, the facilitator

TABLE 25.2
High-Fidelity Presimulation, Intrasimulation, and Postsimulation Activities

Learner activities	*Presimulation*
	-Complete assigned readings
	-Review scenario
	-Reflect on/practice skills required for scenario
	-Procure/organize required materials/equipment
	Intrasimulation
	-Arrive promptly at scheduled time
	-Dress in designated clinical attire (including name badge)
	-Bring *all* essential equipment (e.g., stethoscope, otoscope, watch with second hand, etc.)
	-Address/treat mannequin as a "real" patient
	-Communicate with patient/patient/team members as in an actual clinical situation
	-Be aware of personal emotions, responses, behavior during the simulated scenario
	Postsimulation
	-Participate in the debriefing
	-Complete/submit required evaluation materials
Instructor–Facilitator activities	*Presimulation*
	-Procure the necessary equipment and supplies
	-Develop and disseminate schedule for learners to attend/participate
	-Develop/obtain and refine the scenario script with a grading rubric and evaluation criteria
	-Discuss/become familiar with details of the simulated scenario/case study/activity
	-Practice using the technology/device
	-Understand the expected learner outcomes
	-Practice monitoring/evaluating learner's skill level/activities
	-Pilot test the scenario/case study/activity (whenever feasible) to become proficient with activity nuances
	Intrasimulation
	-Arrive a few minutes before the simulation activity is scheduled to begin
	-Have all essential equipment/supplies available (e.g., grading rubric, script(s), etc.)
	-Dress in the designated attire (e.g., lab coat, scrubs, etc.)
	-Orientate/demonstrate simulation technology to familiarize learners to this teaching strategy/tools
	-Assess learners' knowledge/familiarity/comfort level with using simulation technology
	Postsimulation
	-Facilitate debriefing and evaluation procedures
	-Review/summarize activity and feedback
	-Revise case study/activity as needed for future use
	-Provide feedback/disseminate information on outcomes to appropriate venues/administrators, etc.
	-Clean and store equipment as recommended by the manufacturer
	-Resupply materials as appropriate

begins by introducing himself/herself and, if appropriate, provides an introduction to the activity. If more than one learner is required for the simulation scenario, the facilitator assigns each to a specific role(s). A grading rubric for the scenario is used to evaluate and document the learner's competencies or lack thereof.

POSTSIMULATION ACTIVITIES

Debriefing is a critical element of simulation activities. Unless feedback and debriefing are provided, the learner can learn something incorrectly, sometimes termed as negative transfer of learning. During the debriefing, misinformation can be corrected; improper techniques can be noted while appropriate interventions or techniques should be demonstrated. One cannot overstate the importance of feedback to enhance learners' ability to integrate correct behaviors into their skill set. Simulation gaps in knowledge can be identified by the learner that would otherwise remain undetected. While debriefing, learners are asked to reflect on their own skills and knowledge and identify what was done well and what needs improvement. Since multiple activities occur during a simulation activity, the learner may be focused only on the assigned role, and debriefing can be used to review key points about the exercise. This could include discussion about the sequencing of events, psychomotor and communication skills, required documentation, as well as feelings that occurred during the procedures. It is important to provide learners with an opportunity to evaluate their experience and use of the technology as an instructional strategy. Verbal learner feedback (evaluation) of the process and outcomes is part of the debriefing, but could be separate in the form of paper and pencil or computerized surveys. Learner feedback (evaluation) could be part of a course evaluation if the simulation was an instructional component.

BENEFITS AND OUTCOMES

Studies have shown that students who participate in simulations attain desired knowledge, demonstrate competence skills, and gain increased confidence in their abilities to perform a specific skill or in a given situation (Bambini, Washburn, & Perkins, 2009; Bruce et al., 2009; Cannon-Diehl, 2009; Cheraghi, Hassani, Yaghmaei, & Alavi-Majed, 2009; Dillard et al., 2009; Hicks, Coke, & Li, 2009; Lambton, 2008; Sinclair & Ferguson, 2009). The majority of studies have been done in educational settings with limited research on outcomes of simulation in continuing education of nurses. There have been no large-scale studies that present compelling evidence to support the use of simulation as an alternative to clinical practice (Sanford, 2010). However, neither has the value of learning in the actual clinical setting been supported by research (Tanda & Denham, 2009). Ongoing research is needed to assess the transfer of knowledge and skills from the simulated setting to the clinical setting. Research is also required to determine if learning outcomes with simulation are equal to, or better than, learning in an actual clinical setting.

Use of simulation in nursing education is a relatively new instructional methodology. The rationale for using simulation as an educational strategy includes the absence of risk to a "live" patient; the ability to provide standardization of cases and clinical scenarios; the promotion of critical thinking, clinical decision making, and psychomotor skills; the provision of immediate and constructive feedback to the learner; and the integration of knowledge and behavior. Through realistic simulation scenarios, essential elements of patient safety can be emphasized such as prevention of medication errors and appropriate documentation, facilitating effective communication and team work. In nurse transition-to-practice programs, the leaner is exposed to critical or emergency care situations. The simulated context provides an opportunity for the novice nurse to learn and refine skills, and develop competence in caring for an actual patient with a particular condition.

Individuals are better prepared for delivering safe and effective care when simulation is experienced during transition to practice. Learning to function within the health care team during a residency or internship develops leadership, communication, and collaborative skills as well as leading to optimal patient outcomes. The challenge for the instructor is to embrace simulation as an instructional strategy and to learn how to effectively use the technology to develop nurses' clinical competence. In rural settings, the instructor needs to be creative and tailor scenarios to the rural context. To reiterate, patient simulation technology is exciting but it is only as effective as the faculty who use it. Essentially, when used effectively, the benefits to learners outweigh the costs of the equipment and faculty training.

Regardless of the context, be it rural or urban, the future of nursing education must be developed with a vision that includes innovative strategies, such as low- and high-fidelity simulation. Simulation may be useful in preparing additional nurses to enter the workforce and retrain experienced nurses for other specialty areas. As the U.S. population ages, two crucial issues must be considered:

■ The demand for nurses will increase.
■ Nursing care will become more complex.

In summary, simulation and simulated experiences can be useful in both academic and clinical settings to enhance learning and to improve the quality of rendered nursing care. In rural contexts, simulation could be useful for assessing and maintaining nurses' competence with select diagnoses or conditions that are infrequently encountered in the facility, hence an approach to address quality of care and patient safety.

REFERENCES

Bambini, D., Washburn, J., & Perkins, R. (2009). Outcomes of clinical simulation for novice nursing students: Communication, confidence, clinical judgment. *Nursing Education Perspectives, 30,* 79–82.

Bruce, S. A., Scherer, Y. K., Curran, C. C., Urschel, D. M., Erdley, S., & Ball, L. S. (2009). A collaborative exercise between graduate and undergraduate nursing students using a computer-assisted simulator in a mock cardiac arrest. *Nursing Education Perspectives, 30,* 22–27.

Cannon-Diehl, M. R. (2009). Simulation in healthcare and nursing: State of the science. *Critical Care Nursing Quarterly, 32,* 128–136.

Cheraghi, F., Hassani, P., Yaghmaei, F., & Alavi-Majed, H. (2009). Developing a valid and reliable self-efficacy in clinical performance scale. *International Nursing Review, 56,* 214–221.

Decker, S., Sportsman, S., Puetz, L., & Billings, L. (2008). The evolution of simulation and its contribution to competency. *Journal of Continuing Education in Nursing, 39,* 74–80.

Dillard, N., Sideras, S., Ryan, M., Carlton, K. H., Lasater, K., & Siktberg, L. (2009). A collaborative project to apply and evaluate the clinical judgment model through simulation. *Nursing Education Perspectives, 30,* 99–104.

Florida Center for Nursing. (2010). *Addressing the nursing shortage through simulation: White paper.* Orlando, FL: Author. Retrieved March 30, 2011 from http://www.flcenterfornursing.org/files/FCN_Addressing_Nursing_Shortage_Simulation_Feb_2010.pdf

Fowler-Durham, C., & Alden, K. (2008). Enhancing patient safety in nursing education through patient simulation. In R. Hughes (Ed.), *Patient safety and quality: An evidence based handbook for nurses* (chap. 51). Rockville, MD: Agency for Healthcare Quality and Research (AHRQ). Retrieved March 30, 2011 from http://www.ahrq.gov/qual/nurseshdbk/

Hicks, F. D., Coke, L., & Li, S. (2009). The effect of high-fidelity simulation on nursing student's knowledge and performance: A pilot study. *NCSBN Research Brief.* Retrieved 9/4/11 from http://www.phoenix.edu/colleges_divisions/nursing/articles/2011/01/nursing-education-high-fidelity-simulation-labs-offer-high-impact-training.html

Institute of Medicine (IOM). (2000). *To err is human: Building a safer health care system: A report to the Committee on Quality of Health Care in America.* Washington, DC: Institute of Medicine.

Jefferies, P. (Ed.). (2007). *Simulation in nursing education: From conceptualization to evaluation.* New York, NY: National League for Nursing.

Lambton, J. (2008, October). Simulation as a strategy to teach clinical pediatrics within a nursing curriculum. *Clinical Simulation in Nursing*, 4(3), e79–e87.

Li, S. (2007). *The role of simulation in nursing education: A regulatory perspective.* Presented at the American Association of Colleges of Nursing Hot Issues Conference. Denver, CO. Retrieved March 30, 2011 from https://www.ncsbn.org/ The_Role_of_Simulation_in_Nursing_Education(1).pdf

Sanford, P. (2010). Simulation in nursing education: A review of the research. *The Qualitative Report*, 15(4), 1006–1011. Retrieved March 30, 20011 from http://www.nova.edu/ssss/QR/QR15-4/sanford.pdf

Sinclair, B., & Ferguson, K. (2009). Integrating simulated teaching/learning strategies in undergraduate nursing education. *International Journal of Nursing Education Scholarship*, 6, 1–11.

Tanda, R., & Denham, S. A. (2009). Clinical instruction and student outcomes. *Teaching and Learning in Nursing*, 4, 139–147.

Webster's New World Dictionary. (2011). New York, NY: Simon & Schuster. Retrieved 9/4/11 from http://www.yourdictionary.com/simulate

SELECTED ANNOTATED BIBLIOGRAPHY

Benhuri, G. (2010, July). Teaching community telenursing with simulation. *Clinical Simulation in Nursing*, 6(4), e161–e163. doi: 10.1016/j.ecns.2009.11.011

Abstract: Nurse educators may use homecare simulation experiences to enhance the learning of nursing students and help fill the need for community clinical practice. Simulation experience gives students a safe opportunity to expand the skills and critical thinking needed for community health nursing, in addition to increasing self-confidence. This article presents a two-part scenario that adds telenursing technology to a homecare simulation experience for students to become comfortable with the technology. By understanding telenursing, students may learn that telenursing is a way to provide appropriate care to a large number of clients, potentially inspiring community nursing as a career option.

Burns, H. K., O'Donnell, J., & Artman, J. (2010, May). High-fidelity simulation in teaching problem solving to 1st-year nursing students: A novel use of the nursing process. *Clinical Simulation in Nursing*, 6, e87–e95. doi: 10.1016/ j.ecns.2009.07.005

Abstract: *Background*: The efficacy of using high-fidelity simulation to facilitate 1st-year nursing students' learning of problem-solving skills has not been established.

Method: The authors tested the efficacy of using high-fidelity simulation to facilitate understanding of problem-solving skills among 1st-year nursing students. Knowledge and attitude changes were evaluated using pre- and posttests.

Results/Conclusions: Of students who completed the pre- and postsimulation assessments, 82% showed a significant gain in knowledge. All students (114) showed a significant positive difference for multiple attitudinal items, including critical thinking skills, overall nursing knowledge, confidence, and communication. Facilitating acquisition of problem solving through the use of high-fidelity simulation is effective and welcomed by all participants in this study cohort. More research is needed to determine the long-term effects of this method.

Gantt, L. T., & Webb-Corbett, R. (2010). Using simulation to teach patient safety behaviors in undergraduate nursing education. *Journal of Nursing Education,* 49(1), 48–51. doi: 10.3928/01484834-20090918-10

Abstract: The purpose of this article is to describe how our college of nursing began to integrate patient safety instruction into simulation experiences for undergraduate nursing students. A system for evaluating and grading students was developed. Data on student safety behaviors were collected before and after the implementation of instruction designed to improve adherence to hand washing and patient identification procedures. In the first semester in which data were collected, students did not demonstrate satisfactory performance of either hand hygiene or patient identification 61% of the time. After instruction, students still did not perform these procedures consistently 38% of the time. Lessons learned and future plans for addressing these problems with basic patient safety behaviors are discussed.

Gore, T., Hunt, C. W., & Raines, K. H. (2008, October). Mock hospital unit simulation: A teaching strategy to promote safe patient care. *Clinical Simulation in Nursing,* 4(3), e57–e64. doi: 10.1016/j.ecns.2008.08.006

Abstract: Patient safety is a priority in nursing care. Nursing educators must prepare future registered nurses with the skills necessary to deliver safe, effective care. The purpose of this article is to report on the use of a mock hospital unit with human patient simulation (HPS). Participants were 24 first-semester baccalaureate nursing students out of a class of 79 juniors, and the project took place prior to the students' first actual clinical experience. The students were assigned to three faculty and, during 4 h, cared for patients with various diagnoses. On completion of the HPS teaching project, faculty and students viewed the simulation as a positive experience with several beneficial outcomes. Beginning in fall 2008, the use of HPS as a teaching strategy will expand to include the entire junior class.

Greenawald, D. A. (2008, July). LIVE! From the Sim Lab: Broadcasting a simulated patient-care scenario as a teaching-learning strategy in a nursing fundamentals clinical lab. *Clinical Simulation in Nursing,* 4(2), e11–e14. doi: 10.1016/j.ecns.2008.06.004

Abstract: At one baccalaureate program, the faculty and staff feel strongly that simulation experiences are such an effective teaching elearning strategy that they warrant inclusion in the very first clinical nursing course, an on-campus weekly 2-hour Fundamentals of Nursing lab experience. The innovative use of real-time broadcast technology and simulated patient care scenarios has proved to be a winning combination for these novice nursing students and at the same time has made optimal use of limited lab time and resources. LIVE! From the Sim Lab was highly effective in demystifying the simulation experience for students and introducing them to the patient care scenario format for practice and evaluation.

Hayden, J. (2010). Use of simulation in nursing education: National survey results. *Journal of Nursing Regulation,* 1(3), 52–57.

Abstract: While simulation in nursing programs continue to increase, it is important to understand the prevalence of this new technology in nursing education, how this technology is utilized, and how educators are preparing to teach with this educational tool. This article reports on the results of a survey conducted by National Council of State Boards of Nursing of 1,060 prelicensure nursing programs in the United States as a means of describing use of simulation.

Kaakinen, J., & Arwood, E. (2009). Systematic review of nursing simulation literature for use of learning theory. *International Journal of Nursing Education Scholarship, 6*(1), 1–20. doi: 10.2202/1548-923X.1688

Abstract: The purpose of this systematic analysis of nursing simulation literature between 2000 and 2007 was to determine how learning theory was used to
design and assess learning that occurs in simulations. Out of the 120 articles in
which designing nursing simulations was reported, 16 referenced learning or
developmental theory as the basis of how and why they set up the simulation.
Of the 16 articles that used a learning type of foundation, only two considered
learning as a cognitive task. More research is needed that investigates the efficacy
of simulation for improving student learning. The study concludes that most
nursing faculty approach simulation from a teaching paradigm rather than a
learning paradigm. For simulation to foster student learning there must be a fundamental shift from a teaching paradigm to a learning paradigm and a foundational learning theory to design and evaluate simulation should be used.
Examples of how to match simulation with learning theory are included.

MacGougan, C. K., & Lam, K. H. (2005). Human patient simulation and distance
education: A review. *Israeli Journal of Emergency Medicine, 5*(2), 13–17.

Abstract: High-fidelity human patient simulation (HPS) and distance education (DE) are two new tools available to medical educators. HPS makes use
of a computerized "patient" mannequin to simulate medical problems. HPS
allows for knowledge integration through experiential learning while optimiz-
ing patient safety. It is not a tool for every learning objective—it is expensive,
labor intensive, and, despite having face validity, has not been validated by
other means. DE facilitates learning between physically separated learners and
educators, by allowing students to access educational materials from anywhere.
Quality materials take time and effort to develop properly, but educators can
spread the cost of development over the increased number of students compared
to traditional methods. Although DE is well suited to knowledge-based topics, it
is not ideal for all curricula. HPS and DE are not substitutes for training on real
patients but represent bridges that make this transition smoother and safer.

Nehring, W. M. (2009). Nursing simulation: A review of the past 40 years. *Simulation
and Gaming, 40*(4), 528–544. doi: 10.1177/1046878109332282

Abstract: Simulation, in its many forms, has been a part of nursing education
for many years. The use of games, computer-assisted instruction, standardized
patients, virtual reality, and low-fidelity to high-fidelity mannequins have
appeared in the past 40 years, whereas anatomical models, partial task trainers,
and role playing were used earlier. A historical examination of these many forms
of simulation in nursing is presented, followed by a discussion on the roles of
simulation in both nursing education and practice. A viewpoint concerning
the future of simulation in nursing concludes the article.

Pattillo, R. E., Hewett, B., McCarthy, M. D., & Molinari, D. (2010, September).
Capacity building for simulation sustainability. *Clinical Simulation in Nursing,
6*(5), e185–e191. doi: 10.1016/j.ecns.2009.08.008

Abstract: The capacity building for simulation sustainability model is presented to assist nursing faculty in the development of simulation resources
and activities. The model gives significant consideration to the economic

concepts of both capacity building and sustainability. The complex systems model was conceived and utilized as our faculty moved forward with planning, implementing, and evaluating simulation activities for our undergraduate curriculum. The conceptual framework and an informal evaluation of the model are described.

Shea, P., Sau, L. C., & Pickett, A. (2006). A study of teaching presence and student sense of learning community in fully online and web-enhanced college courses. *Internet and Higher Education, 9*(3), 175–190.

Abstract: This paper focuses on two components of a model for online teaching and learning—"teaching presence" and "community." It is suggested that previous research points to the critical role that community plays in academic success and persistence in higher education. Through a review of literature it is proposed that teaching presence—viewed as the core roles of the online instructor—is a promising mechanism for developing learning community in online environments. This investigation presents a multi-institutional study of 1,067 students across 32 different colleges that further substantiates this claim. An instrument to access instructor presence ("The Teaching Presence Scale") is presented and validated. Factor and regression analysis indicate a significant link between students' sense of learning community and effective instructional design and "directed facilitation" on the part of course instructors, and highlights interesting difference between online and classroom environments. Alternative hypotheses regarding student demographics associate with variables such as age (the "net generation" effect) and gender are also examined. Despite assertions that younger students are or soon will be too sophisticated to "feel at home" in largely text-based asynchronous learning environments, no significant effects were found by demographic differences examined. Recommendations for online course design, pedagogy, and future research are included.

Smith, G. G., Sorensen, C., Gump, A., Heindel, A. J., Caris, M., & Martinez, C. D. (2011). Overcoming student resistance to group work: Online versus face-to-face. *Internet and Higher Education, 14*(2), 121–128. doi: 10.1016/j.ihedu2010.09.005

Abstract: This study compared student group work experiences in online (OL) versus face-to-face (f2f) section of the same graduate course, over 3 years, to determine what factors influence student group work experiences and how do these factors play out in f2f versus OL environments. Surveys and student journals suggest that communication issues, personal feelings about group members, and their participation play a prominent role in student perceptions about group work. Students in OL sections were more negative about group work than were students in f2f sections. Because of OL norms of working individually an asynchronously, OL students were less satisfied with group work. Also, because of fewer channels of communication, lack of the immediacy of f2f meetings and other differences in the two learning environments, OL students were less able to resolve logistical difficulties associated with group work.

Starkweather, A. R., & Kardong-Edgren, S. (2008). Diffusion of innovation: Embedding simulation into nursing curricula. *International Journal of Nursing Education Scholarship, 5*(1), 1–11.

Abstract: Numerous articles have documented the benefits of using simulation as a teaching method for undergraduate nursing students. Simulation can enhance learning and provides a stimulating environment for technologically proficient students. Yet, there remain a large number of nursing programs and faculty members that are resistant toward implementing simulation as a learning tool. This article provides details on the efforts to embed simulation in an undergraduate program that started with a few interested faculty at a large, multisite nursing program. The Diffusion of Innovation theory was used to guide the expansion of simulation to other faculty groups. The techniques used to embed simulation into the undergraduate curriculum were directed by past research. This process led to a successful integration of simulation which could provide some innovative suggestions for other programs facing similar barriers.

Swanson, E. A., Nicholson, A. C., Boese, T. A., Cram, E., Stineman, A. M., & Tew, K. May 2011 simulation and student outcomes. *Clinical Simulation in Nursing, 10*, e1–e10. doi: 10.1016/j.ecns.2009.12.011

Abstract: *Background*: Teaching strategies need to engage learners and focus on active learning. The nursing faculty shortage challenges us to prepare competent students. Simulation has been suggested as an appropriate teaching strategy.

Method: The basic experimental posttest-only design of this study evaluated effects of three teaching strategies on the outcomes of performance and retention performance of intervention activities, student satisfaction and self-confidence, and educational practice preferences.

Results: Students' scores were significantly higher in retention performance than in first performance. There was a significant interaction effect for time and teaching strategy. Nursing education needs to focus on use of high-fidelity simulation as a teaching strategy.

Waldner, M. H., & Olson, J. K. (2007). Taking the patient to the classroom: Applying theoretical frameworks to simulation in nursing education. *International Journal of Nursing Education Scholarship, 4*(18), 1–14.

Abstract: On completion of their education, nursing students are expected to practice safely and competently. Societal changes and revisions to nursing education have altered the way nursing students learn to competently care for patients. Increasingly, simulation experiences are used to assist students to integrate theoretical knowledge into practice. Reasons for and the variety of simulation activities used in nursing education in light of learning theory are discussed. By combining Benner's nursing skill acquisition theory with Kolb's experiential learning theory, theoretical underpinnings for examining the use of simulations in the context of nursing education are provided.

Walsh, M. (2010). Using a simulated learning environment. *Emergency Nurse, 18*(2), 12–16.

Abstract: Stilwell is a simulation environment designed for postgraduate emergency care staff. It encourages participants to make less obvious diagnoses of patients who have presented to emergency departments, and to consider a wide range of factors when making treatment and management decisions.

Weller, M., Pegler, C., & Mason, R. (2005). Use of innovative technologies on an e-learning course. *Internet and Higher Education, 8*(1), 61–71.

Abstract: This paper examines how four innovative technologies were incorporated into one course at The UK Open University. The technologies were: blogging, audio conferencing, instant messaging, and Harvard's Rotisserie system. Each of the technologies is addressed, and details from the student evaluation are provided. The student feedback on all the technologies was positive. The role of the learning object-based course design is examined and it is suggested that this approach facilitates the incorporation of innovative technologies into a course. The authors suggest that as students become increasingly accustomed to standard communication tools such as asynchronous bulletin boards, there will be a shift toward implementing a range of technologies, each offering particular affordances for different forms of communication.

Willhaus, J. (2010, November). Interdepartmental simulation collaboration in academia: Exploring partnerships with other disciplines. *Clinical Simulation in Nursing, 6*(6), e231–e232. doi: 10.1016/j.ecns.2010.02.011

Abstract: Multidisciplinary collaboration provides opportunities for growth in any simulation program. Simulation coordinators pursuing excellence may find unlikely partners among health care and non-health-care professionals. Nonnursing collaborations can offer students, faculty, and simulation coordinators fresh views about simulation in an interdisciplinary climate. Examples of cooperative work with instructors and researchers in radiology, sports medicine, and criminal justice studies are described. Sports medicine students participated in scenarios involving a school-aged child with a spontaneous pneumothorax, a coach who was having a stroke, a pregnant yoga instructor experiencing an asthma attack, and a football player who had been momentarily unconscious after a tackle. Nursing students were asked to participate in criminal justice scenarios because of their understanding of simulation principles.

Woo, Y., & Reeves, T. C. (2007). Meaningful interaction in web-based learning: A social constructivist interpretation. *Internet and Higher Education, 10*, 15–25.

Abstract: Interaction is an essential ingredient in any learning process. However, every interaction does not lead to increased learning. When interaction has a direct influence on a learner's intellectual growth, we can say the interaction is meaningful. The precise meaning of meaningful interaction is strongly related to the learning theories underlying the development of particular environments. The primary goal of this paper is to reconceptualize online interaction in terms of meaningful learning based on the learning theory known as social constructivism. Analyzing interaction through this theoretical framework may yield design principles needed to improve the quality of web-based learning environment. A secondary goal of this paper is to present the implication of meaningful online interaction from researchers and developers.

26

Program Evaluation and Outcome Measurement

Deana L. Molinari and Angeline Bushy

Evaluation is critical to the success of any innovation. The success of creation and implementation cannot be revealed without process and outcome measurement. Evidence (data) is essential to refine instructional strategies or clinical experiences, and to substantiate cost–benefit ratios for program sustainability. This chapter focuses on transition-to-practice outcome measurement relative to patient safety and program quality and fiduciary decisions in rural contexts.

Determining success, or the lack of it, is the art of measuring quality. There are different ways of defining and measuring success. Although there are barriers to addressing quality improvement of health care in rural America, there are solutions. Measurement of quality is also vital to the development of nursing transition-to-practice programs as the processes contribute to desired outcomes of such initiatives. Two reasons for measuring success are fiscal, that is, "money decreases" and "money increases." Poorly designed systems can result in errors that cost money while efficient systems can produce profits (Institute of Medicine, 1998; 2001). Thus, outcome improvements within a system are another motivation for measuring quality. Sometimes the mere process of analyzing can increase patient and employee/worker satisfaction associated with achieving desired outcomes. Metaphorically, measuring can be described as the wrapping paper for the gift of quality health care.

There are two types of value measurements—technical performance and interpersonal performance. Technical performance is designed to compare standards or best practices with the care that is provided. Interpersonal performance is designed to measure how care is

323

accomplished by people (i.e., employees). The essence of nursing is interpersonal performance. Since interpersonal actions are more difficult to ascertain, measurement studies and proofs (outcomes) are limited. Nonetheless, it is essential that nurses address the barriers of measuring nursing effectiveness. Undervaluing nursing care will ultimately lead to the use of more unlicensed personnel to deliver health care services (Campbell-Heider, 1998).

QUALITY

Quality improvement is defined as the study of improving systems. *Continuous quality improvement* is a method that emphasizes future outcomes while seeking to improve service provision. *Quality assurance* provides the mechanisms to effectively monitor patient care provided by health care professionals using cost-effective resources. Although the terms are sometimes used interchangeably, the combined influence of the two approaches is exponentially effective. Health care is dynamic and daily changes emerge associated with the "quality" approach to measuring success. Concomitantly, standards of practice are developed that also require health professionals to quickly modify practice at the risk of not being reimbursed for their services.

Measuring Quality

Professional organizations collaborated to produce quality standards and corresponding indicators that addressed s communities, health care systems and its providers. The National Quality Forum (NQF) determined national priorities for performance improvement, established standards for measuring performance, and strongly recommended attainment of these priorities (National Quality Forum, 2004; 2008). The NQF emerged because of the multiple perspectives of how quality is, or should be, defined and the manner in which quality should be measured. To expedite achievement of the national goals, a consensus approach was encouraged. The NQF further specified three types of quality measurement: Patient outcomes, process outcomes, and structure outcomes (Montalvo, 2007). Essentially, the NQF standardized definitions of quality and associated measurement are based on the NQF recommendations; subsequently, the American Nurses Association (ANA) developed the National Database of Quality Indicators (NDNQI) to measure patient-centered, nursing-centered, and system-centered variables (see Table 26.1).

Ideally, nursing-sensitive, patient-focused outcomes should improve when a greater quantity or quality of nursing care is provided.

TABLE 26.1
Categories of Outcome Measures With Select Clinical Indicators

CATEGORY	CLINICAL INDICATORS
Patient centered	▪ Failure to rescue surgical inpatients with treatable serious complications
	▪ Pressure ulcer prevalence
	▪ Falls prevalence
	▪ Falls with injury
	▪ Restraint prevalence (vest and limb only)
	▪ Urinary catheter-associated urinary tract infection
	▪ Central line catheter-associated blood stream infection rate
	▪ Ventilator-associated pneumonia
Nursing centered	▪ Smoking cessation counseling for acute myocardial infarction
	▪ Smoking cessation counseling for heart failure
	▪ Smoking cessation counseling for pneumonia
System centered	▪ Skill mix (registered nurse, licensed vocational/practical nurse, unlicensed assistive personnel, and contracted individuals)
	▪ Nursing care hours per patient day
	▪ Practice environment scale
	▪ Voluntary turnover

Among the first of adverse events that were identified as "nursing-sensitive indicators" were pressure ulcers, falls, and intravenous infiltrations. The indicators of these events are technical skills with outcomes that are relatively easy to measure. Patient injuries, medication errors, and nosocomial infections are other events that are sensitive to nursing care (Kohn, Corrigan & Donaldson, 2000). Evidence shows that number of nurses on duty and their education levels can make a difference in when these events occur.

Process outcomes refer to nursing actions including assessment and interventions. Job satisfaction is in the process outcome category. The type of nursing staff on a unit can impact on satisfaction levels. The final category, structure of nursing care, is measured by the number of nurses, their skill levels, mix of skills, and education of the staff (Kanai-Pak, Aiken, Sloane, & Poghosyan, 2008). Effectiveness of a nurse transition-to-practice program falls within these two quality measurement categories—process and outcomes.

RURAL TRANSITION-TO-PRACTICE PROGRAMS

Facilities that implement nurse transition-to-practice programs without incorporating quality assessment will not know whether or not the initiative was worth the cost or if it made a difference in retention and quality of care rendered by the participants (Burton, 2011). Measurement data that indicate outcomes can be a useful tool in determining whether or not a program should continue. Administrators as well as employees are emotionally and cognitively impressed by measures to find solutions when numbers are perceived as unacceptable. (Cebul, 2011).

Health care administrators reviewing performance measures are better able to adjust care, share success, and probe for the causes for less than ideal care. All these activities contribute to improved patient care outcomes. Measure results are often shared with boards of trustees, employees, and consumers who, in turn, use the information to make choices, ask questions, and, ultimately, will advocate for the health care facility. Facilities use the data to market their services. External regulatory entities disseminate and rate outcomes to educate consumers. Likewise, governmental third-party payers determine reimbursement rates for a particular condition or diagnosis. Insurance companies, in turn, use facility-specific data as a preassessment for reimbursement rates, bonuses, or as condition for nonpayment.

The study of nurses' transition-to-practice concentrates on measuring both the process and the structure of practice. The analysis of the care processes reveals effectiveness of patient care protocols. Data further indicate whether or not an action was completed. For example:

- Determining of new employees complete a mentored orientation and a thorough competence assessment before caring for their own caseload.
- Assessing if new nurse employees are coached through a yearlong residency.

Process measures focus on outcomes as well as actions. Residencies are measured by the number and kinds of medication errors, patient satisfaction levels, and employee retention rates. The 15 nursing-sensitive indicators were designed to determine the effectiveness of an employee. The number of new employees on committees and even the number of phone calls to physicians during the night shift can serve as measures for structure outcomes (Graben, 2008).

Joseph Higgins, a rural nurse informaticist in Idaho, invented and tested a dashboard tool to keep nurses informed of personal pain assessment practices. The hospital's goal was to ensure that patients were reassessed for pain after receiving a *pro re nata* (PRN) medication in a timely fashion. The tool gathers information from nurse charting in the electronic health record. The data are converted into a graphic display for easy analysis. Nurse managers use the tool to compare the time and frequencies when patients are reassessed. The tool informed individual nurses, units, the hospital, and other interested parties of practice patterns. The data gathered become part of performance evaluations for individual nurses, hospital units, and the facility as a whole.

Nursing-sensitive indicators such as falls could be evaluated using root-cause analysis procedures to determine the date, time, and location of the event, patient diagnosis and status, staffing mix, and educational level of staff (Needleman et al., 2001). Using root cause analysis, a system can be analyzed thoroughly for opportunities to improve performance and patient outcomes. When video is combined with data, a more sensitive performance story can be told. For instance, a patient fall from a wheelchair while waiting for an x-ray can be analyzed as a number-1 fall, a performance deficit-lack of prevention, or as a facility design issue-long halls preventing visual monitoring. Data depend on the analyzer's motivations and goals, hence the need for standardized measures and standards. For example, the goal of one hospital was to conduct an initial discharge planning interview within 24 hours of a patient's admission to the facility. Monitoring technology collected the time social workers and nurses reported interviewing new admits about their initial discharge issues. Barriers were identified. Staffing duties were altered to meet the desired outcome. The various specialty units competed with each other to be the first and most successful in achieving the outcome. Likewise, nurse managers learned new care strategies from each other. Ultimately, in that acute care facility, the patients benefited and nurses were held accountable for achieving the goal of early-discharge planning.

Measurement can reveal unknown issues. For instance, a comparison of hospital performance in the care of myocardial infarction (Curry et al., 2011) indicates that protocols are not enough to save lives as a "strong organizational culture" was associated with variances in death rates of as much as 9.5 percentage points. Another example is described in Chapter 19. The study of rural nurse preferences and organizational issues identified violence against nurses was identified as a retention issue. Although findings were unexpected, a national view indicates nurses are three times as likely to experience violence as other professions (Raines, 2011) In fact, some states and many health care facilities mandate violence protection education programs. Even with educational intervention, there is little change in the number of violent incidents against nurses indicating that new approaches are still needed. The National Institute of Occupational Safety (NIOSH) provides an online best-practices course to train health care workers in violence prevention (CDC, 2004). Administrators of rural health care facilities may want to examine violence from a communication and social networking viewpoint to prevent incidents or mediate events (American Nurses Association, 2011).

Studying nursing practice in relation to patient outcomes can offer deferent factors with which to solve problems. Traditionally, nurses measured the individuals' professional activities (Mullenbach, 2010). However, the focus on patient outcomes can provide additional insights by measuring health status improvements, time, functional abilities, quality of life, and care costs. Facility data are then compared with standards of excellence as established by the NQF. Using this information, policy developers and decision makers can tailor evidence-based protocols for improving delivery and efficiency of care.

Maas, Johnson, and Morehead (1996) coined the phrase "nursing-sensitive indicators" to reflect patient outcomes that are affected by nursing practice. Needdleman (2002) notes that most outcome research stresses on the negative impact that nursing has on patient care. Several nursing processes are rarely measured: specifically, communication, collaboration, documentation, and teamwork, as these concepts and behaviors lack a standard definition and cannot be readily isolated in administrative databases. Another challenge of measurement is the lack of data codes for individual nursing performance measures such as assessment, therapeutic communication, and collaboration. If a nursing activity is not coded or recorded, recorders are not aware that the activity has taken place; therefore, the concept cannot be measured or valued.

Associated with data input, information systems do not have the capability to extrapolate data on nurses' contribution to adverse effects like surgical wound infection or septicemia, or for that matter, positive outcomes, such as prevention of an infection. Most technology monitoring tools are not yet sensitive to nursing-centered actions because as a result of lack of standardization and their resulting payment codes, there are few national nursing-sensitive indicators. Lack of a core set of nursing measures, along with variability in risk adjustment and indicator unit of analysis, hinders nurses from becoming accountable for the care they provide to patients. Health care facilities in rural settings find that lack of standardization is compounded by lack of information technology needed to ask relevant questions and obtain meaningful answers. Another issue for hospitals with the designation of critical access is associated with measuring the practices of small facilities. Critical access hospitals serve different purposes, stress another purpose with different goals, employ different strategies, and measure outcomes with different tools than larger urban-based tertiary care facilities. The question, therefore, is: How can standards of practice that are determined for a 300-bed facility be implemented in a 15-bed facility in a more remote and sparsely populated region?

Philosophically, rural and urban differences related to nurse staffing patterns and viewing quality indicators comprehensively, rather than analyzing a single indicator in isolation. Staffing within a large facility with many resources and variables cannot be viewed in the same manner as a very small facility that operates with minimal staff and fewer technological resources. Additionally, outcome measures are retrospective surveillance approaches at a macroscopic level. In other words, information systems are not designed to measure one unit's activities or a single individual's performance. Eventually, these issues will be addressed as nurse informaticists develop programs that are designed to use data for remedial education and performance evaluations, as well as patient safety systems. Analysis of data that demonstrates how nursing activities positively impact on patient care outcomes will have even greater impact on quality of care than simply measuring the influence of adverse events. See Chapter 18 focusing on appreciative inquiry for additional information related to this topic.

Rural-specific quality data are the most effective method to dispel the misperception of residents in small rural communities that "bigger is better." Outcome information particular to local institutions is key to marketing the benefits of local health care. Rural residents will seek health care where they believe the best quality is found. Patients travel great distances to obtain services at urban centers if there is a perception of poor local outcomes. Hospitals that cannot prove their quality of care have low retention rates of nurses and physicians. In turn, lack of quality health care provides a deterrent to economic sustainability and community expansion. Ascertaining and measuring quality are critical for the survival of small rural health care facilities. "The science of measuring healthcare performance has made enormous progress over the last decade, and it continues to evolve. The high stakes demand ... collective perseverance. Measures represent a critical component in the national endeavor to assure all patients of appropriate and high-quality care" (National Quality Forum, 2009).

According to Buckley, Joyce, Garcia, Jordan, and Scher (2010) undergraduate nurses are not taught adequate information about quality improvement mechanisms to effectively improve patient care or nursing care. Therefore, new graduates need to be taught about this topic at the bedside; the same holds true for middle-management nurse leaders (Bushy, 1991). Along with lack of knowledge about the process, rural quality improvement is hampered by insufficient personnel to monitor, collect, and analyze data; insufficient funds to purchase useful and appropriate health information technology, coupled with interprofessional role overloads and conflicts, a small/low volume sample size, lack of relevant rural quality standards, and confidentiality issues associated with small-town social structures (Pagan-Sutton, Silver, & Gupta, 2009). Nevertheless, there are recommended solutions for rural quality improvement programs, including:

- Making use of the resources found in 53 quality improvement organizations. The federally contracted agencies assist rural facilities to improve performance on clinical process measures, promote the implementation and use of health information technology, and advance organizational safety culture.
- Networking and building rural partnerships or accessing existing collaborations can save money while building up resources (Kemp, 2002). Collaborative partnerships with rural hospitals or providers could include entities such as Medicare Peer Review Organizations/Quality Improvement Organizations (PRO/QIO), a state office of rural health, a state department of health, or a state hospital association. Collaborating on quality projects can standardize goals and methodologies while increasing organizational power (Cebul, Rebitzer, Taylor, & Votruba, 2008).
- Surviving involves incremental advances by a small health care facility (Nebraska Office of Rural Health, 2009). Urban advances in quality improvement have been relatively fast associated with funding mandates based on quality. Rural communities initially were exempt and thus did not begin publishing quality outcomes for several years. The financial drive to prove quality outcomes will hasten the rate of improvements.
- Sharing resources encourage effective communication, skill sharing, training, coaching, and empowerment methods. Resources could include the integration of computer systems, statisticians, research designers, publications, and interfacility quality studies.

Health care organizations spend significant time and resources on nurse recruitment, orientation, and training. Yet, new nurse graduates account for more than half of the turnover rate in some hospitals according to a study published in 2007 by Johns Hopkins University School of Nursing. Reducing turnover rates requires use of quality improvement practices (Rhéaume, Clément, & Lebel, 2010). Retention and nurse turnover are studied at the macrolevel in terms of a nursing shortage; and, at a microlevel in terms of an individual nurse and institution (National Advisory Council on Nurse Education and Practice, 2010). The study of new nurse graduates, supportive programs for newly hired nurses, and organizational systems has been ongoing for decades (Ulrich 2010). The quality improvement approach ties nurses' activities to health care outcomes. Eventually, when the body of work about a topic is of sufficient size, standards and even legislation may change. For instance, California introduced regulations on minimum staffing levels after studies indicated adequate staffing saved lives (Aiken, Clarke, Sloane, Lake, & Cheney, 2009; Applebaum, Fowler, Fiedler, Osinubi, & Robson, 2010; Perrine, 2009; Van Bogaert, Meulemans, Clarke, Vermeyen, & Van de Heyning, 2009; Van den Heede et al., 2009). Recent studies indicate that increased staffing reduces patient mortality rates (Horsham, 2010).

In summary, this chapter focuses on evaluation approaches to assess the process and outcomes of transition-to-practice programs. Evidence (data) is essential to refine instructional strategies and clinical experiences, substantiate cost–benefit ratios, determine the impact on quality and safety as well as staff recruitment, retention, and productivity.

REFERENCES

Aiken, L. H., Clarke, S. P., Sloane, D. M., Lake, E. T., & Cheney, T. (2009). Effects of hospital care environment on patient mortality and nurse outcomes. *Journal of Nursing Administration*, 38(5), 223–229.

American Nurses Association. (2011). *Workplace violence*. Retrieved Mary 16, 2011 from http://www.nursingworld.org/MainMenuCategories/ANAPoliticalPower/State/StateLegislativeAgenda/WorkplaceViolence.aspx

Applebaum, D., Fowler, S., Fiedler, N., Osinubi, O., & Robson, M. (2010). The impact of environmental factors on nursing stress, job satisfaction, and turnover intention. *Journal of Nursing Administration*, 40(7), 323–328.

Buck, C. (n.d.). *Application of six sigma to reduce medical errors*. Retrieved 9/45/2011 from http://asq.org/healthcar esixsigma/pdf/reduce_medical_errors.pdf

Buckley, J. D., Joyce, B., Garcia, A. J., Jordan, J., & Scher, E. (2010). Linking residency training effectiveness to clinical outcomes: A quality improvement approach. *Joint Commission Journal on Quality and Patient Safety*, 36(5), 203–208.

Burton, M. (2011). Revisioning transition-to-practice issues. *Kentucky Nurse*, 59(1), 1.

Bushy, A. (1991). Quality assurance in rural hospitals. *Journal of Nursing Administration*, 21(10), 34–39.

Campbell-Heider, N. (1998). Collaboration and independent practice: Ongoing issues for nursing. *Nursing World*, 3(5). Retrieved 9/4/2011 from http://nursingworld.org/DocumentVault/NTI/Vol3No5May1998.aspx

Cebul, R. D. (2011). *The difference a good measure can make*. Retrieved January 2011 from http://www.qualityforum.org/Measuring_Performance/ABCs/The_Difference_a_Good_Measure_Can_Make.aspx)

Cebul, R. D., Rebitzer, J. B., Taylor, L. J., & Votruba, M. E. (2008). Organizational fragmentation and care quality in the U.S. health care system. *Journal of Economic Perspectives*, 22(4), 93–113. Also in NBER Working Paper Series. Working paper 14212. http://www.nber.org/papers/w14212.

Center for Disease Control. (2004). *Workplace violence prevention strategies and research needs.* National Institute of Occupational Safety. Retrieved March 2011 from http://www.cdc.gov/niosh/docs/2006-144/pdfs/2006-144.pdf

Curry, L. A., Spatz, E., Cherlin, E., Thompson, J. W., Berg, D., Ting, H. H., Decker, C., Krumholz, H. M., & Bradley, E. H. (2011). What distinguishes top performing hospitals in acute myocardial infarction mortality rates? *Annals of Internal Medicine, 154*(6), 384–390.

Graben, M. (2008). *Lean hospitals.* www.superfactory.com.

Horsham (2010). California's mandated staff ratios reduce mortality. *Nursing, 40*(6), 21.

Institute of Medicine. (2001). *Crossing the quality chasm: A new health system for the 21st century.* Institute of Medicine. Washington, DC: National Academy Press.

Institute of Medicine Report: To err is human: Building a safer health system. (1999). Washington, DC: National Academies Press.

Kanai-Pak, M., Aiken, L. H., Sloane, D. M., & Poghosyan, L. (2008). Poor work environments and nurse inexperience are associated with burnout, job dissatisfaction and quality deficits in Japanese hospitals. *Journal of Clinical Nursing, 17*(24), 3324–3329. doi: 10.1111/j.1365-2702.2008.02639.x

Kemp, K. (2002). *Networking for rural health: Quality improvement in rural hospitals: How networking can help.* Academy for Health Services Research and Health Policy.

Kohn, L. T., Corrigan, J. M., & Donaldson, M. S. (2000). *To err is human: Building a safer health system.* A report of the Committee on Quality of Health Care in America. Institute of Medicine. Washington, DC: National Academy Press.

Maas, M., Johnson, M., & Moorehead, S. (1996). Classifying nursing-sensitive patient outcomes. *Journal of Nursing Scholarship, 28*(4), 295–301.

Montalvo, I. (2007). The national database of nursing quality indicators TM (NDNQI®). *OJIN: The Online Journal of Issues in Nursing, 12*(3), Manuscript 2. doi: 10.3912/OJIN.Vol12No03Man02)

Mullenbach, K. F. (2010). Senior nursing students' perspectives on the recruitment and retention of medical-surgical nurses. *Medsurg Nursing, 19*(6), 341–344.

National Advisory Council on Nurse Education and Practice. (2010). *Addressing new challenges facing nursing education: Solutions for a transforming healthcare environment.* http://bhpr.hrsa.gov/nursing/NACNEP/reports/eighth.pdf

National Quality Forum. (2004). *National voluntary consensus standards for nursing-sensitive care: An initial performance measure set.* http://www.qualityforum.org/Projects/n-r/Nursing-Sensitive_Care_Initial_Measures/Nursing_Sensitive_Care__Initial_Measures.aspx

National Quality Forum. (2008). Health Information Technology Expert Panel Report: Recommended Common Data Types and Prioritized Performance Measures for Electronic Healthcare Information Systems.

National Quality Forum. (2009). *How do we know? We measure.* Retrieved April 10, 2011 from http://www.qualityforum.org/Measuring_Performance/ABCs_of_Measurement.aspx

Nebraska Office of Rural Health. (2009). *A roadmap for improving the quality of care in CAHs: Recommendations from the April 15 Planning Summit.* https://www.ruralcenter.org/tasc/resources/roadmap-improving-quality-care-critical-access-hospitals

Needleman, J., Buerhaus, P. I., Mattke, S., Stewart, M., & Zelebinsky, K. (2001). *Nurse staffing and patient outcomes in hospitals.* Harvard School of Public Health. Retrieved from at http://bhpr.hrsa.gov/dn/staffstudy.htm

Needleman, J., Buerhaus, P., Mattke, S. et al. (2002). Nurse staffing levels and the quality of care in hospitals. *New England Journal of Medicine, 346*(22), 1715–1722.

Pagan-Sutton, P., Silver, L., & Gupta, J. (2009). *Achieving success in QIO and rural hospital partnerships.* Retrieved February 25, 2009 from http://www.norc.org/NR/rdonlyres/93069917-D956-4E87-8A2E-8EC1F3ABC287/0/WalshQIORevised ReportFeb09_final.pdf

Perrine, J. L. (2009). Strategies to boost RN retention. *Nursing Management, 40*(4), 20–22. doi: 10.1097/01.NUMA.0000349685.24165.21

Raines, L. (2011). *Hospitals have a higher rate of workplace violence.* A.J.C. Retrieved March 10, 2011 from http://www.ajc.com/jobs/hospitals-have-a-higher-848571.html?sms_ss=email&at_xt=4d67d52324ed86e7%2C0

Rhéaume, A., Clément, L., & Lebel, N. (2010). Understanding intention to leave amongst new graduate Canadian nurses: A repeated cross sectional survey. *International Journal of Nursing Studies, 48*(4), 490–500.

Savitz, L. A., Jones, C. B., & Bernard, S. (2005). Quality indicators sensitive to nurse staffing in acute care settings. *Advances in Patient Safety, 4.* Retrieved 9/4/2011 from http://www.ahrq.gov/downloads/pub/advances/vol4/Savitz.pdf

Ulrich, B., Krozek, C., Early, S., Ashlock, C. H., Africa, L. M., & Carman, M. L. (2010). Improving retention, confidence, and competence of new graduate nurses: Results from a 10-year longitudinal database. *Nurse Economics, 28*(6), 363–376.

Van Bogaert, P., Meulemans, H., Clarke, S., Vermeyen, K., & Van de Heyning, P. (2009). Hospital nurse practice environment, burnout, job outcomes and quality of care: Test of a structural equation model. *Journal of Advanced Nursing, 65*(10), 2175–2185. doi: 10.1111/j.1365-2648.2009.05082.x

Van den Heede, K., Sermeus, W., Diya, L., Clarke, S. P., Lesaffre, E., Vleugels, A. et al. (2009). Nurse staffing and patient outcomes in Belgian acute hospitals: Cross-sectional analysis of administrative data. *International Journal of Nursing Studies, 46*(7), 928–939.

27

Specialty Topics: Genetics, Genomics, and Informatics in Rural Nursing

Christine F. Mladenka and Deana L. Molinari

Regardless of the practice setting, be it a rural or an urban insti-
tution, nurses need to have an understanding of specialty topics
such as genetics, genomics, and informatics when implementing
patient care. This chapter highlights essential information for
rural bedside care, and includes web resources for developing
transition-to-practice programs.

Every transition-to-practice initiative contains both core content and threaded concepts. Core content pertains to the knowledge needed for patient care whereas threaded concepts pertain to the knowledge needed to practice the nursing role. Examples of core classes are crisis assessment and management whereas examples of threads include clinical reasoning, genetics, and informatics. Clinical reasoning is covered elsewhere in the text. Informatics, genetics, and genomics were recognized more recently as basic nursing competencies.

The American Association of Colleges of Nursing (AACN) included genetics and genomics throughout the revised *Essentials of Baccalaureate Education for Professional Nursing Practice in 2008.* Historically, very little genetics and genomics information were included in formal nursing education. As more genetic and genomic discoveries impact on patient care, professional nurses in all areas of health care should be prepared to address patient questions, concerns, and issues regarding genetic risk, susceptibility, and the complexities of genetic testing and interpretation (Consensus Panel on Genetic/Genomic Nursing Competencies, 2009). According to the Consensus Panel (2009), present-day health care requires competent nursing practice to meet six responsibilities that include the incorporation of genetic and genomic content and skills.

The websites for the International Society of Nurses in Genetics (ISONG) (www.isong.org), the National Coalition for Health Professional Education in Genetics (NCHPEG) (www.nchpeg.org), and the Genetics Education Program for Nurses (http://www.cincinnati-childrens.org/ed/clinical/gpnf/default.htm) provide educational opportunities on the impact of genetics and genomic on care standards and on patient health (International Society of Nurses in Genetics (ISONG), 2010b). Moreover, many professional nursing organizations include educational opportunities on genetic and genomic content in their annual conferences. Rural nurses manage several factors affecting professional genetic/genomic education and services. Accessibility is impacted by financial constraints, distance, acceptance of specialty services, and reluctance to travel to an urban community where specialty services are available (Bushy, n.d.).

Genetic services are specialty services that are not typically available to rural patients. Moreover, formal genetic education is often lacking. Therefore, patient needs may go unmet. The Institute of Medicine (IOM, 2009) identified similar access barriers in smaller communities that include lack of a consistent definition of genetic services, provider knowledge and training deficiencies, inadequate insurance coverage, patient communication or value issues, and geographic disparities. The IOM recommends that these barriers be addressed to ensure that all individuals have access to genetic counseling, testing, and personal information so that all have the opportunity to make personal health care decisions (IOM, 2009).

The ISONG is an international nursing specialty organization "dedicated to fostering the scientific and professional growth of nurses in human genetics and genomics worldwide" (ISONG, 2010a). Through newsletter communication, annual conferences, and credentialing efforts, ISONG promotes the role of nursing in providing genetic health care to meet individual, family, community, and population needs. Registered nurses and advance practice nurses can earn certification as specialists in genetics through the Genetic Nursing Credentialing Commission (GNCC) in cooperation with ISONG (GNCC, 2007). Benefits of the certification for nurses and advance practice nurses include recognition of competence and clinical expertise to address genetic health needs based on the evidence of meeting standards set by ISONG and American Nurses Association (ANA) (GNCC, 2007; ISONG, 2006, 2010b).

The NCHPEG is a national organization whose mission is "to promote health professional education and access to information about advances in human genetics to improve the health care of the nation" (National Coalition for Health Professional Education in Genetics (NCHPEG), 2010b). Nursing is represented by ANA, Sigma Theta Tau, and six other nursing organizations and plays an important role in this effort.

Both ISONG and NCHPEG support basic core competencies that include each professional should (a) examine one's competence of practice on a regular basis, identifying areas of strength and those in need of professional development related to genetics and genomics; (b) understand that genomic information can have social and psychological implications for individuals and families; and (c) know when and how to provide referrals for individuals and families to genetic and genomic professional services (Consensus Panel on Genetic/Genomic Nursing Competencies, 2009; NCHPEG, 2007). As in the case of other nursing specialties, the professional nurse who practices in a rural setting needs to recognize his or her limitations in genetics/genomics, assist the patient and their family, understand and cope with the implications of genetic/genomic impacts on their health, and know when, where, and how to refer patients and their families to genetic professional services proximal to their community. The Consensus Panel on Genetic/Genomic Nursing Competencies (2009) adds other essential competencies for the professional nurse delineated into four categories.

INFORMATICS

Informatics was defined by the ANA in 1994 as a combination of nursing, computer, and information science "for identifying, collecting, processing, and managing data and information to support nursing practice, administration, education, research, and expansion of nursing knowledge (Staggers & Thompson, 2002). It supports the practice of all nursing specialties, in all sites and settings, whether at the basic or advanced level. The practice includes the development of applications, tools, processes, and structures that assist nurses with the management of data in taking care of patients or in supporting their practice of nursing."

A revised definition focused on nursing control rather than technology. "Nursing informatics is a specialty that integrates nursing science, computer science, and information science to manage and communicate data, information, and knowledge in nursing practice. Nursing informatics facilitates the integration of data, information, and knowledge to support patients, nurses, and other providers in their decision making in all roles and settings. This support is accomplished through the use of information structures, information processes, and information technology."

The Technology Informatics Guiding Educational Reform (TIGER) group conducted a research study and developed competencies for basic computer skills, information management, and information literacy. A list of 100 workforce competencies can be found at http://tigercompetencies.pbworks.com/w/page/22247287/FrontPage. The purpose of the list is to provide understanding of the skills, knowledge, and attitudes for entry-level and advanced practice (Staggers, Gassert, & Curran, 2002). Six articles were found useful for operationalizing definitions and measuring informatics competence (Carter-Templeton, Patterson, & Russell, 2009).

Online certificate programs and master's degree programs are available in relation to the complex topic. Advanced understanding in informatics is a pressing need for today's nursing workforce in research, practice, administration, and education disciplines (Staggers & Lasome, 2005). Every role requires basic skills; therefore, specific content and skills are required for graduation from academic programs (Hassett, 2006). The TIGER group also developed competencies for nurse educators (The Technology Informatics Guiding Educational Reform Group, 2009). A recent National League for Nursing survey revealed a lack of educator understanding of the topic.

Curriculum topics may include:

- Electronic literature searches for evidence-based practice.
- Basic computer skills: software, networks, types, and application to nursing care.
- Information systems: definitions, types, bedside practice applications.
- Electronic health records, information sharing, discharge planning, and community networks.
- Confidentiality and security issues.
- Expert systems and artificial intelligence (AI).
- Bioethical issues and legal responsibilities.
- Health literacy and health promotion.
- Social and professional networking.
- Technology as critical thinking structure.
- Media as change medium.
- Lifelong learning and specialization.

In summary, professional nurses need to consider and incorporate the role of genetics, genomics, and informatics in every aspect of practice wherever they work and provide quality patient care. See Table 27.1 for online resources regarding genetic and genomic

TABLE 27.1
Genetic/Genomic Internet Resources

	ACTIVE AS OF JANUARY 2011
DNA Interactive	http://www.dnai.org/
Genetic Alliance	http://www.geneticalliance.org/
Genetests	http://www.ncbi.nlm.nih.gov/ sites/GeneTests/
Genetics Home Reference, U.S. National Library of Medicine	http://ghr.nlm.nih.gov/
International Society of Nurses in Genetics	http://www.isong.org/
National Coalition for Health Professional Education in Genetics	http://www.nchpeg.org/
National Human Genome Research Institute (NHGRI)	http://www.genome.gov/
National Newborn Screening and Genetics Resource Center	http://genes-r-us.uthscsa.edu/
U.S. Department of Energy Genomic Websites	http://genomics.energy.gov/
University of Utah—Genetic Science Learning Center	http://learn.genetics.utah.edu/

information. Competencies for new graduates measure the ability to interview families about genetic concerns, the ability to recognize pharmacological issues, and the importance of patient-centered care related to individual and ethnic genetics. Informatics is another way of saying information management. The TIGER group documents competencies for both instructors and nurses. Both specialty topics are threaded through all patient safety and quality care concepts.

REFERENCES

American Association of Colleges of Nursing (AACN). (2008). *The essentials of baccalaureate education for professional nursing practice.* Retrieved from http://www.aacn.nche.edu/education/pdf/BaccEssentials08.pdf

American Nurses Association. (1994). *The scope of practice for nursing informatics.* Washington, DC: ANA. Publication NP-907.5M 5/94.

Bushy, A. (n.d.). Rural nursing: Practice and issues. *American Nurses Association Continuing Education Program.* Retrieved from http://www.nursingworld.org/mods/mod700/rurlfull.htm

Carter-Templeton, H., Patterson, R., & Russell, C. (2009). An analysis of published nursing informatics competencies. *Student Health Technology and Informatics, 146,* 540–545.

Consensus Panel on Genetic/Genomic Nursing Competencies. (2009). *Essentials of genetic and genomic nursing: Competencies, curricula guidelines, and outcome indicators* (2nd ed.). Silver Spring, MD: American Nurses Association.

Genetic Nursing Credentialing Commission (GNCC). (2007). Retrieved from http://www.geneticnurse.org/

Hassett, M. (2006). Case study: Factors in defining the nurse informatics specialist role. *Journal of Healthcare Information Management, 20*(2), 30–35.

Institute of Medicine (IOM). (2009). *Innovations in service delivery in the age of genomics. Workshop summary.* Washington, DC: National Academies Press.

International Society of Nurses in Genetics (ISONG). (2006). *Genetics/genomics nursing: Scope and standards of practice.* Silver Spring, MD: American Nurses Association.

International Society of Nurses in Genetics (ISONG). (2010a). *Our vision.* Retrieved from http://www.isong.org/ISONG_about.php

International Society of Nurses in Genetics (ISONG). (2010b). *Professional practice.* Retrieved from http://www.isong.org/ISONG_professional_practice.php

National Coalition for Health Professional Education in Genetics (NCHPEG). (2007). *Core competencies for all health care professionals.* Retrieved from http://www.nchpeg.org/index.php?option=com_content&view=article&id=94&Itemid=8

National Coalition for Health Professional Education in Genetics (NCHPEG). (2010b). *Mission statement.* Retrieved from http://www.nchpeg.org/index.php?option=com_content&view=article&id=83&Itemid=57

Staggers, N., Gassert, C., & Curran, C. (2002). A Delphi study to determine informatics competencies for nurses at four levels of practice. *Nursing Research, 51*(6), 383–390.

Staggers, N., & Lasome, C. (2005). RN. CIO: An executive informatics career. *CIN: Computers, Informatics, Nursing, 23*(4), 201–206.

Staggers, N., & Thompson, C. B. (2002). The evolution of definitions for nursing informatics: A critical analysis and revised definition. *American Medical Informatics Association, 9*(3), 255–261. doi: 10.1197/jamia.M0946. Retrieved from http://www.ncbi.nlm.nih.gov/pmc/articles/PMC344585/

The Technology Informatics Guiding Educational Reform Group. (2009). *TIGER Informatics Competencies Collaborative (TICC).* Final Report Retrieved from: http://tigercompetencies.pbworks.com/f/TICC_Final.pdf

Appendix A

The Perceptive, Affective, Cognitive Critical Thinking Model

Deana L. Molinari

Critical Thinking Model

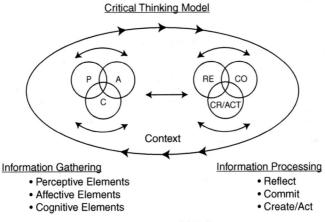

Information Gathering
- Perceptive Elements
- Affective Elements
- Cognitive Elements

Information Processing
- Reflect
- Commit
- Create/Act

External and Internal Processes

Perceptive, Affective, and Cognitive Critical Thinking Model by Molinari, Abbeglanb and Mills, 1997

CRITICAL THINKING MATRIX				
DATA DIMENSION:: SOURCE	SELF	CLIENT	STAKEHOLDERS	CONTEXT
Perceived Goals				
Information Gathering				
Contextual Elements				
Perceptive Elements				

(Continued)

CRITICAL THINKING MATRIX				
DATA DIMENSION:: SOURCE	SELF	CLIENT	STAKEHOLDERS	CONTEXT
Affective Elements				
Cognitive Elements				
Information Processing				
Reflection				
Info Quality/Quantity				
Risk of Error Analysis				
Restraining/Driving Forces				
Integrates/Synthesizes				
Commitments				
Thinking/Practice Frameworks				
Hypotheses				
Resources				
Evidential Elements				
Create/Act				
Decision Evaluation Plan				
Communicates (oral/written)				

CRITICAL THINKING SUMMARY AND MODEL

The Perceptive, Affective, Cognitive Model of Critical Thinking describes the process of gathering and processing information for reflective decision making. This process is enables clinical reasoning. Clinical reasoning is the purpose for critical thinking and not the same task. The information gathered and processed is applied to the reasoning process for practice decisions. Critical thinking processes occur to some degree in all meaningful choices.

The model characterizes thinking as a nonlinear process of information gathering and processing impacted by both an individual's internal and external context. Information-gathering processes require assessing internal perceptive, affective, and cognitive elements as well as external perceptive, affective, and cognitive elements. There are many information repositories for these elements. All thinking is situational so the context contains important information. Individuals like the patient, family, caregivers, health providers, can powerfully impact the context. Organizational, professional, science, community, evidence, and standards all contain information important to the current situation. Other information such as geographical location, time, amount of health care resources, values, health status, and expectations also impact thinking.

Nurses are encouraged to perform quick self-assessments of each information repository for three types of information.

Perceptive elements refer to information that can be gathered from ones senses. A self-assessment is for the purpose of discovering how prepared one is to perform the thinking task and to reveal bias. Physical conditions like low blood sugar, full bladder, or aching back can be distracting and require control before assessing the environment. Assessments of patients, families, care providers, and organizations are also needed. If someone is unable to communicate or is uncomfortable, the information provided will be of less quality than needed for quality care.

At times organizations', governments', and professions' perceptions can impact decision making. Perception of insufficient funds, personnel, authority, or other resource is felt for a certain situation, the care decision will be different than when adequate resources are perceived.

Affective elements include an individual's/group's/organization's/community's emotional status, emotional history, bias, values, emotional management habits, and beliefs about emotional issues. Nurses commonly assess patients and others for these elements. Nurses less frequently assess themselves for emotional elements that may impact decision making.

Each of these processes contains thinking processes which are necessary for a quality outcome. A simple measuring device enables a facilitator to identify strengths and weaknesses in the information observation and management.

Common terms and measurement mean all participants understand what the concept means. Although clinical reasoning models are also described, outcomes are measured using practice competencies. Patient-centered care, teamwork and collaboration, evidence-based practice, quality improvement, safety, and informatics are the practice competencies measured.

Appendix B

Rural Nurse Role Competencies
Adapted by Idaho State University School of Nursing

Rural Nurse Residents are expected to achieve the competencies described in this document. The competencies are based on the Rural Competencies by Professional Development Centre & Nova Scotia Department of Health, rural nursing literature, standards of practice, national standards, consultation with rural nurse experts, and directors of nursing.

The competencies are arranged under five general areas (Critical Thinking, Clinical Practice, Relationship Centered Practice, Professionalism and Leadership). The expected Performance Criteria and Behavioral Indicators have been identified for learners.

*The use of the term **client** throughout this document can include the **patient, family, groups, populations or entire communities**.*

Nurse supervisors use the document to plan education and evaluate performance at the one year employment anniversary.

Total Score:_____
Comments
Summary: _____

_____
_____
_____
_____
_____
_____
_____
_____
_____
_____
_____

CRITICAL THINKING AND CLINICAL REASONING

The nurse analyzes, synthesizes and evaluates knowledge for the practice of rural nursing

COMPETENCIES	PERFORMANCE CRITERIA	BEHAVIORAL INDICATORS
1. Acquires the knowledge necessary for practice	Applies critical thinking to clinical reasoning challenges	▓ Meets established assessment criteria for examinations and assignments Acceptable _____ Unacceptable _____ Comments:
2. Participates in activities that contribute to an understanding utilization of research in practice	Applies an awareness of the relationships between research/evidence/best practices to quality decision making	▓ Questions evidence on which rural nursing practice is based ▓ Identifies areas of rural nursing clinical practice requiring further clarification ▓ Performs information searches on the PDA without assistance ▓ Reflects upon literature in relation to clinical practice ▓ Relates research findings to rural practice ▓ Utilizes evidence daily in the performance of duties ▓ Questions patient care orders and seeks information to verify best practice Acceptable _____ Unacceptable _____ Comments:
3. Employs critical thinking models to guide professional decision making	▓ Assesses issues/ situations ▓ Assesses personal opinions, knowledge, assumptions ▓ Identifies alternative actions/choices and their potential outcomes based on available information ▓ Selects optimal actions/ choices ▓ Evaluates outcomes	▓ Gathers all relevant information (including internal assessments of capability, feelings, bias) and reflects before making decisions – Explores personal values/assumptions and reflect on the influence on client care (experience/history, culture, spiritual, client/family matters) – Explores personal expectations of the nurse's role and its relationship to client, family, team, community in client care ▓ Analyzes situations ▓ Identifies issues ▓ Lists alternatives ▓ Sets priorities for actions and choices ▓ Utilizes the expertise of an inter professional team ▓ Makes decisions ▓ Communicates rationale ▓ Envisions outcomes and compares to expected results

4. Reflects on the impact personal actions have on client outcomes

- Evaluates the effectiveness of decision making
- Identifies other courses of action where appropriate
- Questions decisions and usual hospital practices
- Can identify literature and resources to support decision making (e.g., quality improvement, EBP)

Acceptable _____ Unacceptable _____
Comments:

Assesses events/experiences in one's own practice

- Describes the experience, event
- Examines the event in detail
- Describes feelings associated with the event
- Identifies and applies resources needed to nourish self

Acceptable _____ Unacceptable _____
Comments:

Reflects on the event/experience

- Compares the event/experience to past experiences and knowledge
- Identifies new knowledge gained through the experience
- Identifies strengths and areas of improvement

Acceptable _____ Unacceptable _____
Comments:

Develops a plan to improve one's own practice

- Identifies internal and external resources to meet needs
- Identifies barriers to changing practice
- With help of preceptor/colleagues, seeks solutions to barriers in achieving goals

Acceptable _____ Unacceptable _____
Comments:

Evaluates the results of one's reflections

- Identifies the impact that reflection has on improving one's practice and decision making
- Utilizes knowledge and former experiences in rural nursing practice to guide future practice

Acceptable _____ Unacceptable _____
Comments:

CLINICAL PRACTICE

The nurse provides competent and safe nursing care that is responsive to changing situations of clients in the rural setting

COMPETENCIES	PERFORMANCE CRITERIA	BEHAVIORAL INDICATORS
1. Demonstrates clinical reasoning based on family/patient preferences, evidence, professional and organizational policies	Applies professional development content to the work place	▦ Demonstrates an understanding of normal health states across the lifespan ▦ Demonstrates an understanding of common health problems across the lifespan ▦ Demonstrates knowledge of risk factors based on developmental stage ▦ Shares information and ideas relevant to clinical experiences with preceptor/colleagues ▦ Explains the rationale for nursing actions ▦ Defines common, urgent, and emergent health problems seen in a rural healthcare setting ▦ Demonstrates knowledge of commonly used medications and dosages across the lifespan ▦ Seeks out and uses patient/families preferences ▦ Bases care planning and interventions on for interventions, education and support Acceptable _____ Unacceptable_____ Comments:
	Engages in evidence-based practice	▦ Uses research, literature and experts as resources to guide rural clinical practice ▦ Demonstrates knowledge of local or external human and literary resources Acceptable _____ Unacceptable_____ Comments:
	Self reflects on clinical experiences	▦ Compares current experience to past knowledge ▦ Identifies impact one's own practice and the care received by the team has on client outcomes ▦ Identifies ways of changing practice Acceptable _____ Unacceptable_____ Comments:

2. Completes a comprehensive client health assessment	▦ Identifies need for more information based on client assessment, laboratory data, etc.
Makes clinical decisions within a collaborative team for positive client outcomes	▦ Utilizes community resources to gather information (e.g., police, EMS, family, caregivers, community witnesses to events)
	▦ Determines what data is relevant (e.g., past history, lab data, diagnostic tests)
	▦ Able to set priorities for client care based on client data, workload and available resources
	▦ Questions information gathered
	▦ Able to communicate verbally and in writing pertinent history and physical assessment findings to validate decision making
	▦ Communicates appropriately with leadership gradients
	▦ Communicates clearly and completely during handoffs and transitions
	Acceptable _____ Unacceptable _____
	Comments:
Continued: Completes a comprehensive client health assessment	▦ Discusses health history including medications with client or caregiver
Collects data from various sources to provide a history of the client's past and current health status	▦ Consults with rural health team members
	▦ Consults with family/caregiver/ others to obtain collateral information as appropriate
	▦ Obtains pertinent data from previous health record (e.g., locates record both in rural community and tertiary center)
	▦ Analyzes lab data and diagnostic tests relevant to client's past and current health status
	Acceptable _____ Unacceptable _____
	Comments:
Performs a comprehensive assessment: biological; physical; psychological; social; functional; cultural; and spiritual health	▦ Utilizes inspection, percussion, palpation and auscultation according to provided guidelines
	▦ Performs a mental status examination as appropriate
	▦ Obtains information regarding: family history; personal history; psychological status; functional status; social, spiritual, cultural circumstances
	▦ Identifies client beliefs; community beliefs
	▦ Selects appropriate assessment tools based on client's age/health condition and own scope of practice
	▦ Assesses client taking into consideration the determinants of health
	Acceptable _____ Unacceptable _____
	Comments:

(Continued)

349

CLINICAL PRACTICE (*Continued*)

COMPETENCIES	PERFORMANCE CRITERIA	BEHAVIORAL INDICATORS

2. Completes a comprehensive client health assessment continued	Assesses the rural client's health capacity. (strengths and weaknesses)	▦ Identifies:
		  – personal attributes
		  – health beliefs
		  – coping resources
		  – motivation for treatment
		  – family support
		  – community resources
		Acceptable _____ Unacceptable_____
		Comments:

Completes a comprehensive client health assessment continued	Assesses the meaning of the health and illness experience from the rural client's/family's perspective	▦ Determines the client's perception of what brought them to the rural healthcare setting ▦ Determines the client's perception of their health status ▦ Identifies client's generation level ▦ Considers generational characteristics which could influence interactions ▦ Discusses the meaning of health and illness with the client ▦ Discusses the client's health beliefs and practices (e.g., acupressure, diet, nutritional supplements) ▦ Acknowledges the client as a valued partner in all aspects of care Acceptable _____ Unacceptable_____ Comments:
Completes a comprehensive client health assessment continued	Organizes assessment findings within a holistic framework	▦ Considers all components of assessment findings including age, physical findings, client/family culture, community culture, spirituality, lab data, etc. ▦ Prioritizes findings in a biopsychosocial framework ▦ Identifies problem as common, urgent or emergent health problems Acceptable _____ Unacceptable_____ Comments:
Completes a comprehensive client health assessment continued	Validates assessment findings	▦ Validates health history with client and/or caregiver ▦ Obtains the client's permission to validate assessment findings with family/significant others ▦ Reports assessment findings to the health care team as appropriate Acceptable _____ Unacceptable_____ Comments:

3. Analyzes assessment data to formulate nursing diagnoses and/or collaborative problems Utilizes assessment data from pertinent sources to identify actual/potential nursing diagnoses and/or collaborative problems	▣ Uses assessment findings collected in the comprehensive assessment to differentiate between normal findings and signs and symptoms ▣ Clusters signs and symptoms ▣ Identifies actual and potential nursing diagnoses ▣ Identifies collaborative problems with the healthcare team, client, family, and community ▣ Identifies wellness nursing diagnoses ▣ Identifies determinants of health which are pertinent for the client (e.g., education, employment) ▣ Determines learning needs for client and family Acceptable _____ Unacceptable _____ Comments:
4. Formulates a plan of care aimed at attaining expected client outcomes Guides care with primary, secondary and tertiary knowledge of health	▣ Possesses appropriate care knowledge for common, urgent, and emergent health problems within scope of practice ▣ In collaboration with preceptor, able to prioritize client care in unpredictable situations ▣ Matching client's need with appropriate medical intervention. (e.g., medical directives; physician; EHS life-flight crew; community paramedic team ▣ Stabilizes patient for life flight or transfer Acceptable _____ Unacceptable _____ Comments:
Develops a plan of care	▣ Considers client diversity (age, gender, cultural or ethnic background, spirituality, sexual orientation, socioeconomic status, community values, marginalization, and nature of health problems) ▣ Determines the client's definition of family and includes members in care planning and implementation ▣ Guides the impact of care with the client and the client's family involvement ▣ Discusses stressors (e.g., socioeconomic factors, child care, employment, healthcare insurance, role in family) ▣ Collaborates with the client/other health care professionals to assist with alleviating stressors ▣ Determines needs of clients receiving end-of-life care ▣ Collaborates with health care team to provide quality care Acceptable _____ Unacceptable _____ Comments:

(Continued)

351

CLINICAL PRACTICE *(Continued)*

COMPETENCIES	PERFORMANCE CRITERIA	BEHAVIORAL INDICATORS
	Identifies realistic goals to guide the plan of care	▨ Uses principles of primary health care in developing plan of care (e.g., accessibility and client participation) ▨ Identifies and supports client's short-term goals ▨ Identifies and supports client's long-term goals ▨ Identifies patient/family education wanted and needed ▨ Develops learning plans based on patient readiness and patient goals Acceptable _____ Unacceptable _____ Comments:
	Identifies expected outcomes	▨ Determines realistic outcomes which are individualized to client ▨ Includes outcomes which are specific and clearly stated ▨ Includes outcomes which are measurable Acceptable _____ Unacceptable _____ Comments:
	Selects evidence-based interventions to achieve expected client outcomes	▨ Identifies independent nursing interventions (e.g., vital signs q4h, assessment q4h) ▨ Identifies collaborative interventions (e.g., diagnostic tests, medications, consult to district/ tertiary care centre) ▨ List interventions with rationale based on current evidence ▨ Discusses with preceptor the usefulness of care protocols to guide practice in the rural setting Acceptable _____ Unacceptable _____ Comments:
5. Implements a care plan to achieve identified client outcomes	Coordinates the delivery of client care	▨ Prioritizes elements of care based on threat to client ▨ As necessary, calls for appropriate healthcare provider in urgent/emergent situations ▨ Acts in appropriate manner to urgent/emergent situations ▨ Negotiates delivery of care in collaboration with the client ▨ Collaborates with rural health team members and other health care facilities ▨ Encourage family involvement ▨ Practices culturally competent care ▨ Arranges for follow-up care prior to discharge ▨ Facilitates client transfer Acceptable _____ Unacceptable _____ Comments:

Continued: Implements a plan of care to achieve identified client outcomes	▪ Performs prioritized nursing care in a timely fashion
	▪ Implements independent nursing interventions (e.g., vital signs q1h, glucose monitoring in an appropriate time frame)
Implements interventions that are consistent with the plan of care (e.g., common/urgent/ emergent) within the expected time frame	▪ Implements collaborative interventions (e.g., changing medication based on client responses)
	▪ Recognizes changing client status (e.g., client becoming urgent or emergent)
	▪ Initiate code management and/or rapid response team mechanism
	▪ In consultation with preceptor utilizes delegated medical functions and/or medical directives based on assessment findings
	▪ Supports clients' strengths and resources for self-care
	▪ Implements education plans and evaluates effectiveness
	Acceptable _____ Unacceptable _____
	Comments:
5. Implements a plan of care to achieve identified client outcomes (cont'd)	▪ In collaboration with the client/family, develops health promotion goals, objectives, strategies
Provides health promotion and disease prevention information to the rural client	▪ Incorporates principles of health promotion in the plan of care
	Acceptable _____ Unacceptable _____
	Comments:
Coordinates individualized client education	▪ Assesses client's overall learning needs in relation to their developmental stage
	▪ Assesses client's readiness to learn
	▪ Selects appropriate teaching strategies to address individual client learning needs
	▪ Assesses clients understanding of information
	▪ Creates an environment that encourages questioning
	▪ Provides evidence-based health information to clients
	Acceptable _____ Unacceptable _____
	Comments:
Promotes rehabilitative care, chronic care and palliative care as necessary	▪ Initiates timely rehabilitative measures for clients in the community and facility
	▪ Initiates measures to facilitate care of the client with chronic illness
	▪ Initiates palliative measures in collaboration with client, family, and health care team
	▪ Facilitates adaptations needed in the client's environment (home, hospital) to support rehabilitation, palliation or chronic care
	Acceptable _____ Unacceptable _____
	Comments:

(Continued)

353

CLINICAL PRACTICE (Continued)

COMPETENCIES	PERFORMANCE CRITERIA	BEHAVIORAL INDICATORS
6. Evaluates the effectiveness of the implemented plan of care in relation to expected client outcomes	Compares client responses to interventions with expected outcomes	▓ Collects data at specified time intervals ▓ Identifies expected and unexpected responses to interventions ▓ Communicates evaluation findings to appropriate rural health care professionals Acceptable _____ Unacceptable _____ Comments:
	Modifies plan of care based on client outcomes and evidence-based practice	▓ Analyzes the reason for the identified differences between actual and expected outcomes ▓ Discusses revisions to plan of care with client/family and appropriate rural health care professionals ▓ Implements change to plan of care ▓ Documents changes to plan of care ▓ Evaluates outcomes based on change to plan of care Acceptable _____ Unacceptable _____ Comments:
7. Contributes to a safe practice environment	Assesses environment for clients' and health professionals' safety	▓ Monitors client safety and utilizes continual assessment to detect early changes in the client's status ▓ Notifies preceptor of malfunctioning equipment ▓ Identifies safety hazards and notifies preceptor ▓ Refuses to accept the role of primary care provider in preceptor/experienced charge nurse absence ▓ Knows resources required to manage potential unsafe situations ▓ Values and seeks clients' perspectives on their care (e.g., validates medications) ▓ Incorporates institution's policy and procedures ▓ Explains emergency codes (e.g., disaster activation in rural facilities) ▓ Identifies actual and potential nursing diagnoses related to client safety ▓ Reviews appropriate use of medication with the client considering potential problems (e.g. polypharmacy) ▓ Administers medications accurately and safely, monitoring therapeutic responses, reactions, untoward effects, toxicity, and potential incompatibilities with other medications or substances

	■ Implements standard safety procedures (e.g., WHMIS, body mechanics, electrical safety) ■ Implements principles of infection control ■ Performs skills as per program checklist ■ Evaluates with the preceptor the effectiveness of rapid responses to unsafe situations and modifies plans as necessary Acceptable _____ Unacceptable _____ Comments:
8. Uses appropriate communication technology for managing client information	■ Documents pertinent information accurately and in a timely manner ■ Records assessment data on correct flow charts/records within the specified time frame (e.g., q1h vital signs) ■ Records nursing diagnoses and/or collaborative problems on correct flow charts/records if appropriate ■ Documents the teaching/learning process in a timely fashion Acceptable _____ Unacceptable _____ Comments:
Records client information as per agency policies	
Communicates client information to appropriate health care professional	■ Communicates assessment findings to preceptor and other health care professionals in a timely manner ■ Shares client's perceptions/concerns with preceptor/health care professionals as required ■ Communicates verbal report to other health care professionals as required utilizing systematic approach with assistance of the preceptor/experienced charge nurse (e.g., Life Flight report, SBAR- Situation-Background-Assessment-Recommendation technique) ■ Complies with principles of confidentiality (e.g., awareness that the client's neighbor may be in the next bed/client may be the nurses' cousin) Acceptable _____ Unacceptable _____ Comments:

RELATIONSHIP CENTERED PRACTICE

The nurse develops relationships that support the uniqueness of the client/family and community building client capacity within the rural setting

COMPETENCIES	PERFORMANCE CRITERIA	BEHAVIORAL INDICATORS
1. Establishes therapeutic relationships with clients that respect diversity	Respects the individuality and human worth of rural clients	▮ Incorporates client characteristics into plan of care: – Age, gender – Cultural, ethnic background – Spirituality / religion – Sexual orientation – Socioeconomic status – Community value – Interpretation of present and past healthcare illnesses and experiences Acceptable _____ Unacceptable _____ Comments:
	Uses therapeutic communication techniques	▮ Listens actively to client ▮ Maintains eye contact ▮ Validates concerns ▮ Open, honest, empathetic ▮ Appropriate use of touch, posturing, facial expressions ▮ Focuses on the problem significant to the client – Makes no assumptions – Uses open ended questions – Avoids talking in generalities – Makes what is implicit explicit – Assures client of confidentiality – Allows client appropriate time to express oneself Acceptable _____ Unacceptable _____ Comments:

Maintains professional boundaries	▓ Identifies the difference between a professional and a non-professional relationship (e.g., recognizes issues regarding to living and working in the same community) ▓ Identifies warning signs that professional boundaries are in question or may be crossed ▓ Describes the CRNNS Decision-Making Framework for Appropriate Professional Behavior Acceptable _____ Unacceptable _____ Comments:
2. Promotes the client's/ family's autonomy, participation and choice in health and health care	
Assesses the rural client's ability/ capacity for participation	▓ Identifies threats to client ▓ Validates client's perception of their health status ▓ Validates client characteristics that will influence level of participation in care ▓ Validates and respects the client's choice for level of involvement in care ▓ Determines whether client has living will/advanced directives ▓ Determine with client the level of family involvement ▓ Recognizes cultural influences on communication/understanding and healthcare choices ▓ Recognizes that community beliefs and resources influence healthcare choices Acceptable _____ Unacceptable _____ Comments:
Engages the client to enhance their decision-making	▓ Provides information on treatment/health status ▓ Discusses the impact medication, treatment, etc. has on client's health ▓ Provides information regarding care, referrals, follow-up, and health promotion ▓ Respects client choice regarding self-care practices Acceptable _____ Unacceptable _____ Comments:
Supports the client(s) to draw on their own capacities for self-care/health promotion	▓ Respects the client's knowledge regarding their health (e.g., incorporates client's knowledge into the plan of care) ▓ Respects the client's control of health and health care ▓ Assists the client to identify personal capabilities ▓ Assists the client to identify resources to support health care needs (e.g., support groups, financial assistance) ▓ Assists client to access health related resources (e.g., the Internet, book mobile, library and other community resources) Acceptable _____ Unacceptable _____ Comments:

(Continued)

357

RELATIONSHIP CENTERED PRACTICE (Continued)

COMPETENCIES	PERFORMANCE CRITERIA	BEHAVIORAL INDICATORS
	Facilitates client's coping strategies related to the illness/ environment	■ Identifies stressors with the client ■ Considers the impact client diversity has on coping strategies ■ Interprets with the client responses to distress such as fear, anger, anxiety, helplessness, hopelessness, grief and denial ■ Supports effective client coping strategies ■ Supports the client's choices to maintain their self-esteem, power and hope ■ Facilitates the development of new coping strategies Acceptable _____ Unacceptable_____ Comments:
	Intervenes on behalf of the client	■ Assists the client to meet their care needs ■ Shares client perceptions with the rural health care team ■ With the help of the preceptor, facilitates a meeting between the client and physician and / or other health care professionals as necessary Acceptable _____ Unacceptable_____ Comments:

PROFESSIONALISM

The nurse follows ethical, legal and professional standards

COMPETENCIES	PERFORMANCE CRITERIA	BEHAVIORAL INDICATORS
1. Complies with professional, ethical, and legal guidelines relevant to rural nursing practice	Utilizes the ethical and legal principles that guide rural nursing practice	▪ Identifies potential legal and ethical risks in the rural setting ▪ Acts congruently with state and national Nursing Standards ▪ Acts congruently with relevant institutional policies (e.g., Policy/Procedures/Protocols) ▪ Acts congruently with ANA Code of Ethics (e.g., informed consent, confidentiality) ▪ Continually seeks to improve practice (e.g., professional development, reflection, data gathering analysis, evidence-based practice) Acceptable _____ Unacceptable _____ Comments:
	Articulates the delineation between the practice of nursing and other healthcare professionals	▪ Distinguishes between independent nursing actions and collaborative actions ▪ Maintains competency to perform the above ▪ Practices within a nursing scope of practice ▪ Accepts responsibility when delegating activities to the appropriate rural health care team member ▪ Evaluates outcomes of delegated activities Acceptable _____ Unacceptable _____ Comments:

(Continued)

359

PROFESSIONALISM (*Continued*)

COMPETENCIES	PERFORMANCE CRITERIA	BEHAVIORAL INDICATORS
2. Engages in activities and behaviors that foster a professional image	Demonstrates professional attitudes towards rural clients, colleagues, health care professionals and community members	▨ Uses appropriate personal and interpersonal professional behaviors ▧ Uses effective communication skills ▧ Shows respect when interacting with clients, colleagues, health care professionals and community members ▧ Values that each person provides a unique perspective ▧ Identifies self to clients, colleagues, health care professionals and community members ▧ Identifies the impact of working with multigenerations ▨ Recognizes the impact one's own generational value system has on one's actions ▨ Uses appropriate strategies in working with multigenerations ▨ Supports client's informed choices regarding care (e.g., right to refuse) ▨ Demonstrates openness to new learning experiences ▨ Describes professional practice role to clients, colleagues, and other rural health care professionals ▨ Gives feedback constructively Acceptable _____ Unacceptable _____ Comments:
2. Engages in activities and behaviors that foster a professional image (cont'd)	Demonstrates responsibility for own actions and decisions	▨ Demonstrates that actions and decisions are evidence-based ▨ Seeks help from preceptor/program staff when needed ▨ Notifies appropriate individual of knowledge gaps or errors ▨ Exercises accountability for actions ▨ Demonstrates professional judgment and accountability ▨ Notifies preceptor when ill, late, etc. ▨ Reports to work on time on time Acceptable _____ Unacceptable _____ Comments:

Takes personal responsibility for maintaining continued competence	▣ Interacts with colleagues to enhance one's practice in the rural setting ▣ Seeks constructive feedback from preceptor ▣ Participates in self-assessment ▣ Reflects on own practice ▣ Discusses individual learning needs with preceptor ▣ Identifies methods to meet these needs ▣ Negotiates specific learning experiences with preceptor ▣ Discusses future professional continuing education with preceptor Acceptable _____ Unacceptable _____ Comments:
Contributes to the professional development of others in the rural setting	▣ Shares knowledge and skills with peers/preceptor ▣ Contributes to an environment that is conducive to the education of others ▣ Fosters capacity team building ▣ Contributes in committees to develop practice standards Acceptable _____ Unacceptable _____ Comments:
Supports the continuing development of rural nursing practice	▣ Describes the unique role of rural nursing to colleagues and other health care professionals ▣ Describes the role of rural nursing practice within the profession of nursing ▣ Recognizes the role of specialty nursing groups and their contribution to rural nursing Acceptable _____ Unacceptable _____ Comments:

LEADERSHIP
The nurse promotes professional nursing practice in the rural setting

COMPETENCIES	PERFORMANCE CRITERIA	BEHAVIORAL INDICATORS
1. Contributes to collaborative relationships with the healthcare team	Provides pertinent information to rural health care professionals to enhance the decision-making process	▓ Articulates, verbally and in writing, concise assessment and treatment findings ▓ Gives rationale regarding medication, treatment, and referrals ▓ In consultation with preceptor, provides written information regarding care, referrals, and follow-up Acceptable _____ Unacceptable _____ Comments:
	Consults with other rural health care professionals regarding the plan of care for the client	▓ Describes the roles and responsibilities of each member of the rural health care team ▓ Identifies with the preceptor the need for a consultation ▓ Attends family conferences/meetings when appropriate ▓ Participates in inter professional rounds ▓ Discusses client care with appropriate health care professionals ▓ Works collaboratively, recognizing the knowledge and abilities of all team members to ensure excellent delivery of care within rural communities Acceptable _____ Unacceptable _____ Comments:
	Involves other rural health care professionals in the delivery of care	▓ Coordinates client care in collaboration with preceptor/ multidisciplinary team ▓ Respects and assists the healthcare professional as needed while practicing within own scope of practice Acceptable _____ Unacceptable _____ Comments:

2. Contributes positively towards a quality professional practice environment	Uses effective interpersonal skills	■ Respects individual contribution
		  – Uses assertive, open, two-way communication
		  – Listens actively
		  – Encourages questions
		  – Uses conflict management skills effectively
		  – Utilizes the facility's conflict resolution model as appropriate
		  – Discourages workplace bullying-lateral violence
		Acceptable _____ Unacceptable _____
		Comments:

2. Contributes positively towards a quality professional practice environment (cont'd)	Recognizes the impact the practice environment has on own/other's performance	■ Identifies factors in the environment that cause stress (e.g., workload issues, caring for family and known community members)
		■ Identifies personal coping mechanisms to deal with stressors
		■ Acts as a role model and resource to clients and colleagues (e.g., offers workload assistance/support to colleagues)
		■ Demonstrates ability to assess patient acuity and nursing skill mix required
		■ With assistance of preceptor, delegates responsibilities to appropriate team members
		■ Recognizes leadership behaviors in the practice setting that affect one's own/other's performance
		■ Practices qualities that assist in growth and development of future rural nursing leaders
		  – constructive feedback
		  – ongoing empathetic, non-threatening support
		  – models respectful and professional behavior
		  – inspires a vision for positive change
		Acceptable _____ Unacceptable _____
		Comments:

(Continued)

LEADERSHIP   (*Continued*)

COMPETENCIES	PERFORMANCE CRITERIA	BEHAVIORAL INDICATORS
	Provides input into decisions regarding resource utilization	▧ Identifies essential equipment/resources required in rural settings (i.e., OBS delivery pack; pediatric & adult resuscitation/trauma equipment; disaster response equipment; infectious diseases outbreak supplies) ▧ Identifies inadequacies in client care supplies ▧ Reports inadequacies/broken equipment to the appropriate person ▧ Considers cost and appropriateness when identifying resources for client care ▧ Identifies the role of the rural nurse in product and equipment evaluation ▧ Considers inadequacies in community resources Acceptable _____ Unacceptable _____ Comments:
	Provides input into decisions regarding health promotion and injury prevention	▧ Knowledge of Principles of Primary Healthcare ▧ Knowledge of the community's determinants of health ▧ Knowledge of community resources ▧ Identify community groups ▧ Identify community leaders ▧ Articulates potential role in community activities, projects and programs. (e.g., bike safety) ▧ Encourages community members to be active in development of rural health programs Acceptable _____ Unacceptable _____ Comments:
3. Utilizes technology to advance patient care, institutional, professional and community advancement	Demonstrates proficient use of communication, informatics and practice technologies	▧ Utilizes personal digital assistant for best practices, drug information, calculation, and patient education ▧ Evaluates web based information appropriately ▧ Utilizes electronic health record and pharmacy systems appropriately for patient care ▧ Utilizes database searches for literature reviews ▧ Practices appropriate communication standards when using electronic communication systems Acceptable _____ Unacceptable _____ Comments:

INDEX

A & P. *See* Anatomy and physiology
AACN. *See* American Association of
　　Colleges of Nursing
AAN. *See* American Academy of
　　Nursing
AB Tech. *See* Asheville-Buncombe
　　TechnicalCommunity
　　College
Accessibility Remoteness Index of
　　Australia (ARIA), 96
ACE-HC. *See* Alaska Coalition of
　　Educators–Health Care
ADN. *See* Associate of degree in nursing
ADRN. *See* Associate degree registered
　　nurse
Adult learning theory, 297
Advanced practice registered nurses
　　(APRNs), 9
Affirming emotions, 230
Agency for Health Care Policy and
　　Research (AHCPR), 7
Agency for Healthcare Research
　　and Quality
　　(AHRQ), 163
AHCPR. *See* Agency for Health Care
　　Policy and Research
AHEC. *See* Area Health Education
　　Center
AHRQ. *See* Agency for Healthcare
　　Research and Quality
AI. *See* Appreciative inquiry (AI)
Alaska, 177, 178. *See also* Competency
　　development initiative
　　challenge for hospitals, 182
　　health care delivery system,
　　　177–178
　　native health care system, 179
　　nursing experience
　　　in, 178–181
　　patient evacuation, 178

Alaska Coalition of Educators–Health
　　Care (ACE-HC), 182
Alaska Native Medical Center
　　(ANMC), 178
Alaska State Hospital and Nursing
　　Home Association
　　(ASHNHA), 182
American Academy of Nursing
　　(AAN), 110
American Association of Colleges of
　　Nursing (AACN), 83, 109
　　on curriculum, 137
　　genetics and genomics, 335
　　postbaccalaureate nurse
　　　residency, 110
American Nurses Association
　　(ANA), 324
　　continuing education, 26
　　informatics, 337–338
　　recommendation, 27
American Nurses Credentialing Center
　　(ANCC), 63
American Organization of Nurse
　　Executives (AONE),
　　123, 228
ANA. *See* American Nurses Association
Anatomy and physiology
　　(A & P), 251
ANCC. *See* American Nurses
　　Credentialing Center
ANMC. *See* Alaska Native Medical
　　Center
Anticipatory principle, 230
AONE. *See* American Organization of
　　Nurse Executives
Appreciative inquiry (AI), 227,
　　228, 233
　　beliefs, 229
　　change management, 228
　　concepts, 231

365